Health/Nursing Informatics and Technology

Health/Nursing Informatics and Technology
(Computer for Nurses)

As per the Revised Syllabus for BSc Nursing

Semester II

R Sreevani PhD (N)
Professor and Head
Department of Psychiatric Nursing
Dharwad Institute of Mental Health and Neurosciences (DIMHANS)
Dharwad, Karnataka, India

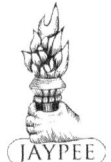

JAYPEE BROTHERS MEDICAL PUBLISHERS
The Health Sciences Publisher
New Delhi | London

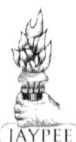 **Jaypee Brothers Medical Publishers (P) Ltd.**

Headquarters

Jaypee Brothers Medical Publishers (P) Ltd
EMCA House
23/23-B, Ansari Road, Daryaganj
New Delhi - 110 002, India
Landline: +91-11-23272143, +91-11-23272703
+91-11-23282021, +91-11-23245672
Email: jaypee@jaypeebrothers.com

Corporate Office

Jaypee Brothers Medical Publishers (P) Ltd
4838/24, Ansari Road, Daryaganj
New Delhi 110 002, India
Phone: +91-11-43574357
Fax: +91-11-43574314
Email: jaypee@jaypeebrothers.com

Overseas Office

J.P. Medical Ltd
83 Victoria Street, London
SW1H 0HW (UK)
Phone: +44 20 3170 8910
Fax: +44 (0)20 3008 6180
Email: info@jpmedpub.com

Website: www.jaypeebrothers.com
Website: www.jaypeedigital.com

© 2023, Jaypee Brothers Medical Publishers

The views and opinions expressed in this book are solely those of the original contributor(s)/author(s) and do not necessarily represent those of editor(s) and publisher of the book.

All rights reserved. No part of this publication may be reproduced, stored or transmitted in any form or by any means, electronic, mechanical, photocopying, recording or otherwise, without the prior permission in writing of the publishers.

All brand names and product names used in this book are trade names, service marks, trademarks or registered trademarks of their respective owners. The publisher is not associated with any product or vendor mentioned in this book.

Medical knowledge and practice change constantly. This book is designed to provide accurate, authoritative information about the subject matter in question. However, readers are advised to check the most current information available on procedures included and check information from the manufacturer of each product to be administered, to verify the recommended dose, formula, method and duration of administration, adverse effects and contraindications. It is the responsibility of the practitioner to take all appropriate safety precautions. Neither the publisher nor the author(s)/editor(s) assume any liability for any injury and/or damage to persons or property arising from or related to use of material in this book.

This book is sold on the understanding that the publisher is not engaged in providing professional medical services. If such advice or services are required, the services of a competent medical professional should be sought.

Every effort has been made where necessary to contact holders of copyright to obtain permission to reproduce copyright material. If any have been inadvertently overlooked, the publisher will be pleased to make the necessary arrangements at the first opportunity.

Inquiries for bulk sales may be solicited at: jaypee@jaypeebrothers.com

Health/Nursing Informatics and Technology

First Edition: **2023**

ISBN: 978-93-5696-121-0

Contributors

A Giridhar
Canara Bank
Regional Office
Hubballi, Karnataka, India

Dayanand BO
RN Yeovil District Hospital
NHS Foundation Trust
Higher Kingston
Yeovil, Somerset, England

Irasangappa Mudakavi
Clinical Instructor
All India Institute of Medical Sciences
Jodhpur, Rajasthan, India

Jithendra HY
Lecturer
Government College of Nursing
Mysuru, Karnataka, India

P Srinivasan
Assistant Professor
College of Nursing, AIIMS
Mangalagiri, Andhra Pradesh, India

Paramesha AE
Professor
Government College of Nursing
Mysuru, Karnataka, India

Prasanth Bevoor
Nursing Officer
Dharwad Institute of Mental Health and Neurosciences
Dharwad, Karnataka, India

Sunanda GT
Assistant Professor
Department of Nursing
Dharwad Institute of Mental Health and Neurosciences
Dharwad, Karnataka, India

Preface

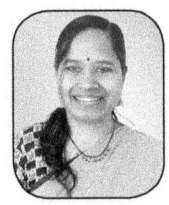

Nursing and computer science may seem like two fields that are unlikely to intersect with one another very often. However, behind every nurse providing care in clinics and hospitals across the country is a wealth of technology and data. Professionals responsible for developing these technologies and analyzing this data are known as health/nursing informatics professionals. Health/nursing informatics incorporates the fields of nursing, computer science, and information science in order to manage medical data and develop and maintain data systems that are designed to improve patient outcomes as well as boost the overall performance of a healthcare organization.

A better overall outcome is probably the most important reason why health informatics is so important. Electronic health records (EHRs) help doctors provide safer, cheaper and higher quality care. Because coordinated care teams have access to the same information, they are able to work more efficiently, make better diagnoses and commit fewer errors. It also eliminates a lot of manual jobs thereby saving additional time in clinics, hospitals and even for the patient. Health informatics just provides a better overall outcome for everyone involved.

With information and communication technologies becoming omnipresent in the healthcare systems globally and nurses constituting a majority of the health sector workforce, they are expected to be adequately skilled to work in a technology-mediated environment. It is however observed that nursing students use several information and communication technology tools primarily for academic purposes and rarely for clinical practice. It is thus necessary to integrate nursing informatics into undergraduate nursing education which is the cornerstone to nursing education and practice. The challenges mostly include limited information and communication technology skills among faculty and students; poor teaching strategies; and a lack of standardization of nursing informatics competencies. Successful integration of nursing informatics into undergraduate nursing education depends on restructuring nursing informatics content and teaching strategies, capacity building of the faculty and students in information and communication technologies, political commitment, and collaborative partnership.

Responding to these challenges, the Indian Nursing Council, New Delhi while revising the undergraduate nursing curricula during the year 2020 introduced *Health/Nursing Informatics and Technology* as one of the subjects for Semester II. The course has been designed to equip novice nursing students with knowledge and skills necessary to deliver efficient informatics-led healthcare services.

For those interested in a career in nursing and also with a passion for information technology and analytical science, nursing informatics is a rewarding option to consider. I have made an earnest attempt to not only encompass all that has been envisaged in the syllabus but also go beyond where necessary to provide a holistic view of the topics/subjects. I am confident that this publication will lay a proper foundation for all the future health/nurse informaticists.

R Sreevani

Acknowledgments

I thank the Almighty God, who bestowed upon me the spiritual strength and perseverance to make it all happen.

I would like to thank the publishers M/s Jaypee Brothers Medical Publishers (P) Ltd, New Delhi, India, especially Sri Jitendar P Vij (Group Chairman), Mr Ankit Vij (Managing Director) and Mr MS Mani (Group President), for believing in me and encouraging me to come out with this edition in a short time.

Nobody has been more important to me in the pursuit of this title than the members of my family. I would like to thank my grandparents, parents and in-laws, whose love and guidance are with me in all my endeavors. If I am anything today, it is because of what they were to me yesterday. Most importantly, I wish to thank my loving and supportive husband, Mr Giridhar who has contributed immensely to this edition and my two wonderful children, Pranith and Daivik for their unending love and inspiration.

I am very grateful to Dr Madhu Choudhary (Director–Educational Publishing), Ms Pooja Bhandari (Production Head), Ms Sunita Katla (Executive Assistant to Group Chairman and Publishing Manager), Ms Samina Khan (Executive Assistant to Director–Educational Publishing), Ms Alisha Talwar (Development Editor), Mr Rajesh Sharma (Production Coordinator), Ms Seema Dogra (Cover Visualizer), Mr Vakil Khan (Proofreader), Mr Akshay Thakur (Typesetter), Mr Shravan Kumar (Graphic Designer) of M/s Jaypee Brothers Medical Publishers (P) Ltd, New Delhi, India, for all their support to work in this project and make it a success.

I wish to present my special thanks to Mr Venugopal (Regional Head–Business Development, DigiNerve) for providing encouragement and always being there when I needed him the most.

Contents

Unit 1: Introduction to Computer Applications for Patient Care Delivery System and Nursing Practice — 1

- Computer *1*
- Use of Computers in Teaching and Learning *6*
- Role of Computers in Research Process *12*
- Role of Computers in Nursing Practice *13*
- Role of Computers in Nursing Administration *18*
- Windows, MS Office: Word, Excel, Powerpoint *20*
- Internet *30*
- Literature Search *36*
- Statistical Packages *43*
- Hospital Management Information System *50*

Unit 2: Principles of Health Informatics — 59

- Elements in Health Informatics *60*
- Health Information System *61*
- Applications of Health Informatics *63*
- Objectives of Health Informatics *64*
- Need for Health Informatics *64*
- Principles of Health Informatics *64*
- Benefits of Health Informatics *64*
- Limitations or Disadvantages *67*
- Trends for the Future *68*
- Use of Data, Information and Knowledge for More Effective Healthcare and Better Health *68*

Unit 3: Information System in Health Care — 74

- Architecture of Information System in Modern Healthcare Environment *79*
- Clinical Information Systems *83*

Unit 4: Shared Care and Electronic Health Records — 90

- Ethical Issues in Electronic Health Records *97*
- Challenges of Capturing Rich Patient Data in A Computable Form *100*
- Electronic Health Records Standards for India *103*
- Implementing Electronic Health Records in India *106*

Unit 5: Patient Safety and Clinical Risk — 115

- Patient Safety *115*
- Adverse Events in Health Care *116*
- Importance of Patient Safety Initiative *117*
- Relationship Between Patient Safety and Health Information Technology *118*
- Functions and Applications of Risk Management Process *128*
- Healthcare Risk Management and Technology *135*

Unit 6: Clinical Knowledge and Decision-making — 140

- Health Care Knowledge Management *143*
- Standardized Software Languages/Terminologies Used in Health Informatics *149*

Unit 7: E-Health: Patients and the Internet — 158

- Use of Information and Communication Technology to Improve Personal and Public Health *162*
- Digital Health Services in India *168*
- Ayushman Bharat Digital Mission *175*
- Public Health Informatics *176*
- Role of Nurse *179*

Unit 8: Using Information in Healthcare Management — 183

- Nursing Information and Nursing Information System *183*
- Nursing Informatics *188*
- Evaluation, Analysis and Presentation of Healthcare Data to Inform Decisions in the Management of Healthcare Organizations *194*

Unit 9: Information Law and Governance in Clinical Practice — 201

- Privacy and Confidentiality in Electronic Health-related Data *210*
- Nurses' Responsibilities in Legal and Ethical Aspects of Digital Health *213*
- Telenursing Practice Guidelines in India *214*

Unit 10: Health Care Quality and Evidence Based Practice — 220

Index *227*

Syllabus

PLACEMENT: II SEMESTER **THEORY:** 2 Credits (40 hours)
PRACTICAL/LAB: 1 Credit (40 hours)

DESCRIPTION: This course is designed to equip novice nursing students with knowledge and skills necessary to deliver efficient informatics-led healthcare services.

COMPETENCIES: On completion of the course, the students will be able to:
1. Develop a basic understanding of computer application in patient care and nursing practice.
2. Apply the knowledge of computer and information technology in patient care and nursing education, practice, administration and research.
3. Describe the principles of health informatics and its use in developing efficient healthcare.
4. Demonstrate the use of information system in healthcare for patient care and utilization of nursing data.
5. Demonstrate the knowledge of using Electronic Health Records (EHR) system in clinical practice.
6. Apply the knowledge of interoperability standards in clinical setting.
7. Apply the knowledge of information and communication technology in public health promotion.
8. Utilize the functionalities of Nursing Information System (NIS) system in nursing.
9. Demonstrate the skills of using data in management of health care.
10. Apply the knowledge of the principles of digital ethical and legal issues in clinical practice.
11. Utilize evidence-based practices in informatics and technology for providing quality patient care.
12. Update and utilize evidence-based practices in nursing education, administration, and practice.

COURSE OUTLINE
T – Theory, P/L – Lab

Unit	Time (Hrs) T	Time (Hrs) P/L	Learning outcomes	Content	Teaching/learning activities	Assessment methods
I	10	15	Describe the importance of computer and technology in patient care and nursing practice	**Introduction to Computer Applications for Patient Care Delivery System and Nursing Practice** • Use of computers in teaching, learning, research and nursing practice	• Lecture • Discussion • Practice session • Supervised clinical practice on EHR use • Participate in data analysis using statistical package with statistician	(T) • Short answer • Objective type • Visit reports • Assessment of assignments

Health/Nursing Informatics and Technology

Unit	Time (Hrs) T	P/L	Learning outcomes	Content	Teaching/learning activities	Assessment methods
			Demonstrate the use of computer and technology in patient care, nursing education, practice, administration and research.	• Windows, MS Office: Word, Excel, PowerPoint • Internet • Literature search • Statistical packages • Hospital management information system	Visit to hospitals with different hospital management systems	(P) Assessment of skills using checklist
II	4	5	Describe the principles of health informatics Explain the ways data, knowledge and information can be used for effective healthcare	**Principles of Health Informatics** • Health informatics—needs, objectives and limitations • Use of data, information and knowledge for more effective healthcare and better health	• Lecture • Discussion • Practical session • Work in groups with health informatics team in a hospital to extract nursing data and prepare a report	(T) • Essay • Short answer • Objective type questions • Assessment of report
III	3	5	Describe the concepts of information system in health Demonstrate the use of health information system in hospital setting	**Information Systems in Healthcare** • Introduction to the role and architecture of information systems in modern healthcare environments • Clinical Information System (CIS)/Hospital Information System (HIS)	• Lecture • Discussion • Demonstration • Practical session • Work in groups with nurse leaders to understand the hospital information system	(T) • Essay • Short answer • Objective type
IV	4	4	Explain the use of electronic health records in nursing practice Describe the latest trend in electronic health records standards and interoperability	**Shared Care and Electronic Health Records** • Challenges of capturing rich patient histories in a computable form • Latest global developments and standards to enable lifelong electronic health records to be integrated from disparate systems	• Lecture • Discussion • Practice on simulated EHR system • Practical session • Visit to health informatics department of a hospital to understand the use of EHR in nursing practice • Prepare a report on current EHR standards in Indian setting	(T) • Essay • Short answer • Objective type (P) • Assessment of skills using checklist
V	3		Describe the advantages and limitations of health informatics in maintaining patient safety and risk management	**Patient Safety and Clinical Risk** • Relationship between patient safety and informatics • Function and application of the risk management process	• Lecture • Discussion	(T) • Essay • Short answer • Objective type

Unit	Time (Hrs) T	Time (Hrs) P/L	Learning outcomes	Content	Teaching/learning activities	Assessment methods
VI	3	6	Explain the importance of knowledge management Describe the standardized languages used in health informatics	**Clinical Knowledge and Decision Making** • Role of knowledge management in improving decision-making in both the clinical and policy contexts • Systematized nomenclature of medicine, clinical terms, SNOMED CT to ICD-10-CM Map, standardized nursing terminologies (NANDA, NOC), Omaha system	• Lecture • Discussion • Demonstration • Practical session • Work in groups to prepare a report on standardized languages used in health informatics • Visit health informatics department to understand the standardized languages used in hospital setting	(T) • Essay • Short answer • Objective type
VII	3		Explain the use of information and communication technology in patient care Explain the application of public health informatics	**e-Health: Patients and the Internet** • Use of information and communication technology to improve or enable personal and public healthcare • Introduction to public health informatics and role of nurses	• Lecture • Discussion • Demonstration	• Essay • Short answer • Objective type • Practical exam
VIII	3	5	Describe the functions of nursing information system Explain the use of healthcare data in management of health care organization	**Using Information in Healthcare Management** • Components of nursing information system (NIS) • Evaluation, analysis and presentation of healthcare data to inform decisions in the management of healthcare organizations	• Lecture • Discussion • Demonstration on simulated NIS software • Visit to health informatics department of the hospital to understand use of healthcare data in decision making	(T) • Essay • Short answer • Objective type
IX	4		Describe the ethical and legal issues in healthcare informatics Explains the ethical and legal issues related to nursing informatics	**Information Law and Governance in Clinical Practice** • Ethical-legal issues pertaining to healthcare information in contemporary clinical practice • Ethical-legal issues related to digital health applied to nursing	• Lecture • Discussion • Case discussion • Role play	(T) • Essay • Short answer • Objective type
X	3		Explain the relevance of evidence-based practices in providing quality healthcare	**Healthcare Quality and Evidence-based Practice** Use of scientific evidence in improving the quality of healthcare and technical and professional informatics standards	• Lecture • Discussion • Case study	(T) • Essay • Short answer • Objective type

Terminology

- **Administrative data:** It refers to information that is collected, processed and stored in automated information systems. This data includes admission details, claims information, physician office visits, etc.
- **Ancillary information system:** It includes laboratory information system, pharmacy information system and the radiology information system.
- **Anonymization of data:** It is a method of information sanitization which involves removing or encrypting personal identity data in a data set. The main goal is to ensure the privacy of subject's information. It minimizes the risk of information leaks when data is moving across boundaries.
- **Asynchronous telemedicine:** In this the sender takes information or a digital image, stores the information and sends it to the receiver through a computer. The receiver reviews the data according to his convenience. It is used during non-emergent situations with consultation being made in the next 24 to 48 hours and sent back. Teleradiology, telepathology and teledermatology are a few examples.
- **Automated dispensing cabinets:** These are computerized drug storage devices that allow medications to be stored and dispensed near the point of care while controlling and tracking drug distribution.
- **Automated medication dispensing cabinets (ADC):** These are computerized management systems for medications and supplies that store medication at the point of care with controlled dispensing and tracking of medication distribution. These are used as medication inventory management tools that help in automating the medication dispensing process. This minimizes the workload on the central pharmacy thereby keeping a better track of medication dispensing and patient billing. Automated dispensing cabinets reduce medication preparation errors in critical care setting.
- **Automatic staff scheduling:** Automated nurse scheduling systems are termed as shift modules. The system generates daily, weekly, monthly schedules, duty allocation charts, swapping schedules and training details for nurses. This saves a considerable amount of time for the nurses and results in cost reduction. Shift modules are designed to handle absences, overtime, staffing levels and cost-effective staffing.
- **Barcode technology:** These are electronic systems that integrate electronic medication administration records with barcode technology. The barcodes have information on patient's name, drug, dose, route, and time of administration. Barcode scanners placed in patient's room are linked to computerized databases containing patient's drug regimen. The database may be cross-linked to other health information systems such as a patient identification master file, an electronic medication administration record, an order entry system, or even a pharmacy database. The nurse scans the barcode on the medication package and the patient's identification wristband allowing the system to determine whether there is a match. Following a confirmation signal the nurse administers the medication. If there is an alert the nurse stops the process from going forward thus preventing a potential medication error. It is intended

to prevent medication errors by ensuring that the right patient receives the right medication at the right time.
- **Biometric data:** Data provided from various types of devices that monitor weight, pressure, heart rate, oxygen saturation, glucose level, etc.
- **Cardiovascular information system (CVIS):** It integrates all cardiology requests, procedures, images and reports. When CVISs are integrated with other clinical information systems, physicians can extract images and reports from any computer inside and outside of the hospital through a portal. It plays a vital role in monitoring, management, evaluation, and policy development related to cardiac diseases.
- **Central processing unit (CPU):** It is one of the core components of computer system also known as brain of the computer, processor, central processor, or microprocessor. No action can take place without its permission and execution. It communicates with all other components of the computer.
- **Clinical data:** It refers to information about patient care. It is collected from the patient during care or observed or obtained from electronic medical records, hospital information system, image centers, laboratories, pharmacies, physician's notes, physiological monitoring, etc.
- **Clinical decision support systems (CDSSs):** These are IT applications designed to improve clinical decision making and clinical workflow. These tools include notification, alerts and reminders to care providers and patients, clinical guidelines, condition-specific order sets, patient-specific clinical summaries, document templates, investigation and diagnostic support among other tools. CDSSs match patient characteristics against a knowledge base using computer algorithms thereby generating patient management recommendations.
- **Clinical information system (CIS):** It is an information system designed specifically for use in a critical care environment. It can network with the many computer systems in a hospital and draw information from them into an electronic patient record, which clinicians can see at the patient's bedside.
- **Code of ethics:** Collection of principles and rules that govern the ethical conduct of groups of individuals.
- **Computer-assisted learning:** It is defined as the use of computers to support the learning and training of individuals which requires no direct interaction between the user and the human instructor in order to run.
- **Computer:** It is an electronic machine that is used for storing, organizing and finding words, numbers and pictures for performing calculations and controlling other machines.
- **Computerized care documentation:** It is an automate and streamline documentation which allows the healthcare team to enter information about service delivered into patient charts via a computer directly. These systems provide document templates, copy-and-paste functions and automated insertion of clinical data.
- **Confidentiality:** It is defined as restricting of information to persons who are not authorized to access data during either storage, transmission or treatment. It ensures that the information remains protected from unauthorized deletion or modification and undesired modification by authorized users. It relates to non-disclosure of information.
- **Data:** Data is the collection of facts in raw or unorganized form such as numbers or characters. It can be acquired from many different sources. It needs cleaning and processing. Without context and analysis, data has little meaning.
- **De-identification:** It is the process of masking identification data or replacing it with other fictitious names or codes that is unique to the data.

- **Departmental electronic medical record:** It contains patient's medical information entered by a single hospital department (e.g., pathology, radiology, pharmacy).
- **Diagnostic errors:** These refer to a failure in providing an accurate and timely explanation of patient's health problems. Diagnostic errors occur when a diagnosis is delayed, wrong or missed altogether. Diagnostic errors are considered as missed opportunities to make a correct or timely diagnosis based on available evidence.
- **Digital health:** It is an umbrella term for eHealth, telehealth, etc. Digital health has a goal of reaching as many people as possible who need help via the digital channel. Digital health uses tools such as telemedicine, smartphone applications, etc.
- **Digital Information Security in Healthcare Act (DISHA):** This Act enables the digital sharing of personal health records with hospital and clinics and between hospitals and clinics. It is the basis for creation of digital health records in India.
- **eHealth:** It is defined as the delivery of health care using modern electronic information and communication technology when healthcare providers and patients are not in direct contact and their interaction is mediated by electronic means. Health care is provided from a distance.
- **E-Learning:** It is an internet-based form of learning rather than a face-to-face interaction where traditional methods of learning are supported by computer or other electronic devices to provide training, education and learning.
- **Electronic health record (EHR):** It is an electronic version of a patient's wellness history. It is a digital record of health information. It contains past medical history, vital signs, progress notes, diagnoses, medications, immunization dates, allergies, laboratory data and imaging reports. It also contains other relevant information such as insurance information, demographic data and data from personal wellness devices. All authorized clinicians involved in patient care can access the information to provide care to that patient and also share information with other healthcare providers such as laboratories and specialists. EHRs follow patients to the hospital, nursing home or even across the country. This digital version of a patient's health record helps eliminate the problems associated with physical records such as loss and lack of accessibility. It can be stored centrally and accessed at any time, irrespective of where or when the information was collected.
- **Electronic incident reporting:** These are web-based systems that allow healthcare providers involved in safety events to voluntarily report such incidents. Incident reporting is the process of notifying a user or administrator of an abnormal event, process or action identified on a computing device, system or environment. It is part of the security incident and event management process that alerts and logs all security incidents discovered within an information technology environment.
- **Electronic medical record (EMR):** It is the digital version of a patient's chart in clinician offices or hospital. These are online medical records of the standard medical and clinical data from one provider's office. It contains the patient's medical history, diagnoses and treatment by a particular physician, nurse practitioner, specialist, dentist or surgeon. It works well within a practice. They don't travel outside the practice.
- **Electronic medication administration record (eMAR):** It is an electronic medication administration record technology that automatically tracks medications from order to administration using assistive technologies in conjunction with an electronic medication administration record. The physician makes an electronic entry detailing the patient's medication orders. The orders then appear in the pharmacy software package to be edited and verified by a pharmacist. Verified orders are made available in the nursing staff's point-of-care.

- **Electronic physician's orders or E-prescribing or computerized physician order:** These are usually integrated with a clinical decision support system which acts as an error prevention tool. It guides the prescriber on the preferred drug doses, route and frequency of administration. Some CPOE systems have the feature of prompting the prescriber to patient allergies, drug-drug or drug-laboratory interactions. Certain sophisticated systems also prompt the prescriber towards interventions that should be prescribed based on clinical guideline recommendation. Directly entering orders into a computer can reduce errors associated with hand-written orders.
- **Electronic sign-out and hand-off tools:** Sign-out or hand-off communication relates to the process of passing patient-specific information from one nursing official to another, one team of caregivers to the next or from caregivers to the patient and family for the purpose of ensuring patient care continuity and safety. These applications are used as standalone or integrated with electronic medical record to ensure structured transfer of patient information during healthcare provider handoffs.
- **E-mail:** It is considered to be one of the most common and simplest ways to share and receive information, data, and other things over the internet.
- **Emergency department information systems (EDIS):** EDIS system allows patients to be registered into the system with minimal data entry, tracking of patients, quick and easy entry into the computer using touch screens, quick fill templates for clinical documentation and order sets for ordering of laboratories and medications and integration with inpatient systems.
- **Engineering of information systems:** It involves engineering of systems that engage in input of data and its transformation to information using appropriate methods.
- **e-Pharmacy or online pharmacy:** It is a pharmacy that operates over the internet and fulfils the orders through mail, courier or delivery persons.
- **Ethical principle:** Basic or fundamental rule that governs moral conduct in a society and the relationship between individuals.
- **Ethics:** Ethics is that branch of knowledge which deals in 'moral principles'.
- **Evidence-based nursing (EBN):** It is the process of integrating clinical knowledge, judgment, expertise skills and individual preferences with the best available clinical evidence.
- **Evidence-based practice:** It is the conscious, meticulous, explicit and judicious use of current best evidence in making decisions about the care of individual patients.
- **Fiduciary:** 'Fiduciary' is a standard ethical and legal term that describes the relationship of trust between a trustee and a beneficiary. However, the term fiduciary goes much beyond mere trust. The trustee has an obligation to always act in the best interest of the beneficiary even in the absence of specific directions. The trustee also has a duty not to allow personal interests to conflict with his duty towards the beneficiary.
- **Geographical information system (GIS):** It uses map overlay techniques which view data pertaining to demographics, social infrastructure, healthcare institutions and patient's geo-positioned points.
- **Google docs:** These are word documents and spreadsheets that can be created online and stored on a google drive.
- **Google drive:** It is a cloud storage space where data can be saved after a complete document scan making it safer and practical.
- **Graphic processing unit (GPU):** Also called video adaptor, video card or display card it helps to generate high end visuals. This electronic circuit displays high quality images and graphics by performing rapid mathematical calculations. It helps to process 2D and 3D data.

- **Harm:** It refers to bodily or mental injury; loss, distortion or theft of identity; loss of reputation or humiliation; any discriminatory treatment; any subjection to blackmail or extortion; any denial or withdrawal of a service.
- **Health ID:** It refers to identification number or identifier allocated to a data principal.
- **Health informatics:** Medical informatics is the application of computer technology to various fields of medicine such as medical care, medical teaching and medical research.
- **Health information provider:** HIP means hospitals, diagnostic centers, public health programs or other such entities registered with the National Health Infrastructure Registry which act as information providers (by generating, storing and distributing health records) in the digital health ecosystem.
- **Health information system:** It refers to any system that captures, stores, manages or transmits information related to health of the individual or activities of the organization working within the health sector.
- **Health information users:** HIUs are entities that are permitted to request access to the personal data of a data principal with appropriate consent of the data principal.
- **Healthcare virtual assistant:** Is an individual who works remotely and can help healthcare provider with routine tasks such as managing the front office, setting appointments, patient engagements, etc. Virtual assistants work from a remote location not on hospital premises.
- **Healthcare-associated infections (HAIs):** These are infections that people contract while they are receiving health care for another condition. It can happen in any facility including hospitals, ambulatory services and long-term facilities. HAIs are a significant cause of illness and death. They can have serious emotional, financial and medical consequences.
- **Health Insurance Portability and Accountability Act (HIPAA):** It is a United States of America (USA) legislation that provides data privacy and security provision for safeguarding medical information. It sets the standard for patient data protection.
- **Informatics nurse specialist:** A registered nurse with formal, graduate education in the field of informatics or a related field and considered a specialist in the field of nursing informatics.
- **Informatics nurse:** A registered nurse with an interest or working experience in the field of informatics. It also refers to a generalist in the field of informatics in nursing.
- **Information and communication technology (ICT):** It refers to the communication technologies and services used in various applications. It describes these computers, communication and multimedia technologies used to receive, process, store, display and disseminate information.
- **Information processing:** It relates to how the information can be used and what methods can be applied so as to transform healthcare information into useful and usable knowledge.
- **Information:** Information is data organized into meaningful unions, data placed in context with relevance, purpose and meaning. Unlike data, information has various purposes in creating knowledge, decision making and guiding further actions.
- **Informed consent:** It is the permission to accept or reject an intervention or action. It can be obtained only when given by a competent individual on the basis of having been advised and understood all relevant information about that action or intervention.
- **Inpatient clinical information system:** Inpatient clinical information system is much more complex and an intense combination of various workflows. Inpatient visit starts with admission, goes through treatment and procedures and ends with discharge.
- **Integrity:** Integrity assures that the data is accurate and has not been changed or tampered with.

- **Intensive care unit information system (ICUIS):** It provides protocol templates and flow sheets, ensures automatic capture of physiologic parameters from monitors, graphically displays trends to help in decision making, automatically calculates dose adjustments with change in parameters. CISs in ICU reduce time spent by physicians on documentation and increase the time available for direct patient care by providing protocol templates and flow sheets. They support the continuous assessment and adjustment of medication, automatic capture of physiological parameters from patient monitors, and display of patient vital conditions.
- **Inter-departmental electronic medical record:** It contains a patient's medical information from two or more hospital departments.
- **Inter-hospital electronic medical record:** It contains a patient's medical information from two or more hospitals.
- **Keyboard:** It is a primary input device which helps to interact with the computer system. The keyboard layout is similar to that of a typewriter. It has a set of keys such as alphabetical keys, character keys, functional keys, arrow keys and control keys. When we press a key on the keyboard, the computer receives input from the keyboard.
- **Knowledge acquisition:** It includes finding existing knowledge, understanding requirements of organization and searching from multiple sources to acquire knowledge.
- **Knowledge creation:** Knowledge is created by research activities, writing books or articles, etc.
- **Knowledge management:** It is the systematic process and strategy of finding, capturing, organizing, distilling and presenting data, information and knowledge for a specific purpose and serve a specific organization or community.
- **Knowledge:** Information is interpreted and reviewed to generate knowledge. It is combined with intelligence, evidence and qualitative data and presented to form decision making. Knowledge is a set of justifiable beliefs based on data and information. Knowledge itself may be processed to generate decisions. It is needed to produce actionable information that can lead to impact.
- **Laboratory information system:** These are computerized systems that provide accurate and accessible lab sample information in clinical laboratories. A physician may track each step in the testing process, from the administration of tests to the receipt of test results thereby supporting timely decision making and diagnosis.
- **Medication errors:** It is a failure in the treatment process that leads to, or has the potential to lead to patient harm. Medication error can occur in deciding which medicine and dosage regimen to use while prescribing, administering or taking the medication (wrong drug, wrong formulation, wrong label, wrong dose, wrong route, wrong frequency, wrong duration) and monitoring therapy. Medication errors result in significant morbidity and mortality.
- **mHealth:** It is an abbreviation for mobile health which utilizes mobile devices such as cell phone or a tablet to support healthcare practices. With mHealth services patients are able to log, store and monitor their health records on personal mobile devices. These applications are helpful in improving the efficiency of healthcare information delivery.
- **Monitor:** It is an essential part of the computer system. Also termed as the visual display unit, it is made of glass, circuitry, adjustment buttons, power supplies, etc., all enclosed within a casing. The monitor is connected to a computer and display output like text, image or video on the screen. Presently LED (light-emitting diode) and LCD (liquid crystal display) monitors are most commonly being used.
- **Motherboard:** Also called the main board, it is through this circuit board that different electronic components and peripherals of the computer system are connected in order to communicate

with each other towards proper functioning of the computer. The input and output devices are plugged into the motherboard for their functioning. It consists of CPU, RAM, ROM, sound card, video card, network card, ports for input, output and storage devices, etc.

- **Mouse:** It is an input device that helps to communicate with the computer system. It allows the user to move a pointer displayed on the monitor. A computer mouse can be wired or wireless.
- **Computer case:** It is a special box that holds all of the internal components of a computer. It includes motherboard, central processing unit, power supply, drives, memory and writing. The front of the computer case usually provides access to the power on/off button, CD/DVD drives and some ports such as USB, audio jack, etc. On the reverse are the sockets for connecting a monitor, power cord, etc.
- **MS Excel:** It is spreadsheet software that is used to manage and process a larger amount of data. It is organized into grids of rows and columns where rows are indicated by numbers and columns by letters with their intersection termed as the cell.
- **MS PowerPoint:** It is an example of professional-level presentation software of the Microsoft Office suite which is by nature a presentation document but takes the form of a slide show.
- **Non-clinical data:** It refers to information that is not directly related to patient treatment but may still influence the way professionals use healthcare facilities and resources. For example, information about the geographical reach of an organization can help administrators make decisions about whether to extend their healthcare services or not.
- **Nursing informatics:** It is a specialty that integrates nursing science with multiple information and analytical sciences to identify, define, manage and communicate data, information, knowledge and wisdom in nursing practice.
- **Nursing information systems:** These are computer systems that manage and make available clinical data from a variety of healthcare environments in a timely and orderly fashion to aid nurses in improving patient care.
- **Oncology information systems (OISs):** These systems combine radiation, medical and surgical oncology information into a complete oncology specific electronic medical record which helps physicians to manage their patients' entire information from diagnosis through follow-up.
- **Outpatient clinical information system:** It includes clinical administration and outpatient department (OPD) healthcare delivery. Clinical administration includes registration, follow-up visits and billing functions. OPD healthcare delivery system includes OPD electronic medical record tailored for OPD visits. OPD starts with initial registration, goes through physician visit, laboratory investigations and ends with minor procedures or medication prescription.
- **Patient classification systems (PCSs):** PCSs also known as patient acuity system is a tool that provides exact clinical data for forecasting and allocating nursing staff. It classifies patients based on the need for care and nursing activities that are necessary to meet their care needs during a specific period. It assists nurse leaders determine workload requirements and staff needs.
- **Patient electronic portals:** It is a secure online application that provides patients access to their personal health information and 2-way electronic communication with their care provider using computer or mobile device. Patients can log into personal accounts to access secure information about their own medical history. It allows the patient to participate in their own treatment and to know the status of payments or insurance benefits. Often patient portals enable doctors and nurses to send confidential messages to patients, and decide whether to share laboratory reports or simply recap what was discussed at a recent visit.

- **Patient feedback data:** Data provided by patients which may include description of preferences, level of satisfaction, information from systems for self-monitoring of their activity, exercises, sleep, meals consumed, etc.
- **Patient safety:** It is the fundamental element of health care defined as the freedom of a patient from unnecessary harm or potential harm associated with provision of health care.
- **Personal health identifier:** PHI is the data that could potentially identify a specific data principal and can be used to distinguish such data principals from another. PHIs could also be used for re-identifying previously de-identified data.
- **Personal health records (PHR):** It is a health record initiated and maintained by an individual. An ideal PHR would provide a complete and accurate summary of the health and medical history of an individual by gathering data from many sources and making it accessible online. Generally, such records are maintained in a secure and confidential environment such as in a health locker, allowing only the individual or people authorized by the individual to access the medical data.
- **Pharmacy information system** (PIS): It supports the distribution and management of drugs, maintains drug and medical device inventory. PIS manages inpatient and outpatient dispensing of order entry drugs. It allows the pharmacist to identify the physician's order; validate the medication based on drug-to-drug interactions and timing of medications and then dispense the drug for administration. It plays a vital role in preventing dosage errors by providing an individual dosage limit according to patient's age, gender and other factors.
- **Point-of-care diagnostics (POCD):** Also known as remote testing it includes a broad range of products such as biosensors, portable X-rays, handheld ultrasounds and smartphone based POCDs. These devices are generally automated technologies which run on artificial intelligence and machine learning algorithms that enable simplification of complex diagnostic procedures to provide immediate diagnostic results.
- **Privacy:** It refers to the right that someone has to determine for themselves when, how and the level at which accessing personal information is transferred or shared by others. It is the right of an individual to keep information about themselves from being disclosed to others.
- **Pseudonymization:** It is a data management and de-identification procedure by which personally identifiable information fields within a data record are replaced by one or more artificial identifiers or pseudonyms.
- **Public health informatics:** It is the application of informatics to public health practice intelligently and focused on preventive and promotive health.
- **Quality improvement:** It is defined as the combined and unceasing effort of healthcare professionals, patients and their families, researchers, planners and educators to make changes that will lead to better patient health outcomes, better system performance (care) and better professional development.
- **Radiation errors:** It involves over exposure to radiation and cases of wrong-patient and wrong-site identification.
- **Remote monitoring telemedicine:** It uses technological devices to monitor health and clinical signs of a patient remotely.
- **Retained surgical items prevention technology:** Retained items such as sponges, sharps, etc., after surgical procedure are reportable errors that can result in patient harm or death and also increase patient and healthcare costs. Data matrix code (DMC) and radiofrequency identification (RFID) are commonly used technologies to prevent retained surgical items. A RFID system consists of a tag attached to the surgical items and a reader that receives unique

radio-wave signals from the tags. A DMC works on the same principle—a unique data matrix tag on each surgical item is scanned by a barcode reader as it enters and leaves the sterile field. Both systems are designed to count sponges by scanning matrix labels attached to each sponge as they go in and out of the patient's body. Each sponge has a unique identifier that enables the machine to know which type of sponge is missing and then relay that information to the surgical team. A radiofrequency detection system is one that includes a small passive radiofrequency tag attached to every sponge, in addition to a handheld wand or mat that contains a detection system. This allows the surgical team to pass a wand over a patient to determine if there are any sponges left inside the patient.

- **Risk assessment:** It is an aid to decision making regarding the prioritization of management of risks. It involves analysis and evaluation of identified risk and also includes a decision to accept the risk or treat the risk, risk avoidance, risk transference or risk control.
- **Risk identification:** It is the first stage of the entire risk management process which identifies the potential for harm to self or others.
- **Risk management:** It is a systematic approach to identifying, analyzing and responding to risks, maximizing the probability and consequences of positive events, minimizing the probability and consequences of adverse events.
- **Risk:** It is an event happening with potentially harmful outcomes for self and others, e.g., infection, medication errors, IV therapy injuries, patient identification errors, etc.
- **Robotic surgery:** It uses highly advanced computer-controlled instruments to perform complex surgeries in a minimally invasive way that enhances the capabilities of surgeon's hands. It allows surgeons to perform procedures in hard-to-reach areas through small incisions. It can be done solely or performed alongside traditional open surgical procedures.
- **Science of information:** It studies the analysis, collection, classification, manipulation storage, retrieval, movement, dissemination, and protection of information. It also includes how to acquire information systematically from raw data.
- **Scientific research data:** Data from scientific research activities and results of research, drug trials, new inventions, etc.
- **Security:** It is defined as the level at which accessing someone's personal information is restricted and allowed for those authorized only.
- **Smart classroom:** It is a technology enhanced classroom that fosters opportunities for teaching and learning by integrating learning technology such as computers, specialized software, audience response technology, assistive listening devices, networking, and audiovisual capabilities.
- **Smart pumps:** These are intravenous infusion pumps that are equipped with dose calculation software designed to identify and correct pump-programming errors (medication error prevention software). These smart pumps allow clinicians to pre-program standard concentrations and upper and lower dose limits for a variety of drugs. This software alerts the operator when the infusion setting is beyond the pre-configured safety limits.
- **Statistical package for social sciences (SPSS):** It is a product of IBM highly preferred for carrying out all types of quantitative analyses.
- **Synchronous or real-time telemedicine:** In this both the sender and the receiver are online at the same point of time with live transfer of information taking place. It is used when face-to-face consultation is required. While the patient or nurse practitioner or telemedicine coordinator is present at the original site, the specialist is present at the referral site (mostly at urban medical

centers). Video conferencing equipment at both locations allows real-time consultation to take place. All specialties of medicine are conducive to this kind of consultation.
- **Telehealth:** It is the use of electronic information and telecommunication technology to support long-distance clinical health care, patient and professional health-related education and training, public health and health administration.
- **Telemedicine consultation center (TCC):** It is the site where the patient is present. In a telemedicine consultation center, equipment for scanning/converting, transformation and communicating the patient's medical information is available.
- **Telemedicine specialty center (TSC):** It is a site where the specialist is present. He can interact with the patient present at the remote site, view his reports and monitor his progress.
- **Telemedicine system:** It consists of an interface between hardware, software and a communication channel to eventually bridge two geographical locations to exchange information and enable teleconsultancy between two locations.
- **Telemedicine:** It is the delivery of healthcare services by all healthcare professionals using information and communication technologies for the exchange of valid information for diagnosis, treatment and prevention of disease and injuries, research and evaluation and for the continuing education of healthcare providers where distance is a critical factor. It is all done in the interest of advancing health of individuals and their communities.
- **Telenursing:** It is the use of telecommunications technology in nursing to enhance patient care. These include use of electronic channels such as wire and optical to transmit voice, data and video communication signals.
- **Unsafe injections practices:** Unsafe injections practices in healthcare settings can transmit infections including HIV and hepatitis B and C. These pose direct danger to patients and healthcare workers.
- **Unsafe surgical care procedures:** Common errors in surgeries are unnecessary or inappropriate surgeries, anesthesia mistakes, cutting an organ or another part of the body by mistake, instruments and other foreign objects left inside patient bodies, infections, etc. Unsafe surgical care can cause substantial harm.
- **Unsafe transfusion practices:** These practices expose patients to the risk of adverse transfusion reactions and transmission of infections.
- **Website:** It is a collection of web pages or interconnected web pages and related information usually including a home page, available on a common domain name located on the same server, prepared and maintained by an individual, group, or organization to provide a collection of information to its viewers.
- **Work lists:** These are list of nursing tasks and interventions for each patient, generated to provide instructions to nursing and supporting staff.
- **Workload measurement and unit staffing:** Nursing workload management systems assist nursing managers in staffing, budgeting, planning and quality assurance by providing required information.
- **World Wide Web (WWW):** It is a system of internet servers that supports specially formatted documents. It is a leading information retrieval service of the internet.

Introduction to Computer Applications for Patient Care Delivery System and Nursing Practice

INTRODUCTION

The influence of computers in present day era cannot be undermined owing to the fact that all forms of human activities are now being carried out by them. Life in today's world would be unimaginable without computers. They made human lives better and happier. Computers have become an essential part of modern human life. It includes fields of trade and commerce, education, scientific research, social and natural sciences and even health care particularly nursing practice. The use of computers in nursing has increased exponentially. Innovation of computer technology and its use in medicine has also led to introduction of many improved techniques in the field of nursing. Nurses along with doctors are now in a position to develop and implement detailed plans for patient health care. Computers can now help in early detection of diseases and monitoring of patients even from remote locations. Nursing requires the aid of computers for extending better care and treatment of the patient. Healthcare particularly nursing has now truly become inseparable from the use of computer-assisted technology.

COMPUTER

The word computer comes from the word "compute", which means to calculate. Computer is an electronic device that is designed to accept, store and process data, and produce output results. It is used to store and process large amounts of data, provide information to the users and perform calculations rapidly and accurately. Charles Babbage is considered as the father of modern computer.

Meaning

Computer is an electronic machine used for storing, organizing and finding words, numbers and pictures, doing calculations and controlling other machines.

A computer is a machine or device that performs processes, calculations and operations based on instructions provided by a software or hardware program.

A computer is a programmable machine which can respond to a specific set of instructions in a well-defined manner and execute a pre-recorded list of instructions.

Components of Computer

There are five basic elements in a computer which help in processing of data and functioning of a computer (**Fig. 1.1**). These are:
- **Input unit:** A computer responds only when a command is given. These commands can be given through input devices such as keyboard, mouse, punch cards, magnetic tapes, etc. The data entered can be in

the form of numbers, alphabets, images, etc. Input devices convert the data to be processed into a format acceptable to the computer after which it is passed on to the central processing unit.
- **Memory unit:** When data is entered into a computer using input devices, the entered information immediately gets saved in the memory unit of the central processing unit (CPU). Similarly when the output command is processed by the computer, it is saved in the memory unit before giving the output to the user.
- **Control unit:** It is the most essential unit of the computer which manages the functioning of the computer and is the center of all processing actions taking place inside the computer device. This control unit collects the data entered through input devices, leads it on for processing and once done, receives the output and presents it to the user. Basically the control unit receives instructions, interprets them, executes the data and retrieves the data.
- **Arithmetic and logic unit:** It performs all mathematical calculations or arithmetic operations such as addition, subtraction, multiplication, division and other numerical based calculations. It also performs actions like comparison of data and decision-making.
- **Output unit:** When a command is given through an input device, the processing unit converts it into computer understandable language which then processes the data giving out the final result. This result is called the output. The output unit accepts the results produced by the central processing unit and supplies them to the users. The most basic output device is a monitor. When a command is given through keyboard or mouse, information is displayed on the monitor.

Other component of a computer is the software. It refers to a set of programs that controls the processing activity of the computer. There are two types of software: system software and application software.

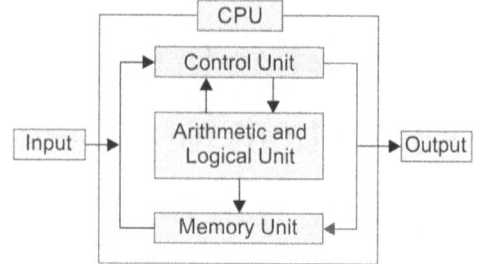

Fig. 1.1: Components of computer

System software is a collection of programs which allows the user to interact with the computer hardware. For example, operating systems like DOS, and BASIC, etc.

Application software consists of programs which perform special functions for the user such as word processing, data processing and spreadsheet programs.

Parts of Computer

Computer is made up of different physical parts and programmed with different languages to carry out a set of algorithms and arithmetic instructions. Each part has an important role to play and helps perform a specific task.

Computer parts are generally divided into internal and external parts. Internal parts refer to built-in components and are placed inside the computer case such as motherboard, CPU, RAM, etc. External parts refer to components that are attached to the computer using one of the ports linked to the motherboard. Example, mouse, keyboard, speakers, webcam, etc. The basic parts of a computer are depicted in **Figure 1.2**.

- **Monitor:** Also called the visual display unit, it is one of the essential parts of a computer system. It is made of glass, circuitry, adjustment buttons, power supplies, etc., all enclosed within a casing. The monitor is connected to a computer and displays output like text, image or video on the screen. LED (light-emitting diode) and LCD (liquid crystal display) monitors are most prevalent these days.
- **Keyboard:** It is one of the primary input devices which helps to interact with the

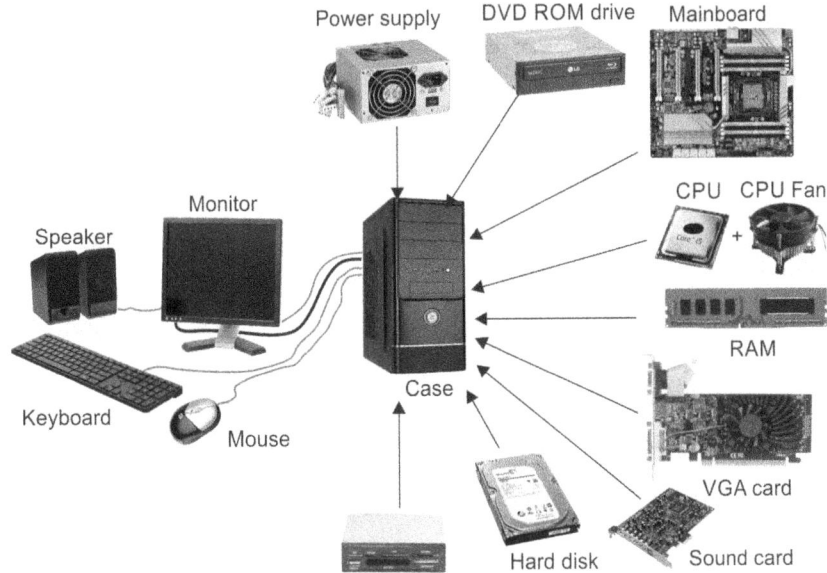

Fig. 1.2: Parts of computer

computer system. A keyboard is one of the ways to communicate with a computer. The keyboard's layout is similar to that of a typewriter. It has a set of keys such as alphabetical keys, character keys, functional keys, arrow keys and control keys. When we press a key on the keyboard, the computer receives input from the keyboard. There are two types of keyboards: mechanical and membrane type.

- **Mouse:** It is an input device which helps to communicate with the computer system. It allows the user to move a pointer displayed on the monitor. A computer mouse can be wired or wireless. A typical mouse usually has three buttons: right, left and middle roller button. Generally, there are two types of mice (plural form of mouse): mechanical and optical. While the mechanical mouse uses a ball and roller, the optical mouse uses laser technology to track the movements of the cursor and allows for accurate precision and smooth movement.
- **Computer case:** It is a special box which holds all of the internal components of a computer. It includes motherboard, central processing unit, power supply, drives, memory and writing. The front of the computer case usually provides access to the power on/off button, CD/DVD drives and some ports such as USB, audio jack, etc. On the back are sockets for connecting a monitor, power cord, etc.
- **Motherboard:** Also called the main board, this circuit board holds all the different electronic components and peripherals of the computer system. These are interconnected so as to allow communication with each other and functioning of the computer. The input and output devices are plugged into the motherboard for function. It consists of CPU, RAM, ROM, sound card, video card, network card, ports for input, output and storage devices, etc.
- **Central processing unit (CPU):** It is one of the core components of computer system also known as brain of the computer, processor, central processor, or microprocessor. No action can take place without its permission and execution. It communicates with all other components of the computer and has three parts: memory unit, control unit, arithmetic and

logic unit. All these components help in the efficient working and processing of data.

- **Graphics processing unit (GPU):** Also called video adaptor, video card and display card help to generate high end visuals. This electronic circuit displays high quality images and graphics by performing rapid mathematical calculations. It helps to process 2D data and 3D data. Higher the memory of the graphic card, higher is the quality of visual effects on the computer screen.
- **Fan:** It is an internal part of a computer system that primarily helps to keep the computer system or its components cool by circulating air. This prevents overheating and physical damage to the computer thereby extending the life of the computer.
- **Memory:** Memory units typically store data and instructions for core system files and configuration. Memory is designed for fast access. The internal memory of a computer is mainly of two types viz. RAM and ROM. Random-access memory (RAM) are one of the basic computer parts which serve as a computer's primary memory for temporary storing of current data or ongoing data. It is also known as volatile memory as it gets erased every time the computer restarts. It has a fast read/write speed and can be accessed quickly by the computer. Read-only memory (ROM) is a non-volatile storage medium that stores essential computer data. It keeps the stored data even after the power is turned off.
- **Storage:** Computers need to store all the data and they either have a hard disk drive (HDD) or a solid state drive (SSD) for this purpose. These storage devices are mainly used to store long-term data. The data saved in these devices is available until it is deleted. HDD are disks that store data which is read by a mechanical arm. SSD are like SIM card faster than hard drives.
- **Speakers:** Speakers are optional parts of a computer. They can be connected to a computer to get audio output while listening to a class. Speakers are attached to the sound card and convert the electromagnetic waves into audible audio waves. These speakers also have amplifiers that enable us to adjust the volume level of sound output. Many monitors and laptop computers come with built-in speakers.
- **Mic:** The mic or microphone is another optional part of the computer. It gives voice input to the computer system. It perceives sounds from the surroundings and converts these sounds into electronic signals. These signals are further converted into digital forms to be stored on the computer. Mic is needed when we need to insert audio into our presentation, do voice conferencing, recording, broadcasting, giving voice command to the computer, etc.
- **Webcam:** This is also an optional part of the computer system mainly used to capture images and videos and send them in digital form to a computer. They must be connected to the computer for proper functioning. Webcam helps to make videos, do video conferencing, live broadcasting, etc.
- Other optional parts of a computer system are CD/DVD drive, uninterruptible power supply device, printer, scanner, etc.

A computer user can control it by input devices such as keyboard, mouse, touch screen and also with voice commands or hand gestures, etc.

Classification of Computers

Based on their power, computers can be classified as follows:

- **Personal computer:** It is a small single-user computer based on a microprocessor. Along with microprocessor a personal computer has a keyboard for entering data, a monitor for displaying information and a storage device for saving data. These are known as all purpose computers.
- **Workstation:** It is similar to a personal computer but with a much powerful microprocessor and a high quality monitor.
- **Minicomputer:** It is a multiuser computer.

- **Mainframe:** It is a powerful multi-user computer capable of supporting many users simultaneously.
- **Super computer:** It is a high-speed computer that can perform millions of instructions per second.

Based on size computers can be classified as follows:
- **Desktop computers:** These are personal computers. A tower, monitor, keyboard and mouse are all common components of a desktop computer.
- **Laptops/net books:** These are more portable than a desktop. A laptop computer is self-contained with an integrated screen, keyboard and mouse pad.
- **Tablet computers:** These are portable computers with screens that are slightly smaller than a laptop. While there is no keypad or a mouse, all user contact is done through touch. Users initiate task or control or input data by swiping, pinching, dragging and rotating icons on the screen.

Features of Computer

Two principal characteristics of a computer are:
1. It responds to a specific set of instructions in a well-defined manner and
2. It can execute a prerecorded list of instructions (a program).
   - It has the ability to accept data, process it, and then produce outputs.
   - It can store data in appropriate storage devices and retrieve whenever necessary.
   - They are designed to execute applications and provide a variety of solutions by combining integrated hardware and software components.

Historical Perspectives of Computers in Nursing

Use of computer technology in nursing emerged in response to the changing and developing technologies in health care industry and nursing practice.

- Prior to 1960s, computers were initially used in health care facilities for basic office functions.
- In 1960s, hospital information systems were developed primarily for carrying out financial transactions and serving billing and accounting systems.
- In 1970s, nurses began to recognize the value of a computer for their profession. Basically, they recognized the computer's potential for improving documentation in nursing practice, quality of care and monitoring patient care.
- In 1980s, nursing informatics became an accepted specialty with many nursing experts entering the field. Starting in 1981, nursing pioneers conducted national and international conferences and workshops to help nurses understand and get involved in this new emerging nursing specialty. Hospital information systems documented several aspects of patient information such as vital signs, medication information, nurses' notes, admission and discharge information. It was during this period that micro computers or personal computers emerged. This revolutionary technology made computers more accessible, affordable and usable by nurses and other health care providers. Personal computers being more user friendly allowed nurses to create their own applications.
- In 1990s computer technology became an integral part of health care settings, nursing practice and the nursing profession. In 1992, nursing informatics was approved by the American Nurses Association as a new nursing specialty with separate scope for nursing informatics practice standards for which a specific credentialing examination was established. During this period local area networks (LANs), wide area networks (WANs), and internet were developed for linking care across health care facilities.
- In 2000s, a change occurred in the new millennium as more and more health care information became digitalized and newer technology emerged. There was

exponential growth in the fields of hardware and software. This growth is reflected in health care and nursing. Electronic patient records were introduced in hospitals. Critical care units were monitored remotely by health providers. Home health care too partnered increasingly with information technology for the provision of patient care.

- With the advent and use of mobile technology (wireless tablet computers, personal digital assistance and smart cellular telephones) information technology too continued to advance.
- Many health care organizations have adopted policies favoring the implementation of digital technology. Presently computers are used not only for diagnosis and imaging techniques but also in home care and long-term facilities.
- Computers can perform a wide range of activities that not only save time but also help nurses in providing quality nursing care.

USE OF COMPUTERS IN TEACHING AND LEARNING

Introduction of computers while changing lives dramatically has also found wide spread application in education. Since the 1950s, people have been trying to use computers, video and telecommunications to transform education. Use of computers has become an important part of nursing education. They help in exchanging information, teaching, learning approaches, scientific research and accessing information. Presently computers are used for a variety of purposes ranging from browsing the web, writing documents, learning, teaching, editing videos, creating applications and playing games, etc.

Computer is an efficient instructional tool providing both students and teachers with more opportunities in adapting, learning and teaching for individual needs. Even distance learning is made productive and effective through internet and video-based classes. Computer programs can influence cognitive, affective and psychomotor skill development. Computers can be used in nursing education for three different purposes: teaching and learning, student evaluation and course record management **(Fig. 1.3)**.

Teaching and Learning

Computer technology has proved to be very successful in the field of education as it changed the nature of classroom teaching dramatically. Computers have not only improved the quality of teaching but also enhanced the learning process with the help

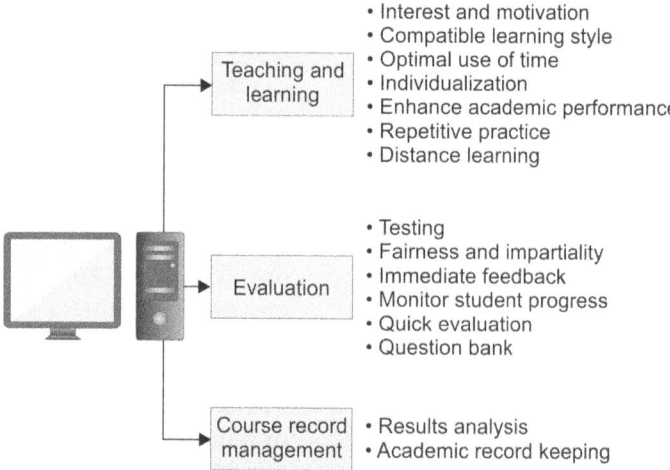

Fig. 1.3: Enhanced academic performance: Monitoring student progress

of various tools such as multimedia projector, power point presentation, etc. in the following ways:

- **Interest and motivation:** The use of multimedia approach to teaching and learning through computers stimulates learners and transforms learning into an active engaging process that promotes problem solving and development of critical thinking skills. Computers make learning process more interesting through visuals, animated graphics, etc. Illustrations along with narrations via computer increase learner's recall and comprehension.
- **Rapid access to information:** Websites allow rapid access to online and printed material. Digital health related materials can be updated quickly allowing educators to create and revise online course content. Students who become competent and literate in use of computers and other digital devices become more successful in their education and practice. Laptops and mobile digital technologies such as smart phones help nurses, nurse students and faculty to access valuable information for managing patient condition.
- **Effective teaching experience:** Advanced educational media technology like projectors, smart boards, computer models and simulation labs are being increasingly used by nursing faculty to provide effective teaching experiences to students. Nursing students are now widely using smart phones, tablets and android applications as a means for educational support. Android apps have made it possible for information to be available on student fingertrips which can increasingly be used in clinical nursing education. Video-assisted teachings with the help of animation are also being widely used in nursing education. Nursing procedures, physical examination, breath sounds and stages of labor can be made clear and thorough with the help of these visual learning technologies.
- **Compatible learning style:** Computers can teach at any level of learning from knowledge and comprehension up through application, analysis and synthesis. They can be programmed to teach problem solving and decision making.
- **Optimal use of learning time:** The learner can without time constraints move as quickly or as slowly as desired to master the content. Also there is no penalty for mistakes committed or low performance speed.
- **Individualization:** Instructors can present to learners more problems with increasing complexity at a pace of learner's own choosing. Here the student is an active participant in the learning process with an opportunity to manipulate information and take action in various situations.
- **Enhanced academic performance:** Computers enhance academic performance of students and faculty by facilitating access to literature, computer-assisted instruction, class room technology, distance learning such as E-books, online libraries and online encyclopedia.
- **Repetitive practice:** Readymade software can provide practice material to students.
- **Distance learning:** Computer and related technologies have been used in distance learning through various ways such as teleconferencing, video conferencing, visuals, multimedia and hypermedia, e-books, recorded videos, online database, online discussion, on-demand call in course, etc. Virtual classrooms play an important role in distance learning wherein students can clarify their doubts without going to one's place.
- **Effective communication:** Students are now able to communicate more frequently with more contacts with the help of computer and advanced educational technology such as multiple digital chat rooms, blogs and social network systems to expand their knowledge.

Evaluation

- **Testing:** For testing, large banks of potential items can be written with the computer

generating different exams for each student depending upon the selection criteria.
- **Fairness and impartiality:** Computer technology ensures fairness and impartiality in the examination. Most exams are now-a-days being conducted by computers all over the world.
- **Immediate feedback:** Computers can be programmed to provide feedback to the educator regarding the learner's grasp of concepts, and speed of learning. Interactive feature of this medium also provides for immediate feedback to the learner.
- **Monitor student progress:** Computers can be used to monitor student progress, evaluate student responses and tailor student remedial work.
- **Quick evaluation:** Students' answers can also be stored electronically and the exam results analyzed quickly. For example, the National Council Licensure Examination (NCLEX-RN) moved from paper and pencil tests to computer tests.
- **Create question bank:** Computers can be used to create a pool of questions.

Course Record Management

- **Results analysis:** Computers are useful in maintaining attendance and student grade results. Computer programs can calculate percentages, sort student scores in order and print results for both students and faculty.
- **Academic record keeping:** Cumulative results can be calculated and stored with ease. Many nursing institutions have now captured all student records in the computer. A computer can keep track of names, addresses, courses taken, grades and all other important data. Nurse educators use computers for academic record keeping too.

Disadvantages

- Lack of computer literacy among all learners
- Lack of easy access to computers
- Deprivation of personal, compassionate one-to-one interaction for the learner.

Forms of Computer Application in Nursing Education

Technology has exerted great influence on teaching learning methods in nursing education. Innovations in teaching and learning like computer-assisted learning, web-based learning, e-learning, smart classroom and other information and communication technology are being increasingly used to promote intellectual development of the learner.

Computer-assisted Learning

Computer-assisted learning (CAL) is a type of e-learning that has been used in nursing education since 1960s. It includes computer-assisted instruction (CAI) and computer-managed instruction (CMI). CAL uses a computer system to perform the teaching function of communicating information to the learner to support learning and training individuals. In computer managed instruction, the computer is programmed to integrate student records, curriculum schedules, time tables and information resources such as combination of text, graphs, sound and video to enhance the learning process.

Internet based learning, online learning, web-based learning are synonymous terms for computer-assisted learning.

Meaning and Definitions

Computer-assisted learning is defined as the use of computers to support the learning and training of individuals. It requires no direct interaction between the user and the human instructor in order to function.

CAL includes a range of computer based packages that focus on providing interactive instructions in a specific subject. The learner responds to instructions and information while the computer monitors the responses, analyzes the learning and provides feedback to the learner.

Computer-assisted learning is an interactive technique whereby a computer is employed to present the instructional material, monitor, analyze learning and provide feedback.

Different Modes of CAL

- CAL consists of a range of computer-based packages such as word processing programs, tutorials and games that focus on providing interactive instructions in a specific subject area, display of information, evaluation of student with embedded quizzes and illustration of abstract idea using computer graphics, multi-media, diagrams, virtual patients and discussion boards.
- This allows the individual to follow self directed access to a particular topic or information of interest and facilitate optimal education resources management. It can be provided either as a standalone or instructor facilitated computer learning activity.
- The main aim is for the computers to play the role of another tutor, peer or examiner so as to provide a holistic insight into the educational process.
- CAL often delivers content through CD-ROM or website, webinar, web based tutorials, or online interactive modules. The content is presented in a linear fashion. It can be learned in a computer lab, at home, or any location with the students having the liberty to use a mobile computing device at any time convenient to them.
- CAL provides text or multimedia content, multiple choice questions, exercises for practice, worksheets, problems, tests, immediate feedback and summarizes student's performance. The different modes of CAL include drill and practice, tutorial, games and simulation (**Fig. 1.4**).
    - *Drill and practice*: This software provides repeated exposure to facts or information, often in a question-answer or game type format. In question-answer type program the computer generates large number of exercises, evaluates

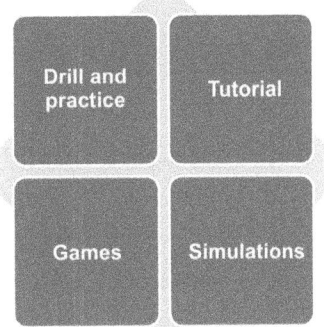

Fig. 1.4: Different modes of computer-assisted learning

responses, provides immediate feedback as to the correctness of the responses and at times gives hints on how to obtain the correct answers if the responses are incorrect. This provides the students an opportunity to practice repeatedly and gain mastery over the skill. These software programs deal with lower order thinking skills such as remembering facts and principles.
    - *Tutorial:* This software presents concepts or skills followed by an opportunity for the students to practice them. It deals with presentation of information in small segments followed by questions mostly using multimedia technology. If an answer is found correct another segment of the explanatory material is generated. Based on the student response the program decides how rapidly the material should be generated and how much it should cover. Students who are absent or need remediation can benefit from a computerized tutorial. This mode is often very interactive and used to teach fundamental/basic subjects.
    - *Games:* In this the learners apply knowledge to win a game. Game mechanics work to engage learners within the digital environment and promote progress within the game experience. Games whether simple or

Advantages	Limitations
• Allows self pacing • Arouses interest and motivation • Provides immediate feedback • Focuses on self directed learning • Helps in rapid learning • Increases subject retention • Enhances practice skills • Maximizes effect of teaching • Lesser geographical constraints • Access to expert faculty and material • Access to flipped class technique • Communication development • Cost and time saving	• Requires special equipment • Requires skilled personnel • Expensive • Requires frequent update of technology • Distracts learner • Limits social behavior

Fig. 1.5: Advantages and limitations of CAL

complex challenge the learner's ability to use higher cognitive function and problem solving strategies.
- *Simulation:* This software provides an approximation of reality without involving the expense of real life or its risks. A simulation is a model of a real life event or object or phenomenon with the learner having the power to manipulate its various aspects. They see the results of their actions and decisions immediately. This presents life-like situations that allow students to learn through experience and take risks without suffering the consequences of poor choices. Simulation program is suitable for teaching all clinical subjects.

CAL uses a variety of multimedia resources offering a personalized learning experience tailored to meet the individual student needs and essential feedback. The advantages and limitations are presented in **Figure 1.5**.

Previous literature has shown that computer-assisted instruction increases cognitive accomplishment among nursing students. Thus addition of computer-assisted programs to existing educational methods would prove to be more effective and useful.

E-Learning (Electronic Learning)

E-learning is an umbrella term that includes various concepts and technologies related to learning such as digital learning, electronic learning, online learning, web-based learning, mobile learning, computer-assisted learning, information technology or information and communication technology (ICT) based learning.

While E-Learning is an internet-based form of learning without any face-to-face interaction, the traditional methods of learning are supported by computer or other electronic devices to provide training, education and learning.

E-learning also termed as network enabled transfer of skills and knowledge is a medium through which the delivery of education is made to a large number of recipients at the same or different times, anytime and anywhere.

E-learning modules related to corona virus disease, maternal and newborn health care modules, skill enhancement modules, etc. are available on the Indian Nursing council (INC) website.

Smart Classroom

With the development of technologies, new strategies of teaching are being introduced in the curriculum, one of which is known as the smart classroom. It uses instructional material, 3D animated modules and videos for the understanding of students.

Smart classrooms are technology enhanced classrooms that foster opportunities for teaching and learning by integrating learning technology such as computers, specialized software, audience response technology,

Unit 1 | Introduction to Computer Applications for Patient Care Delivery System and Nursing Practice

assistive listening devices, networking, and audio/visual capabilities.

In smart classroom, the classroom is integrated with the digital displays, tabs, whiteboards, assistive listening devices, and other audio/visual components that make lectures easier, engaging and more interactive.

Components of Smart Classroom

Smart classroom can be considered as a virtual classroom. Teaching is carried out with the help of smart teaching tools. It helps the teachers to access multimedia content and information that can be used for teaching students more effectively. Components of smart classroom are presented in **Figure 1.6**.

- **Interactive smart/white board:** It uses finest digital ink technology. The four components of interactive white boards are: computer, projector, appropriate software and display panel.
- **Hardware equipment:** It includes desktops, laptops, tablets, iPads, class pads, etc.
- **Tablets and pen:** In these, written words are translated into typed script which is then projected for the whole class to see.
- **Learning management system (LMS):** It is a software application or web-based technology used to plan, implement and assess a specific learning process. It consists of two elements: a server that performs the base functionality and a user interface that is operated by instructors, students and administrators. LMS provides the instructor with a way to create and deliver content, monitor student participation and assess student performance. It also provides students with an ability to use interactive features such as discussion and feedback.
- **Response pad:** These are electronic handheld wireless pads, multi-function touch response supporting multiple touch points.
- **Smart audio:** It includes speaker system, room module, software, infra-red microphone and control unit. It ensures that students are able to hear every word of the lecture.
- **Digital slate:** Students can write notes or highlight information in digital ink.
- **Document camera:** It is capable of projecting both documents and transparencies

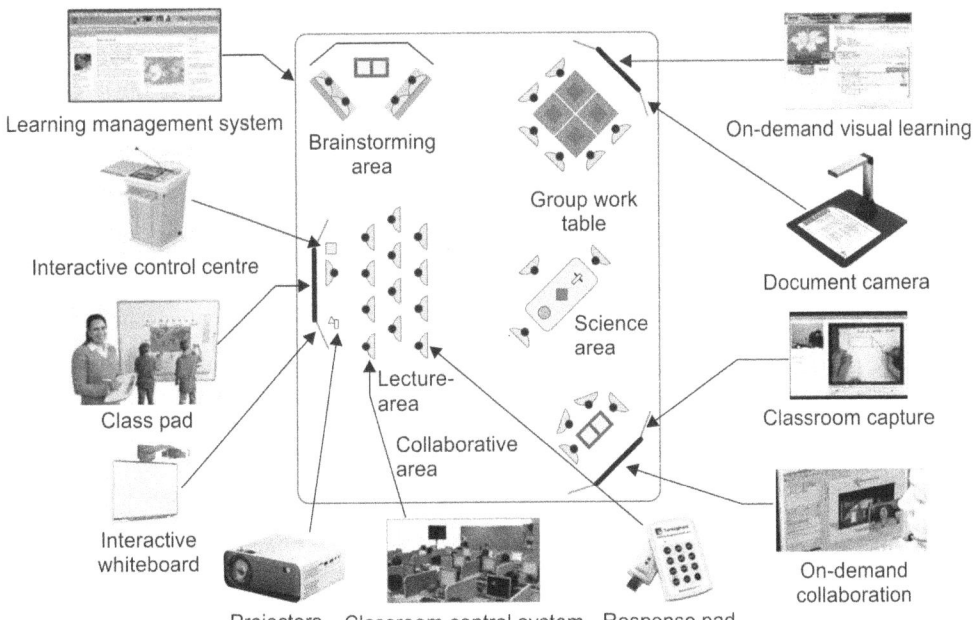

Fig. 1.6: Components of smart classroom

through single device over the classroom. This turns real objects into digital content.
- Other tools include LCD projectors, DVD/VCR combo and microphones.

Computers are highly beneficial in the teaching-learning process as they are cost effective and can provide quality education to a large number of students in shortest possible time.

ROLE OF COMPUTERS IN RESEARCH PROCESS

Computers are an indispensable tool during each stage of the research process. They have revolutionized the way scientific research is compiled and analyzed. The researcher is able to compile vast amounts of data without an element of human error. Thus, the use of computers in scientific research is immensely high and inevitable. Researchers have massive usage of these computers in their work from beginning till the end of their scholarly work.

Importance of Computers in Scientific Research

Research has become a major area in nursing curriculum. Action research and the use of qualitative methodologies in research is getting wider acceptance now.

- **Speed:** Computers can process numbers and information in an exceptionally short time. This helps the researcher to process and analyze the data quickly and utilize the remaining time for conducting further research.
- **Storage:** Computers can store and retrieve huge amounts of data when needed. It overcomes the risk of forgetting and loosing the data.
- **Accuracy:** Computers are incredibly accurate which is very important in scientific research.
- **Organization:** Computers allow easy storage of large amounts of data in an organized manner using simple folders. This not only allows easy retrieval but also saves scarce resources such as time and energy. Computers are more productive and safer compared to paper filing system.
- **Consistency:** Computers are not susceptible to mistakes on account of tiredness or lack of concentration.

Research process consists of a series of steps necessary to carry out research effectively. These series of steps can be organized into five phases. A brief description of use of computers in all these phases is presented in **Table 1.1**.

Technological innovations have integrated the use of computers in research beyond

Table 1.1: Use of computers in various phases of research process

Phases	Use of computers
Conceptual phase: It involves developing a research idea and appropriate design	• They help in searching for relevant papers which allows the researcher to identify the gaps in existing literature • Their use provides a definite advantage over physical search for literature from books, journals and other newsletters in the library which is both tedious and time consuming • They can be used for storing bibliographic references through World Wide Web which allows retrieval of published articles when required • Visual display softwares can be used to create conceptual maps, flowcharts or visual models of research conceptual framework
Design and planning phase: It comprises of selecting the research design and developing study procedures	• They can be used for selection of appropriate research design and facilitating research design planning • Several softwares can be used to calculate the sample size • They help in sample selection from a population using computer software program known as a random number generator. This generates true random numbers which facilitates an unbiased random sample selection for experimental studies

Contd...

Contd...

Phases	Use of computers
Empirical phase: It deals with data collection and preparing the data for analysis	• They help in designing research instruments • Computer programs and internet technology (E-mails, online surveys) can be used for collecting data • Biophysical measurements are monitored only using computers • Computers are also useful for conducting web video recorded interview sessions, narrative led interviews, etc. • Subject related data are stored as word files or excel spread sheets in computers • Computers help in data entry, data editing and data management • Computers allow for greater flexibility in recording and analyzing the data. Data coded in excel sheets can be directly processed using statistical software for analysis.
Analytic phase: In this phase analysis and interpretation of findings takes place	• Data analysis and interpretation can be done with the help of computer softwares which help in calculating averages, percentages, correlation, etc. For example, SPSS, STATA, SYSTAT, etc. • Examples of statistics that can easily be calculated through computers are descriptive statistics, chi-square, correlation, t-tests, ANOVA, etc. • These softwares can also be used for checking the reliability of data, establishing and testing hypothesis, etc. • They can check the accuracy, authenticity and completeness of the data as they are collected. • They help in drafting tables by which a researcher can interpret the results easily. These tables give a clear proof of the interpretation made by the researcher.
Dissemination phase: During this phase research results are shared with others	• The last decade has witnessed a great expansion in nursing literature. The CINAHL, Cochrane, PubMed databases serve as excellent treasures for nurses and nursing students. This has significantly helped in the dissemination of research finding and evidence-based nursing practice across the world. • After interpretation, computer helps in converting the results into a research article or report which can be published. It can be written in a word format or a PDF format. • Computers can also be used for preparing posters and power point presentations for disseminating research study findings. • Articles can be stored or published on website also. • Computers help to access research papers on the internet effortlessly. • International co-operation on scientific projects by forming virtual research teams, aggregating information and sharing of knowledge has been made possible by the use of high speed internet. • For performing Meta-analysis and systematic reviews, data from various studies can be retrieved using specialized softwares.
References: A researcher needs to give source of the literature studied and discussed in references	• References can be written automatically in different styles like APA, Vancouver, etc. which saves considerable time for the researcher. • Some reference managers like 'Medley' can be used to manage the references from where the literature is taken.

imagination. However, it is to be noted that the computers and their applications are only a tool in the hands of the researcher and function as a resource. The researcher should thus exhibit a fine knowledge about the capabilities and limitations of the computer applications and softwares for their optimum use.

ROLE OF COMPUTERS IN NURSING PRACTICE

Scientific advancements in technology introduced various innovations in nursing practice and health care. Computers revolutionized the nursing profession by improving management of clinical and administrative functions of nurses. The clinical and technological advancements led to a nursing specialty called nursing informatics. It is the application of computer and information science to promote and support the practice of nursing and the delivery of nursing care.

A computer assists the nurses with four functions:
- Gathers data base where the computer has resource information such as techniques, drugs, patient preparation and patient education.
- Formulates a list of nursing problems based on assessment data.
- Formulates initial plans for each problem in which the nurse selects from a repertoire of interventions related to each problem and
- Recording progress notes on the problem.

Nurses use computers for assessment and monitoring of patient condition, decision making, care planning, implementing care, patient education and continuing education, documentation of patient information, and communication purpose (**Fig. 1.7**).

Assessment and Monitoring

- Professional nurses use a variety of technological tools for patient assessment. Nurses use bedside handheld monitors to collect a variety of information such as blood glucose levels, clotting time, cardiac output, blood pressure, oxygen saturation, temperature, pulse monitoring, etc.
- This testing enables nurses to receive instant results for planning nursing care. Patient monitoring systems that use wireless technology enable automatic nurse paging capability when patient measurements fall outside normal parameters. For example, when a patient connected to a centralized telemetry system experiences a premature ventricular contraction the monitoring system immediately pages the nurse. These improved techniques enable nurses to act more quickly to abnormal findings.

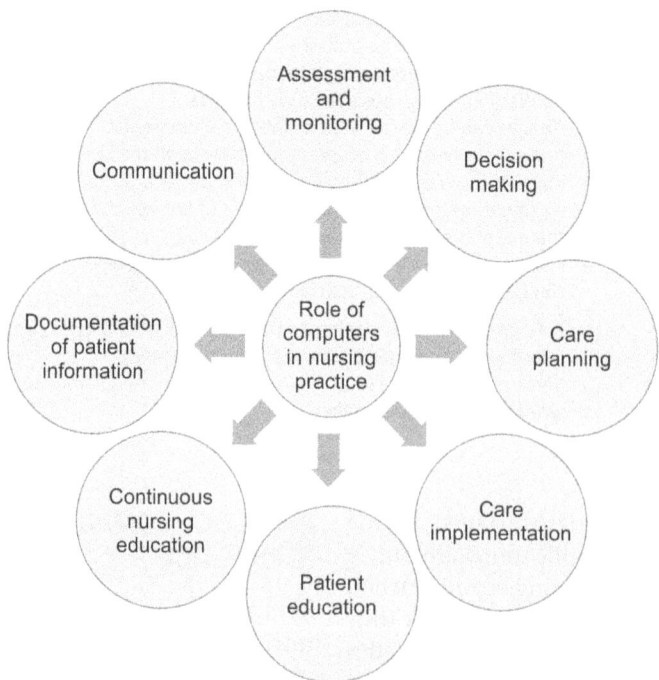

Fig. 1.7: Role of computers in nursing practice

- Wearable gadgets in the form of watches, footwear, chest straps, sensible glasses, etc. designed to collect patient's heart rate, blood pressure and blood sugar levels, etc. are now readily available. These are sensor-based accessories which can collect patient data anytime and anywhere. These help nurses to monitor patient condition.
- Pocket-sized hand-held ultrasound device is predicted to replace the stethoscopes in near future. This can diagnose heart, lung and other problems more accurately than the traditional stethoscopes.

Decision Making

- Computer-assisted decision making is intended to support health care personnel for clinical decision making.
- Clinical decision making support system includes an array of computer-based applications that assist health care clinicians in the day-to-day work of patient care.
- Decision making support systems help nurses define clinical problems, generate potential solutions and select the best solution based on likelihood of success.
- Nurses can also have access to decision making algorithms when clinical practice guidelines and procedures have been entered into the computer system.
- Computer technology enables nurses to access essential nursing tools and key medical references online thus reducing diagnosis time and errors.
- Computer softwares also provide digital assistance to nurses in the form of digital books, medical dictionaries, drug references guides, clinical drug calculation programs, etc.
- Patient helper sofwares enable nurses to enter patient laboratory test results and be cues to the best clinical decision to fit a given situation.
- Nurses and other health care providers also have access to computerized clinical decision-making support systems.
- The use of decision-making support system yields direct benefits for patient and entire health care team and industry. It reduces and prevents patient suffering, adverse events and health care expenses.

Care Planning

- A computer-based patient record facilitates the automation of nursing care planning process.
- Some health care institutions have software that provides the nurse with expected outcomes and nursing interventions related to the identified nursing diagnosis.
- Software programs enable the nurse to input individualized nursing actions to communicate patient care preferences.
- Some institutions place clinical practice guidelines and employee policies onto a mainframe that can be accessed using any computer connected to the local area network.

Implementing Care

- Nurses use software programs and apps to assess, monitor and manage patient problems.
- Computer-assisted therapy helps for planning, monitoring and adjusting dosage regimens of powerful and potentially toxic drugs. For example, digitalis and antibiotics.
- Computerized intravenous pumps enable nurses to program administration rates for ordered medications.
- With patient controlled analgesia pumps being programmed, nurses can select the type of drug and its concentration before inputting an intermittent or continuous infusion rate.
- Some air mattresses use computer components and software to regulate the amount of air inflation.
- Implantable subcutaneous pumps deliver local anesthetic drugs to regulate the rate of subcutaneous drug administration during surgeries.

- Computerized medication dispensing stations prevent nurses from making medication errors which automatically notify the pharmacy when the stocked medications need to be replenished.
- Nurses can also access an array of reference material for patient education, professional information and institutional policies using computers.
- Once a hospital facility assigns an identification number to a patient, nurses can retrieve the patient's health record and verify medication orders before they administer any medications.
- Patient care unit computer terminals are linked to other key departments (X-ray, laboratory, pharmacy, etc). For example, by inputting information regarding patient medication orders into the terminal on the patient care unit, the order is transmitted directly to the pharmacy. This saves a lot of precious time which otherwise would be spent on filling out requisitions and making phone calls leaving the nurse with less time for planning and implementing quality patient care.
- As critically ill patients require large number of therapeutic interventions, many patient variables need to be collected to provide comprehensive care to the patient. In such situations, especially those related to intensive care units, it is now possible to computerize the total management of data recorded on the patient. Data management includes entry, integration and reporting of all vital signs, medications, intake and output volumes and laboratory values. For example, a closed loop system for the direct computer control of infusions of vasodilator has been developed. An intra arterial canula connected to suitable cardiovascular monitor provides the input signal to the computer. A pump which infuses the vasodilator drug to the patient is controlled by the computer to maintain the arterial pressure within predetermined units.

Patient Education and Continuing Nursing Education

- Hospitals while providing educational handouts also use computer programs to teach patients about chronic disease management.
- Preprinted documents such as discharge or preoperative instructions can also be stored in the computer and printed when necessary.
- Internet access permits nurses to stay abreast of current research findings.
- Some nursing organizations offer online continuous education programs for nurses.
- Nurses use computers for a variety of continuing education programs and complete short term online computer courses to obtain advanced degree.

Documentation

- Nursing documentation includes nursing assessment, nursing care plans, treatment charts, nurses' notes, patient charting, discharge plans and other patient progress notes. Computer systems facilitate entering above patient data, record keeping and transmission of patient information among departments.
- Health information system can integrate various aspects of care delivery. For example, when a physician enters an order for a diagnostic test into the computer it is immediately transmitted to the laboratory department. The department schedules the test and sends computer generated information to the nursing unit to notify staff and patient for special patient preparation. Once the test is performed, the business office receives notification for billing. Test results are entered into a computer which are then directly accessible to the health care providers.
- Along with test results nurses also enter patient assessments, interventions and therapeutic effects into the patient record using a computer.

- Hospital information system while tracking patient medical history also double checks the safety of ordered medications for the patient based on drug allergy information.
- Nurses use computers for documentation of electronic health record (EHR). When an organization uses an EHR, all documents related to patient care diagnostic testing, referrals or any other aspect of patient care or management is done on the computer.
- Through electronic health records admission/discharge/transfer can easily be shared among the staff in a short period of time thus reducing the waiting period for the patient and significant others.

Communication/Telemedicine

- Telemedicine enables patients the option of discussing health concerns with nurses, who can then help them decide whether or not they need to get treatment at a medical facility.
- Nurses need technology to assist patients over the phone and record their recommendations using appropriate software.
- Nurses can use software or an app to communicate with other members of the patient's care team and family members as needed.
- Information technology interventions like telecommunication and telemedicine have brought transformation in the existing health care system by lowering health care costs and providing better services. With 3G and 4G broadband access now in every corner of the country telemedicine can be used to transmit images and reports on real time basis, making it an effective tool in providing emergency medical care and specialist access to patients even in small towns and rural areas. This translates into reduced visits, lower costs and quicker diagnosis for remote patients. It also enables training of health care workers located at remote places.
- Electronic mail can be used to send messages about patients' condition to physicians.
- Computers are used not only for diagnosis and imaging techniques but also in home care and long-term facilities.
- Digital video cameras and patient monitoring devices can be linked to complex networks, making off-site patient monitoring and consultations possible. For example, rural critical care units can be linked to a central monitoring location having access to a critical care physician specialist and a critical care nurse to facilitate patient monitoring and make rapid interventions for seriously ill patients.
- Digital video cameras permit home monitoring of patients. For example, a home health agency provides a digital video camera for the patient to connect to the agency. The nurse assesses the patient from the beamed video signal, receives patient vital signs and evaluates patient progress towards expected outcomes. The nurse provides patient education and if required follows up with a home visit.
- In community settings, computers are used for gathering statistics, patient-appointments-identification systems, home care management, and automated remote patient monitoring.

Hospital Information System

- A computerized hospital information system can establish consistent standards in the transmission and storage of data and continuously monitor all transactions. It provides easy access to patient care information.
- Physician and other health care providers can have direct access to all the information of his or her patient through the use of computer.
- A hospital information system generally covers areas like registration, admission/transfer/discharge, billing, medical records, wards, operation theater scheduling, stores/

inventory, pharmacy, diet, CSSD, biomedical maintenance, payroll, accounts, etc.
- Computerized clinical laboratory provides accurate results in a short time. This contributes to efficient patient care system.

Electronic Medical Records

- Computer use has become one of the most successful ways of sharing information in the healthcare system where all computers are linked together by a common network. The application of computer systems to hospitals has provided clinical information in the most convenient form. The speed and efficiency can result in better care for patients. Online medical records significantly reduce the rate of medical information being lost, ultimately resulting in better care.
- Using computers, smartphones and tablets allows nurses to create, manage and update electronic health records with ease.
- Electronic health/medical records help doctors and nurses to communicate more efficiently by eliminating most misinterpretations of written and verbal orders. It makes it easier for medical professionals to record, retrieve and manage patient data for accurate diagnoses.
- Once patient data is captured and recorded, the records are immediately made available for the entire patient care team. This reduces the need for physicians to make trips to the patient's room to retrieve diagnostic data.
- Doctors and nurses can update the patient treatment orders more efficiently.

ROLE OF COMPUTERS IN NURSING ADMINISTRATION

In nursing administration computers are used for planning, organizing, controlling and directing the health care unit.
- In general nursing, managers use computers to collect data needed for planning, budgeting and reporting which ensures quality care.
- Nurse administrators use computers to allocate available resources to provide efficient and effective nursing care. They also use computers for patient classification system, staff scheduling system and inventory.
- An important element of administration is staffing. Some high-tech hospitals make use of computers in assigning nurses to specific patients depending on the degree of severity of the disease condition.
- Computer programs are designed to co-ordinate scheduling of nursing shifts and days off to determine the number of nurses required for the number of patients admitted.
- Many scheduling systems also collect data on individual employees such as the number and types of leaves used or accumulated.
- Staffing and scheduling systems are used to construct daily, weekly or monthly schedules which not only relieve the professional nurse from the time-consuming task but also produce more precise staffing.
- Budgeting and financial tracking are another way in which computers are used in nursing administration.
- A computer-generated inventory system can help the nurse administrators to maintain inventory list, prepare reports, create budgets and maintain personnel records.
- Computers also facilitate budget control besides improving employee satisfaction. This system results in considerable monetary saving.
- Computers are also used to perform administrative function of keeping individual records of nursing personnel.
- Computers provide complete profile of the educational activities carried out by the nursing personnel. This is useful for hospital accreditation purposes as well as keeping track of continuing education credit points earned by each individual staff.

- Computers are used to carry out basic administrative tasks in nursing which were once done on paper.

With increasing demand for efficient healthcare delivery system it can be concluded that computers are now a necessity in order to improve nursing practice encompassing nursing education, nursing research, nursing administration and the nursing process as a whole. Computerized system among health care units should be adopted in time. Health is wealth after all. Strength of the nation comes from the strength of its people.

Advantages

The main advantages of use of computers in nursing practice are that they improve efficiency and effectiveness, enhance accuracy and access of data, prevent medication errors and save time.

Improve Efficiency and Effectiveness

- Through computers, nurses execute their duties and responsibilities with greater efficiency and effectiveness.
- Nursing information system can increase efficiency and accuracy in all phases of the nursing process viz. assessment, nursing diagnosis, planning, implementation and evaluation.
- This method allows nurses to watch their patients more carefully as appreciable amount of time is saved by the computerization of nursing process.

Enhance Accuracy and Access of Data

- Computers record, share and access data accurately thereby supporting the decision making process and implementation of more assertive strategies in health care.
- Software and electronic device apps help nurses update patient records using diagnostic and treatment codes instead of the usual paper charts.
- Electronic health records are more helpful and effective since they are readable and clear compared to the manual handwriting.
- It enhances communication and availability of information, and allows for more convenient resource sharing.
- It makes file sharing easier, is highly flexible and cost efficient.

Prevent Medication Errors

- These programs and apps help the nurses to avoid medication errors and prevent unintended drug interactions.
- The computer can be programmed to record and identify date and time of all entries as well as the initials or the name of the person making the entry. This prevents medical errors and reduces nursing hours spent in non-nursing functions. In addition, these systems have the potential for facilitating research in patient care by keeping records of response to therapy.
- Computer security technology also helps nurses keep patient records confidential.
- Use of computers decreases human errors making health care delivery more reliable and consistent.

Saves Time

Computers can perform a wide range of activities that save time, help nurses provide quality nursing care by reducing clerical work, print forms, centralize patient care data.

Nursing Administration

- Expands the use of nursing staff resources
- Improves quality of patient care and documentation
- Enhances recruitment and retention
- Supports dynamic organization for change.

Limitations/Disadvantages

- They lack decision making power and are not sensitive like the human brain
- Improper data entry can be a major hindrance while using computers
- Use of computers can pose security concerns
- There is a risk of computer viruses and malware corrupting the data
- It requires an expensive set-up.

As nurses work in tandem with other health care professionals to manage and implement health care plans for patients, it is essential for them to acquire basic computer application knowledge and skills.

WINDOWS, MS OFFICE: WORD, EXCEL, POWERPOINT

Windows is a consumer-oriented graphical user interface-based operating system. Though the initial version of Windows 2.1 was released in 1985, the significant one was Windows NT 3.1 which was released in 1993. However, the first popular version that hit the market was Windows 95 which released in August 1995. Since then, Windows operating system which became a popular and successful operating system in the Personal Computers (PC) market made subsequent releases like Windows NT 4.0, Windows 98, Windows 2000, Windows ME (Millennium Edition), Windows XP, XP Professional, Windows Vista, Windows 7, Windows 8, Windows 8.1, Windows 10 (2015) and the latest version Windows 11 released in the year 2021.

Since Windows 10 has reached a wide range of its users and Windows 11 is yet to flourish in the PC market and among the users, this book intends to cover Windows 10 concepts in the later sections where required.

Hardware Requirements for Windows 10

- **Processor:** 1 gigahertz (GHz) or faster processor or SoC
- **RAM:** 1 gigabyte (GB) for 32-bit or 2 GB for 64-bit
- **Hard disk space:** 16 GB for 32-bit OS or 20 GB for 64-bit OS
- **Graphics card:** DirectX 9 or later with WDDM 1.0 driver
- **Display:** 800 × 600

Features of Windows

Windows has various significant features as shown in **Figure 1.8**.

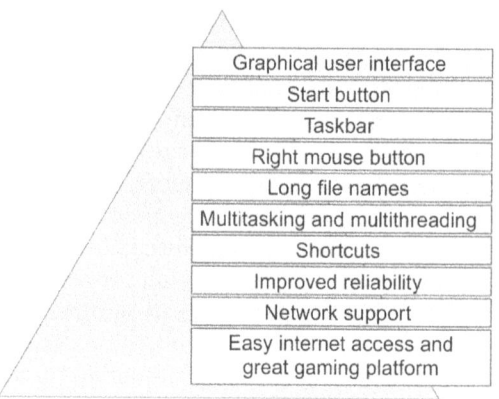

Fig. 1.8: Features of windows

- **Graphical user interface:** As compared to MS-Disk Operating System (MS-DOS), Windows is more powerful, customizable, and efficient as it uses a graphical user interface which makes Windows more user-friendly and beneficial.
- **Start button:** START button has been a permanent feature with Windows which allows the PC users to access their computer programs, start applications, access device settings or shut down the computer.
- **Taskbar:** The taskbar is another significant feature of Windows that provides information about the currently active tasks so that one can switch between tasks and also add quick launch icons in the taskbar.
- **Right mouse button:** Just one click on the right mouse button on any object, file, folder, or desktop opens a pop-up with various commands which makes it easier for the user to complete the task easily.
- **Long file names:** As compared to MS-DOS which permits only 8 letter file name, Windows permits the users to use long file names and with character length of 255 letters.
- **Multitasking and multithreading:** As compared to MS-DOS which was a 16-bit, non-preemptive, single user, single-tasking operating system, Windows has 32-bit and 64-bit versions which enable the user to do multitasking like working on a word document with music playing in the background.

- **Shortcuts:** Windows has a specific feature called the shortcut which helps access tasks with a quick shortcut creation option instead of going through the structural process.
- **Improved reliability:** Windows is a reliable operating system that can handle applications and manage crashed and faulty items better so that users can easily eliminate crashed programs without affecting the rest of the programs installed in the system.
- **Network support:** Windows supports the popular TCP/IP protocol that supports all network transport driver standards. Dial-up networking or wireless through Wi-Fi can be used to connect to the internet service provider.
- **Easy internet access and great gaming platform:** Inbuilt internet functionality of Windows enables users to connect to the internet without major hardware or software requirements. Also the built-in DirectX 12 (DX12) makes the Windows gamers friendly with its high-quality graphics and low power consumption.

Pros and Cons of Windows 10

The various advantages and disadvantages of using Windows 10 are presented in **Table 1.2**.

Advantages

- **Return of the start menu:** The user-friendly start menu is back in Windows 10. In the previous version of Windows 8, the start menu suddenly disappeared causing lot of inconvenience for its users. However, in Windows 10 the start menu and start button are back and one can work as they used to with previous versions such as Windows 7. The new-look start menu makes Windows 10 quite attractive and modern.
- **System updates for a longer period:** Besides being user-friendly, it is the regular system updates that determine the actual usage of a particular version and its active stay among consumers. For instance, Microsoft has phased out versions like Windows 7 and Windows 8 and stopped providing any updates or extensive support. While versions like Windows 8.1 have lost their mainstream support, they are also about to lose their extensive support soon which means no new functions will be added to these operating systems. With Windows 10, it is clear that though mainstream support continued till 2020, extensive support will be available till October 2025. Hence users can continue to enjoy the features of Windows 10, regularly update as and when required, and update their version to Windows 11 before the extensive support for Windows 10 ends.
- **Excellent virus protection:** The version of Windows 10 had shown significant virus protection in comparison to its previous versions. The new and advanced applications in the system make it very difficult for the malicious parties to infect the system with malicious software. For instance, the Windows Hello! functionality of Windows 10 allows unlocking the system with a fingerprint, iris scanner, or face recognition making it safer than the usual password system which might be hacker-friendly. Further, Windows 10 protects files by encrypting them when the system is threatened by malicious software using the BitLocker encryption program. Most of the digital threats are handled by anti-virus software Windows defender which comes activated with this version at every license and also other anti-virus software can be installed when required.

Table 1.2: Advantages and disadvantages of Windows 10

Advantages	Disadvantages
- Return of the start menu - System updates for a longer period - Excellent virus protection - Addition of DirectX 12 - Touch screen - Administrative control - Lighter and faster	- Privacy problems - Compatibility - Removal of certain applications

- **Addition of DirectX 12:** Windows 10 version comes with pre-installed DirectX 12 which can attract gamers as it ensures graphic display of computer games with reduced power consumption. This feature was not available on older versions of Windows.
- **Touch screen:** This option is available for hybrid device users where the exclusive touch view is activated while using the touch screen. It helps the users to switch between laptop and tablet mode in hybrid devices.
- **Administrative control:** Windows 10 control center has been updated and switching applications on and off is highly simplified. It might help the administrators add applications used within an organization and remove those which are not used regularly.
- **Lighter and faster:** This is one of the most important advantages of Windows 10. It works quicker than all its previous versions. The operating system is very efficient and consumes less processing power from the hardware. The laptop's start-up time, opening applications, and battery power consumption have also been improved with Windows 10.

Additionally, Windows 10 has a few other features such as a Microsoft Edge web browser, a Virtual desktop, and Cortana integration which also attract users to Windows 10.

Disadvantages

- **Privacy problems:** The computer behavior being monitored by the analysis tools remains mysterious and unclear about which information Microsoft exactly collects and how the collected data are used.
- **Compatibility:** For users who failed to shift to Windows 10 due to software or hardware requirements and compatibility there is a restriction on updating their version to Windows 10. It is always a good practice to check the compatibility of the system before upgrading to Windows 10.
- **Certain applications:** Due to economics and usage factors certain applications were removed from Windows 10 platform. Windows Media Center and Windows Photo Viewer had been removed from this version, and also there is no standard DVD player available in this version.

Simplest Steps and Basic Tools of Windows

- While beginning to work with windows the initial step is to start the laptop or system which is pre-installed with windows. Further discussion is based on windows 10 and while clicking the start button the windows start and the user can then understand the rest of the tools to work with windows 10. The start-up screen of windows 10 is displayed in **Figure 1.9**.
- Once the windows starts, the desktop begins to work with its in-built variety of tools and understanding that will enable its users to work conveniently. The basics of Windows 10 and desktop tools are presented in **Figure 1.10**.
- **Desktop:** Desktop is the overall look of any window where all the basic icons, menu buttons, taskbar icons, etc. are displayed for easy access for proceeding further with chosen tasks.
- **Start and Start menu:** Start button will show the start menu where we can find all the pre-installed apps through which we can access the apps and carry out tasks as desired.

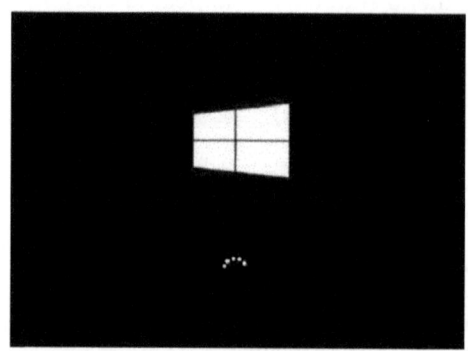

Fig. 1.9: Start-up screen of Windows 10

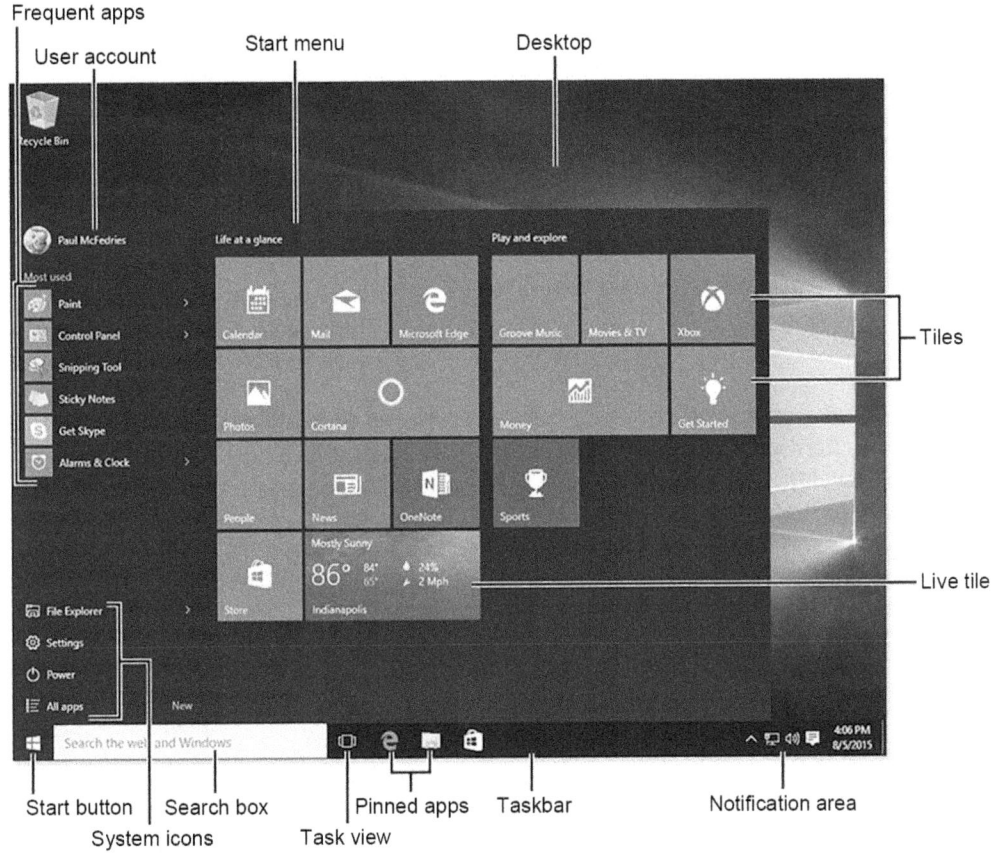

Fig. 1.10: Interface of Windows 10

- **System icons and search box:** System icons are all displayed icons such as settings with a search box in all the newer windows where one can type and get access to apps and drives directly without spending time accessing them through the traditional way.
- **Taskbar:** Taskbar is a horizontal bottom app with icons being displayed by default. Icons can be added by users to keep the apps readily available for easy access. Basic pinned apps by default are Microsoft Edge, file manager, store, etc. The taskbar can also be used to pin other apps which the user might want to access quickly.
- **Task view and notification:** Task view is another pinned icon on the taskbar which has a different functionality rather than just accessing the apps. When the user carries out multiple tasks at one point of time, all tasks can be viewed by clicking the task view icon and shift easily from one task to another without closing the opened task. The shortcut key which can be used to alternate between tasks is Alt+Tab on a system. The other important area on a desktop is the notification area which displays battery, power, network connections, and information mail icons. Further, it has hidden icons that can be explored and an option to add or remove additional icons from the system.

Based on the above basic icons and tools one can use the search button or file manager to explore My PC or directly open apps from the desktop by creating shortcuts of all the desired apps to one's desktop and double click on them. This will open the tasks directly enabling the user to create documents, Excel or PowerPoint. Simply using the right-click button on a mouse or laptop will also display various options where new documents, sheets, and presentations can be created. This basic discussion on windows would help its users to open MSWord, Spreadsheet, and PowerPoint programs. Details on how to create a word, sheet, and presentation are covered in the following sections.

MS Office

- Microsoft office or just called simply office is part of client and server software and services developed by Microsoft.
- These are part of office suites with initial components such as Microsoft Word (word processor), Microsoft Excel (a spreadsheet program), and Microsoft PowerPoint (presentation program).
- While Microsoft office suites developed significantly over the years, it currently covers various programs within office suites namely Word, Excel, PowerPoint, Outlook, OneDrive, OneNote, SharePoint, Teams, and Yammer including access and publishing app features as shown in **Figure 1.11**.

MS Word

- MS Word is one of the most widely used word processor applications which is user-friendly and easy to create word documents on the go. It is computer-friendly, quick, and classy with various collaborative and versatile features that come from the bigger package called MS Office of Microsoft.
- It is not just a word processor but an application that supports desktop publishing features such as newspapers, magazines, brochures, and advertisements.

Features of MS Word

The various features of the MS Word are presented in **Figure 1.12**.

- **Easy:** MS Word is user friendly as it is very easy to create a document, edit, delete, replace or save and store it.
- **Doc-to-print:** MS Word displays the material exactly as it would look like once printed. Also the print output is very much the same way the soft copy of the document would look like.
- **Grammar:** MS Word has a powerful inbuilt spell-check in it which allows simultaneous checking of spellings and making of corrections automatically.
- **Page and margins:** MS Word supports a wide variety of page setup, margins, and sizes. This helps the users to create a custom page as per their requirement, the

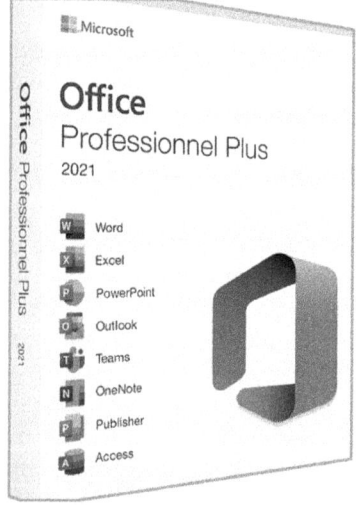

Fig. 1.11: Overview of Microsoft Office

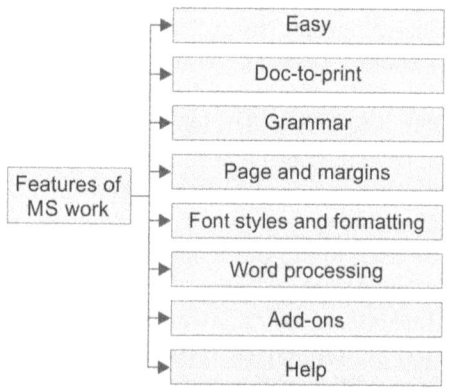

Fig. 1.12: Features of Microsoft Office Word

setting of which can either be applied to the whole document or just a particular part.
- **Font styles and formatting:** MS Word supports various font styles and sizes. One can either choose from a variety of pre-installed fonts or use additional features such as bold, italics, different font colors, underlining, alignment options, etc. In addition to paragraph formatting, word count and other statistics can also be generated with the help of MS Word.
- **Word processing:** MS Word has facilities and features like bookmark, find and replace, headers and footers and auto-text, etc.
- **Add-ons:** Word documents can be aligned and split in one, two or more columns like in a newspaper. Further tables and text boxes can be inserted into the document and additional text added. It supports graphical tools and drawing of objects enabling the user to mix graphical pictures with text. These images can be drawn with the help of tools, created by importing them from a clip art gallery or from websites directly using the copy-paste option. There is an additional feature of mail-merging too.
- **Help:** It is equipped with an in-built as well as an online 'help' feature which enables the user to get the answer related to various queries about any application.

Steps and Basic Tools to begin with MS Word

On opening MS Word by double-clicking on the icon or using the right-click button, one can see the file menu over the ribbon interface. It can be used for various functions like opening an additional new document or saving the document which is done with typing or editing work. The overview of the File menu of MS Office Word (2013, 2011) is shown in **Figure 1.13**.
- While beginning to work with MS Word document processor, one can create a user-friendly document with basic and simple tools which the user needs to understand before creating the document. Further, help section in MS word is also available. Alternately, keeping the cursor over any desired icon would display its function which can be readily understood by any

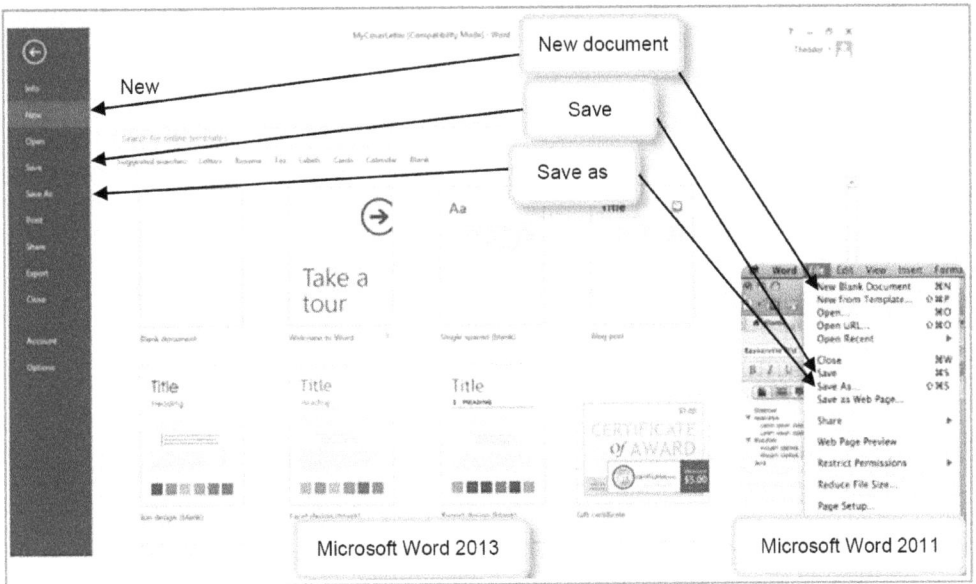

Fig. 1.13: File menu of Microsoft Office Word

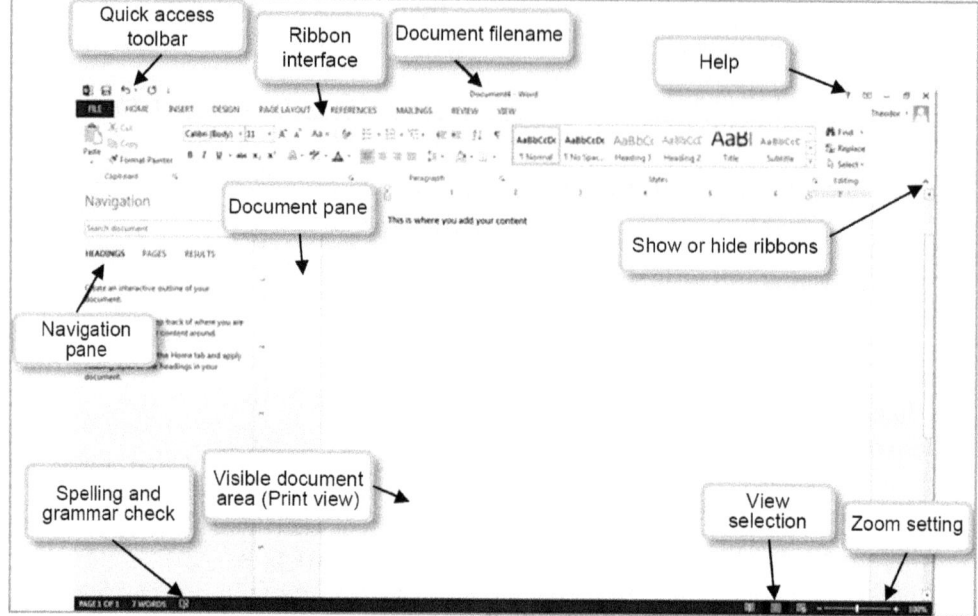

Fig. 1.14: Interface of Microsoft Office Word

beginner or a child with basic knowledge of English language. The overall basic and simple tools are shown in **Figure 1.14**.

- Basic aspect while opening a word document is that it opens a visible document or print area on which one can just type the content, or edit the already typed content, insert images, tables, etc., to make the document complete. This can be saved and stored for later use or a printout taken directly.
- Another important area for creating the document is the ribbon interface area on MS Word where the users can find options like home, insert, draw, design, layout, references, mailings, review and view. The home button gives options for choosing a font, font size, using bold, italics, underline, superscript, subscript, font case, color, text highlighter, paragraph, and alignment options, and select bullets and pointers.
- Insert option will enable the users to choose or insert or create tables, pictures, shapes, charts, SmartArt's, header and footer, text box, symbols, and page numbers which are basics for any document creation.
- Other areas in the ribbon interface include: 'draw' which can be used to draw images; 'design' which can be used to choose theme design and color; 'layout' that helps to format page set-up and paragraph set-up; 'references' used for research-based works such as endnote, citations, and bibliography; 'mailing interface' which helps in creating envelope and labels and merge with mail; 'review' option helps in adding or giving comments while reviewing the prepared materials. Word has a feature for grammar and spell check also.
- All the above-mentioned steps might help the user to create any document in MS Word. This basic understanding is mandatory with which one can understand further elaborative knowledge of MS Word.
- Computer shortcut keys for MS Word are presented in **Table 1.3**.

MS Excel

- MS Excel is a spreadsheet software used to manage and process large amount of data.

Table 1.3: Computer shortcut keys for MS Word

Shortcuts	Uses of Shortcut keys
Ctrl + B	Bold highlighted selection
Ctrl + C	Copy selected text
Ctrl + X	Cut selected text
Ctrl + N	Open a new/blank document
Ctrl + O	Open options
Ctrl + P	Open the print window
Ctrl + F	Open find box
Ctrl + I	Italicize highlighted selection
Ctrl + U	Underline highlighted selection
Ctrl + V	Paste
Ctrl + J	Justify paragraph alignment
Ctrl + L	Align selected text or line to the left
Ctrl + Q	Align selected paragraph to the left
Ctrl + E	Align selected text or line to the center
Ctrl + R	Align selected text or line to the right
Ctrl + (Left arrow)	Move one word to the left
Ctrl + (Right arrow)	Move one word to the right
Ctrl + (Up arrow)	Move to the beginning of the line or paragraph
Ctrl + (Down arrow)	Move to the end of the paragraph
Ctrl + Del	Delete the word to the right of the cursor
Ctrl + Backspace	Delete the word to the left of the cursor
Ctrl + End	Move the cursor to the end of the document
Ctrl + Home	Move the cursor to the beginning of the document
Ctrl + (Left arrow)	Move one word to the left
Ctrl + W	Close document
Ctrl+=	Set chosen text as a subscript
Ctrl+Shift+=	Set chosen text as superscript

- A spreadsheet is organized into grids of rows and columns where rows are indicated by numbers and columns by letters with their intersection named a cell. Thus, A1 is termed as the first cell and so on.
- The sheet we work on is called a worksheet but the work we do and store is called a workbook. A workbook contains many worksheets on which we work. In general, each time we open, close, or save a file in Excel we are opening, closing, and saving the workbook file.
- A spreadsheet document can be lengthy and not delimited by printed pages and contain many printed pages worth of material. Worksheet in Excel contains maximum rows up to row 1048576 and columns up to XFD.

Features of MS Excel

- **Calculations:** MS Excel is extensively used to carry out all sorts of calculations such as summing up a column or row of numbers, calculating averages, etc. The entered data can be automatically calculated as per the pre-installed commands or even by manual calculation commands for all the rows and columns. Any change in the entered data or even changing the value in a single cell results in recalculation of the entire spreadsheet automatically. The formula in spreadsheet software is a mathematical calculation that results in a data value. This value is displayed in the cell in which the particular formula is typed.
- **Graphs and Add-ons:** MS Excel has advanced charting features which can help its users to create graphs and charts with just a few mouse clicks. Based on the data, charts can be created quickly. Even the data in Excel can be easily copied onto any other documents including MS Word.

Steps and Basic Tools to Begin with MS Excel

- On opening MS Excel workbook by double-clicking on the icon or using the right-

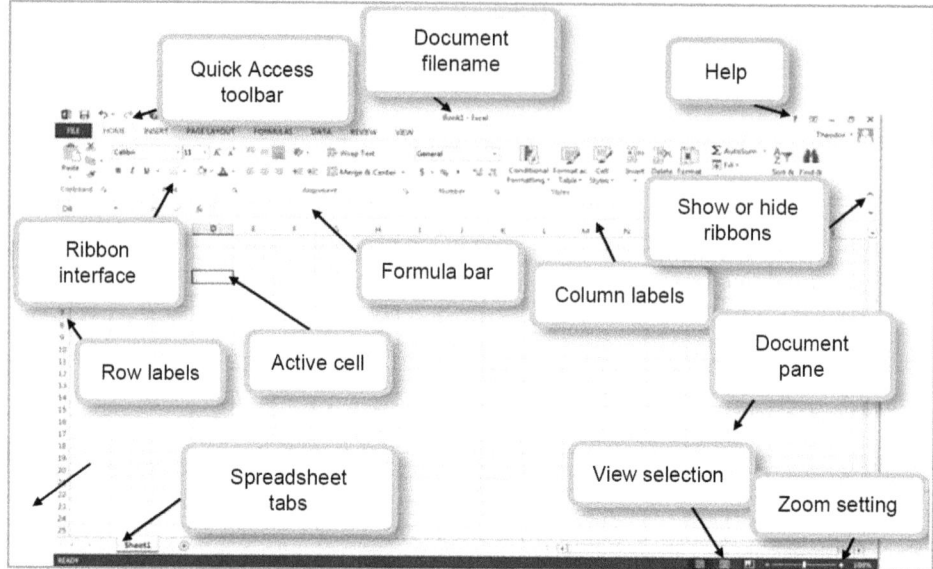

Fig. 1.15: Interface of Microsoft Office Excel

click button, one can see the opened spreadsheet or worksheet on which one can work by entering the data directly or copying the prepared data from MS Word or from other suites that can be pasted on opened worksheet and mathematical work done. Basic tools and interface of MS Excel are shown in **Figure 1.15**.

- While opening the spreadsheet it opens the document pane that contains cells in which data can be entered and mathematical work done. With similar ribbon interface options as in MS Word, work can be carried out easily with similar functionalities of the word like home, insert, page layout, data, review, and view options.
- Also formula option is available in the ribbon interface or in the formula bar, where one can get desired formulas to be applied for the whole document.

MS PowerPoint

- MS PowerPoint is an example of professional-level presentation software of the Microsoft Office suite which is by nature a presentation document which takes the form of a slide show.
- Although one can utilize PowerPoint in many different ways, most of them prefer to use it for making electronic PowerPoint presentations that connect to an overhead projector for making a professional presentation.
- On the flip side, a power point presentation is not useful for large volume of written text or material in the word processor but suitable only for short and to the point content.

Features of MS PowerPoint

- **Visual supplement:** MS PowerPoint though primarily used as a visual supplement to an oral presentation, can also be used as a standalone slide show such as a background during any event or as a reading material to be posted on a web or certain sharing sites like SlideShare.
- **Communication tool:** MS PowerPoint is a supportive tool to communicate ideas in a simple and effective manner during scientific presentations, annual reports, etc. It is mostly used to present simple talking points, less complex topics or headings, preparation of electronic versions of brochures and flyers, grasping the attention

of audience and keeping them engaged during a talk.

- **Graphical and add-ons:** PowerPoint is mostly graphical which makes the presentation completely professional with outlining, drawing, graphing, animations, smart-arts and other management tools. The instructions and tool help features make the user learn various aspects quickly thereby carry out all necessary changes or insertions while creating PowerPoint on the screen.
- **Wider functionality:** It is used to create presentations containing text, graphics, and animations. These can either be presented through projectors or printed out as handouts. The material can also be imported to PowerPoint from Word or other Microsoft applications. It has a large number of ready-made templates and slide formats. Use of SmartArt in PowerPoint is quite significant.

Steps and Basic Tools to Begin with MS PowerPoint

- On opening the MS PowerPoint by double-clicking on the icon or using the right-click button, the file menu over the ribbon interface can be seen. This can be used for various functions like opening an additional new presentation or saving the presentations which are done or being edited. Overview of the file menu of MS Office PowerPoint (2013, 2011) is shown in **Figure 1.16**.
- While beginning to work with MS Word PowerPoint, one can create a user-friendly presentation with basic and simple tools which the user needs to understand before creating the presentations. The overall basic and simple tools are shown in **Figure 1.17**.
- A PowerPoint usually opens with a pre-selected slide design and placeholder textbox, where one can start creating the slides with similar kind of typing and editing options as in MS Word and Excel, such as home, insert, draw, design and other ribbon interfaces.
- Home interface provides options for choosing a slide, creating a new slide, selecting layout and all other basics for creating a presentation which can be made visually attractive by using the ribbon interface options like transitions and animations.

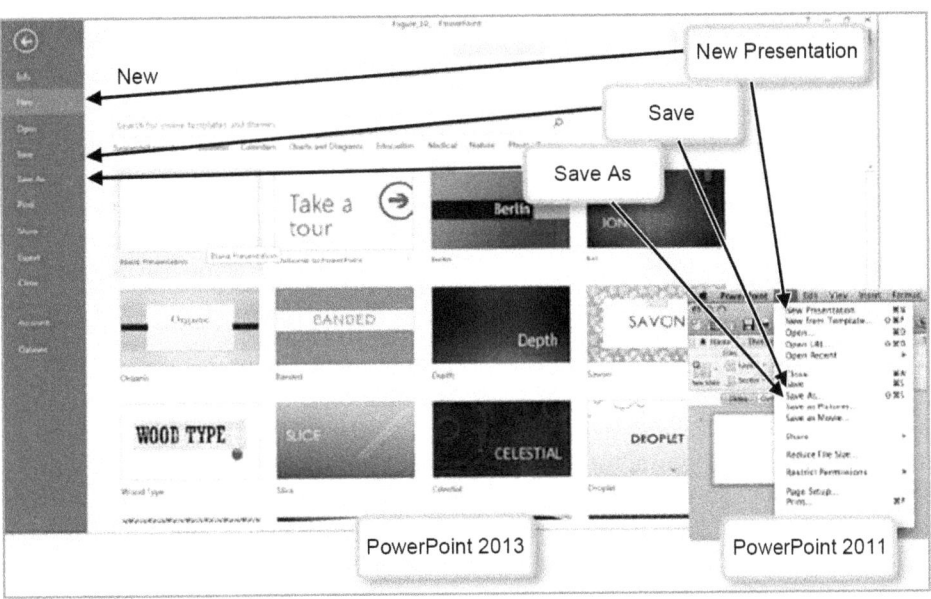

Fig. 1.16: File menu of Microsoft Office PowerPoint

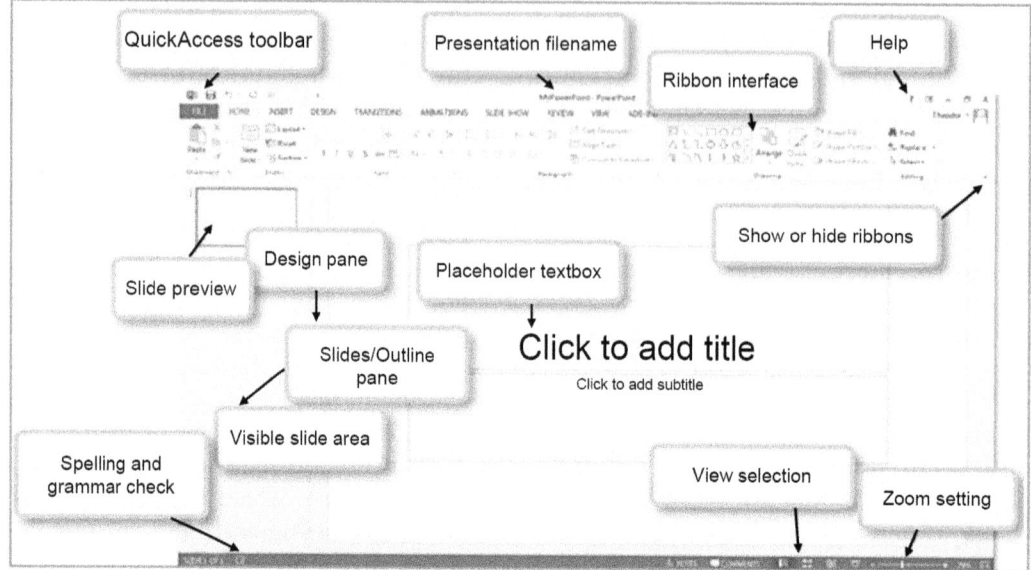

Fig. 1.17: Basics of Microsoft Office PowerPoint

There is also a help section in the PowerPoint. Keeping the cursor over any desired icon would display its function which can be understood by any beginner or a child with basic knowledge of English language.

- Slide show option on the ribbon interface can be used for projecting prepared presentations via projectors to reach mass audiences.

INTERNET

It was telephone communication technology before the invention of computer networks that was being used for connecting people. The internet being a newer communication technology that connects people in many different ways has taken over the work earlier being supported by the landline telephone.

Networking can be referred to as sharing of resources and services. A computer network is a thus a set of interconnected devices sharing resources using a shared link. Shared resources can be anything from data or fax to an email that needs to be shared between the system on a common pathway or medium or transfer medium. Both sending and receiving systems must have proper protocol or common communication guidelines or rules to receive the files from the sender and arrive at the correct destination. To understand the basics of computer networks, one needs to understand the following three aspects: resources (things to be shared), medium (pathway or transmission medium to connect sending and receiving system), and protocols (rules governing computer communication).

The Internet

The internet which is no less than a revolution though started quietly over the years, has grown strongly and involved the entire world. People around the world use internet services these days. A few examples include a college student recording a video on the smart phone and uploading it on the social media, a man walking on the streets using a map to find nearby places, son working abroad connecting to family members on a video call, or a teenager using mobile to download some of his favorite music from the app store or playing some online games.

- Internet is generally thought of as a set of services such as Google, Facebook,

Instagram, Amazon, Netflix, YouTube, WhatsApp, etc. or categorized as 'the Web' or 'email' which is factually incorrect. It is a global computer communication system that has united all of us and made all the services possible. It is a revolution that has changed the way we live and work.

- Usage of internet cannot be simply predicted by the number of devices being connected or the number of people using them as it also reaches out to ships at sea, planes mid-air and vehicles on land. We all are surrounded by the internet in the form of security systems and cameras, money vending machines, android televisions and other household appliances. To conclude, Internet is all pervasive. Without internet each one of us would feel cut-off from easy access to information which otherwise everybody had taken for granted. Moreover, living without WhatsApp, YouTube and all other apps would be quite impossible for the newer generations.
- A computer network is a set of computers linked together for sharing information or resources among themselves but the internet is a "network of networks". It is also termed as information highway, worldwide broadcasting capability, mechanism for information dissemination, and a medium for collaboration and interaction.
- The history of the internet dates back to 1969 when ARPANET using Interface Message Processors (IMP) connected computers at universities. This became the core element in the concept of Internet. It is this single technology that ruled communication system for many years until Vinton Cerf and Robert Kahn (1973) from the DARPA unit wrote a paper that proposed the newer concept called network interconnection and software that passes the data between them. He named it "interconnection of networks" which quickly got shortened to the "internet". Based on this, SATNET (through satellites), PRNET (through mobile packet radio), and later Ethernet (through coaxial cables) came into existence which could deliver data a thousand times faster over the air.
- As protocols used for communication between systems vary a lot, the common internet work protocol TCP/IP (IP address) hides them to overcome the differences. Thus the term internet is used to refer to any network that uses TCP/IP. It means that when a machine is on the internet and if it runs TCP/IP protocol that has an IP address, it can share IP packets to other machines on the internet.

World Wide Web (WWW)

- The World Wide Web (Shortened as Web), a leading information retrieval service of the internet is a system of internet servers that support specially formatted documents. Like all internet services, the World Wide Web is not built into the internet but runs on the computers attached to the internet. The web operates within the internet's basic client-server format.
- Web helps its users to access a wide range of information via documents that are connected by Hypertext or Hypermedia links. These are electronic connections that link related pieces of information and allow its users to access them. Hypertext allows selecting a word or phrase from the text which helps to access additional information pertaining to that selected word or phrase. Hypermedia links to images, sounds, animation, and movies.
- Hypertext document with its texts and hyperlinks is written in *Hyper Text Markup Language* (HTML) and is assigned with an online address called *Uniform Resource Locator* (URL).
- There are various applications called Web browsers via which accessing the World Wide Web is possible. Netscape Navigator, Microsoft Internet Explorer, Google Chrome are a few web browsers. With the use of web browsers users can access view to web pages that contain texts, images, and other media and navigate between them using hyperlinks.

Table 1.4: Difference between internet and web

Internet	Web (www)
• Internet uses a network of networks. • It connects millions of computers globally meaning any computer can connect with any other computer so long as both are connected to the internet.	• Information that flows over the internet via a variety of languages is termed as protocols and a way of accessing information over the medium of the internet is the Web. • The information-sharing model built on top of the internet is called the Web.

- Many of us think and use the terms internet and World Wide Web (the Web) interchangeably though both are quite different. The difference between internet and web is presented in **Table 1.4**.
- Development of the Web began in 1989 by Tim Berners-Lee who created a protocol termed as the Hyper Text Transfer Protocol (HTTP), the only language spoken over the internet to transfer information. The web is just one of the many ways by which information can be transmitted over the internet. The internet can also be used for sending and receiving e-mails, remote sharing and file transfer, etc.

Web Browser: Search Engine

- There are various applications called Web browsers via which accessing the World Wide Web is possible. Some of the most commonly used are Netscape Navigator, Microsoft Internet Explorer, Google Chrome, Mozilla Firefox, Opera, and also Apple's safari. With the use of web browsers users can get access to and view web pages that contain texts, images, and other media and navigate between them using hyperlinks.
- Software giant Microsoft Corporation showed interest in creating its own browser to compete with the already existing web browsers and found Internet Explorer (based initially on Mosaic) in 1995 as an add-on to Windows 95 operating system. It later got integrated within the operating system and became ready for use in 1996. This incidentally became the most popular Web browser in the years to come.
- Although browsers are typically used to access the World Wide Web, they can also be used to access other information through Web servers in private networks or content in file systems.
- Search engines are software designed to carry out web searches for information on World Wide Web. They search web pages, images, articles, research papers, and other types of files based on specified text in the web search query in a systematic way to yield better results (Search Engine Result Pages-SERPs). The text entered in the search box yields results associated with it by running a real-time algorithm or mixture of algorithm and human input. Internet content that cannot be searched by web search engines falls under the category of dark web. Various browsers and search engines are depicted in **Figure 1.18**.
- Many people get confused between a Web browser and a search engine and use them interchangeably. For instance Google Chrome is a browser but Google is a search engine. The difference between a browser and a search engine is presented in **Table 1.5** and the flow of network connection is depicted in **Figure 1.19**.

Internet Connections and Shared Internet

- There are various internet connection facilities available which may vary by Internet Service Provider and/or by region. The one who chooses to use the internet might have to consider aspects such as connection speed or bandwidth, cost, availability, reliability, and convenience.
- While determining the most suitable type of internet connection or speed, it is important to understand the difference between various available routes of accessing the internet to systems or other electronic

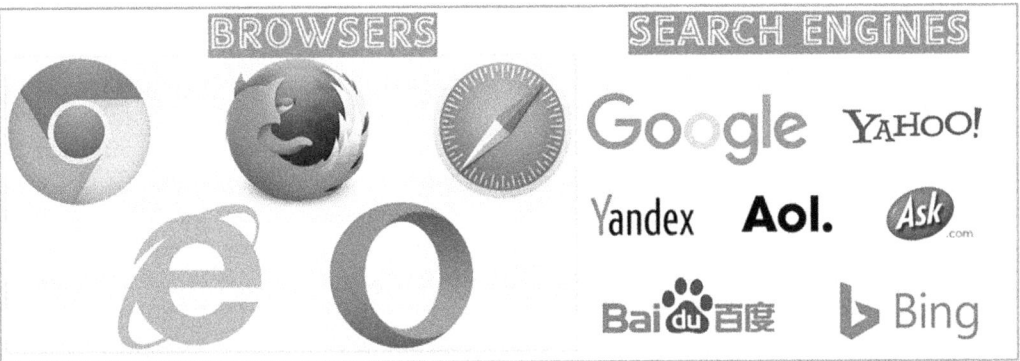

Fig. 1.18: Browsers and Search engines

Table 1.5: Difference between Browser and Search engine

Browser	Search engine
• Browser is a piece of software that retrieves and displays web pages • Browser is a source or infrastructure on which search engine functions. Every browser has a search engine web page as its home page • Example: Chrome, Mozilla, Opera	• Search engine is a website that helps people find web pages from other websites • Search engine is one of the web pages of a browser which helps in searching for other web pages from other websites • Example: Google, Bing, Yahoo

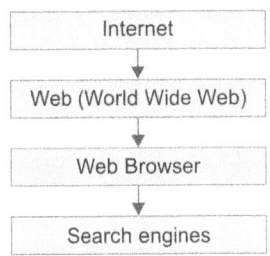

Fig. 1.19: Flow of network connection

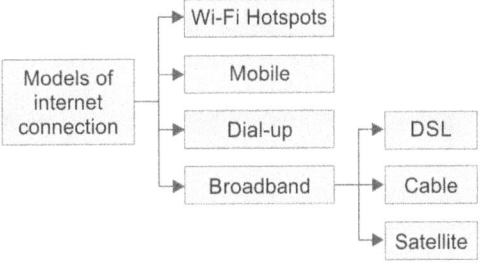

Fig. 1.20: Modes of internet connection

electronic devices to use the internet and exchange data wirelessly through radio waves. These connections can be phone-based, commercial, or free to use mode.

2. *Mobile:* Cell phones and smart phones allow their users to access internet connections with various plans. These have good speeds allowing them to access the internet from anywhere.

3. *Dial-up:* It works by linking one's phone line to a computer to access the internet. This particular connection also called 'analog' was once the most used mode of internet connection. In this form of connection, making or receiving calls is not permitted while receiving a signal for an internet connection due to which it is outdated now.

4. *Broadband:* These are high-speed broad bandwidth internet connections that are provided either by a cable or telephone company which use multiple

devices. A few are described below (**Fig. 1.20**):

1. *Wi-Fi hotspots:* These are sites that provide internet access over a Wireless Local Area Network (WLAN) via a router that connects to the Internet service provider. Hotspot uses Wi-Fi technology to connect with various

data channels to send large quantities of information. For example, DSL and cable are considered high-bandwidth connections.

- **DSL:** This is a 2-wire copper telephone line that provides both internet and telephone to the customer. Unlike in a dial-up connection, the user is at liberty to place calls even while surfing the internet.
- **Cable:** It is a form of broadband connection which uses the cable modem to access the internet over cable TV lines. It is a much faster and more reliable broadband service.
- **Satellite:** Broadband services are delivered directly via a satellite instead of a optical fibre or mobile network. The aggregation of data generated and transmitted by users accessing the internet happens in the sky or space, i.e., the satellite.

Websites (Internet Sites)

- Website is a collection of web pages or interconnected web pages and related information usually including a home page. It is available on a common domain name located on the same server which is prepared and maintained by an individual, group, or organization to provide a collection of information to its viewers.
- Websites can be public or private. While a website which is available to the public falls under the category of the World Wide Web (Web), the one which belongs to private organizations is termed as a private website. It can be accessed only by their employees.
- Information available on websites can be anything and not just limited to news, education, commerce, entertainment, personal narratives, digital libraries, statistics, research, professional journals, publishes articles, biographical information, social networking, etc.
- Users can easily surf through websites and available web pages and navigate between websites and web pages by hyperlinking which can take them to another site, especially to their home page. Users' knowledge about the site and how they evaluate the site matter a lot while accessing any website.
- Though various websites are available, the one chosen might vary between individuals depending upon their needs and preferences. A few internet sites/websites are discussed below **(Fig. 1.21)**:
  1. *Government websites:* These are websites that are created by local or state departments, or national governments of any country to provide information about laws, government statistics, directories, and current affairs and issues among citizens or about government agencies, departments, and other associated details. Few government websites are even created for providing information to tourists about tourism. Most of the website

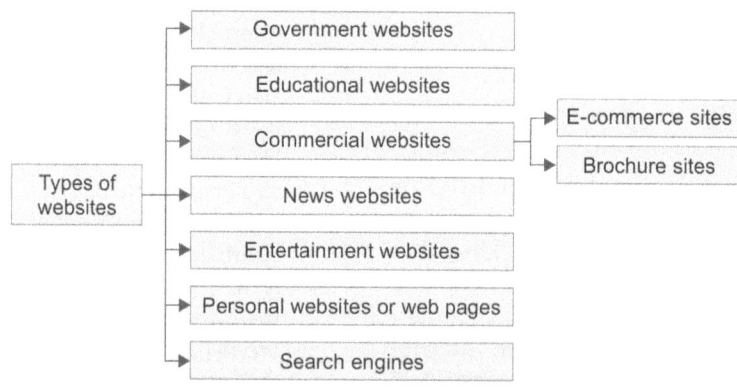

Fig. 1.21: Types of internet sites

addresses end with .gov. For example, india.gov.in, USA.gov, GOV.UK
2. *Educational websites:* These are educational-oriented websites available for the public as well as private entities. They provide information about educational establishments, scholarly works, online courses, home pages of schools and colleges, library catalogs, etc. These website addresses end with .edu.
3. *Commercial websites:* These are websites meant for selling products or services. They are usually created or sponsored by commercial enterprises where information about goods and products is available enabling online sales or online transactions for such sales. These commercial websites can share information about products, sale details, annual enterprise or company reports, histories, and stock reports and may belong to either E-commerce sites or Brochure sites. While E-commerce sites directly sell goods to customers by enabling online sales and transactions like amazon, myntra, etc., brochure websites which are a digital version of printed brochure combine all the information needed in one place by showing products or services the company provides.
4. *News websites:* These are similar to information websites but exclusively associated with disseminating information about news, politics, commentary, etc. These may also carry out commercial operations. These websites are quite common nowadays as all top-rated newspapers and TV news channels like the Times of India, CNN, etc. have their own websites to keep their readers and viewers updated every second. These websites' addresses end with .com.
5. *Entertainment websites:* These are commercial websites ending with .com with the primary purpose of providing entertainment to the viewers or users like music, videos, humor, games, drama, movies, or other similar types of activities.
6. *Personal websites or web pages:* These types of websites are created by an individual or a small group such as a family and may or may not be affiliated to any larger institutions. It may include any information that an individual wishes to add but the reliability and credibility of the information might be questioned and must be used cautiously.
7. *Search engines:* These are primary websites without which it would be impossible to find anything on the World Wide Web. There are many search engines like yahoo, ask, bing, etc. but by many accounts, the most popular search engine remains to be Google.com.

E-mail, G-mail, Google Drive, Docs, Sheets, and Forms

- E-mail is considered to be one of the most common and simplest ways to share and receive information, data, and other material over the internet.
- It requires both the sender and the receiver to have an e-mail address by creating the account on any one of the mailing websites such as yahoo.com, rediff.com, or gmail.com.
- Once the account is created with minimal required information like the user name and password, the sender can access his mailing website. He can enter the credentials to open the mailbox, send or receive information instantly by writing a mail and attaching the desired documents like word, sheets, power points, images, videos and even much larger documents by attaching it to google drive provided the preferred mailing website is Gmail. Out of all other mailing websites, Gmail has become much more familiar and user-friendly with added benefits like google

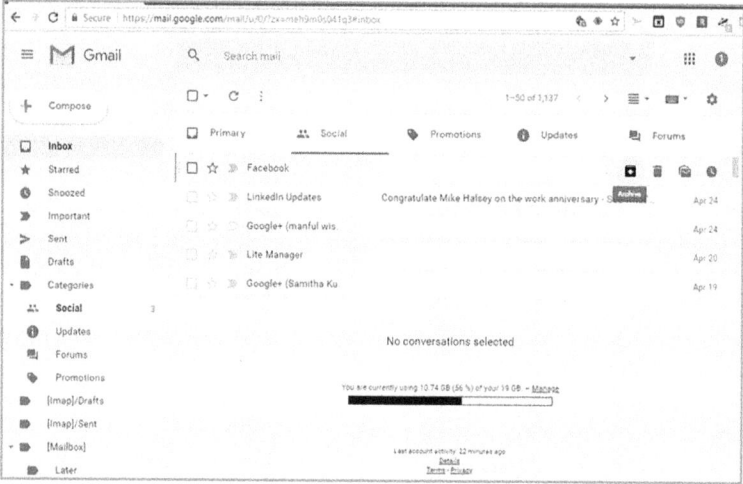

Fig. 1.22: Screenshot of Gmail

forms, docs, spreadsheets, and drives where one can create or store abundant material using cloud storage facilities. Further, one Gmail account is enough to use features like customized use of google search engines, Google drive, docs, forms, and all other facilities attached to it. A screenshot of Gmail is depicted in **Figure 1.22**.

- In certain cases, even the email id is created by educational institutions or working organizations to unite their students and employees and connect each other with their portal email website which has the organization's name in the username of the members like .org, .edu, etc.
- Google drive is a cloud storage space where files can be saved after a complete document scan which makes it safer and practical.
- Google docs and sheets are word documents and spreadsheets respectively which can be created online and stored on a google drive. The shared docs and spreadsheets can be edited and autosaved in the sender's drive. Changes made by anyone can be seen online and also these files can be accessed from any computer over the internet. Similarly, google slides are also available which can be used as a digital replacement for the traditional PowerPoints. All the above-mentioned works on google workspace and online-only tools can be created, stored, edited, tracked, shared, and monitored.
- Finally, the significant one on the Google workspace is Google forms (Forms) which can be used for creating online forms and surveys with multiple question types and analyzing results in real-time. These are research-based tools available on google workspace where a questionnaire can be created to collect the data from around the world via an online survey by sending it to target groups via e-mail, or by shortened URL which can be copy-pasted and sent through various ways. A screenshot of Google form is depicted in **Figure 1.23**.
- Collected data responses through google forms can be seen immediately by sorting individual responses or summaries where graphs and pictorial representations of whole data would be available for interpretation.

LITERATURE SEARCH

Literature search is a key and important step in carrying out authentic research which helps in formulating a research question and planning and performing the study accordingly. Each research needs to be

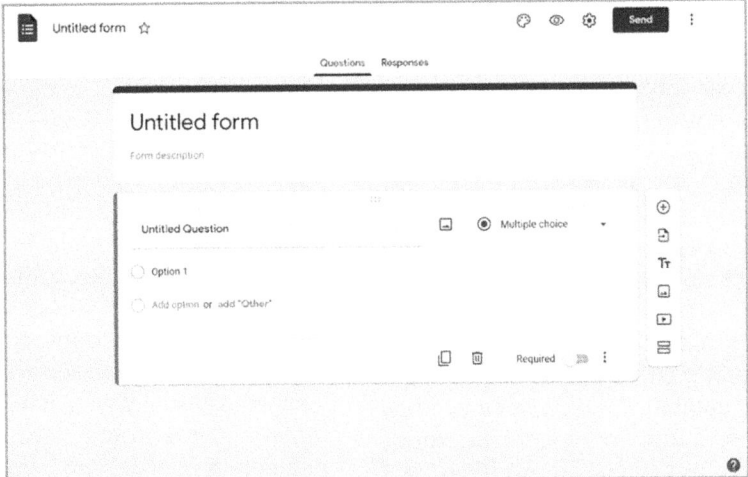

Fig. 1.23: Outlook of Google forms

conducted as per the research question which can be generated only through a proper and organized literature search. One of the biggest tasks in carrying out research is doing a literature search as it is time and energy-consuming. If it is not carried out step-wise it may result in disinterest and discontinuance of further search. As literature search is laborious and availability of published work enormous one needs to devise a proper plan and find a proper search database and strategy to get the correct pieces of evidence.

Meaning

- Literature search is a systematic and well-organized search from the already published data to identify good quality references on a specific topic.
- A literature review is an account of what has already been established or published.

Purposes of Literature Search

1. These are performed to draw information for preparing or making evidence-based guidelines.
2. It is considered as a basic step in research methodology that aids in the preparation of content such as an introduction which needs a proper background, a methodology that includes a selection of design, approach, tools, and planning of the study, discussion which compares the various study findings with the completed study.
3. It can be used as a part of academics.
4. Major purpose remains to be the formulation of research questions based on previously published work with an eye on gaps in knowledge and practice amenable for further or extended research.
   - Conducting a literature search can be time-consuming, but if carried out step-wise doing it can be easy. Primary step is usually the formulation of research problem and planning the area of search.
   - Literature search can be of primary literature and second literature. Primary sources are written by original researchers, the ones who conducted the study whereas secondary sources are systematic reviews and meta-analyses where all primary source literature is inferred and evaluated.
   - This unit does not focus in detail on sources and other basic literature review areas but elaborates on various search strategies and web-based search perspectives to keep it simple and focused in parallel with the aims of nursing informatics.

Methods of Literature Search

- In general, there are various methods of literature search that are used alone or in combination with one or more strategies. Since past many decades physical literature exploration is in practice. With the recent advancement in technology, the internet has become a gateway for carrying out vast amount of medical and nursing literature search.
- Literature search can be protocol-driven where both hand search as well as electronic database can be used to find journals relevant to the research question or reference. This can be done by chasing/tracking them down from identified literature to find more related literature like ancestry and descendancy approaches or use the available theoretical background to frame research protocols. Formulating search strategy is discussed later in this unit after briefly covering available electronic databases for a better understanding of the reader. Various methods of literature search are depicted in **Figure 1.24**.

Electronic Databases

- Conducting literature search or review refers to identifying materials based on a research topic using web-based search engines like google, scholar, etc. or electronic databases.
- There are various databases available for literature searches such as databases for original articles and all other primary sources and databases for evidence-based systematic reviews and other secondary sources. Both web-based and evidence-based databases and literature searches are explained in **Tables 1.6 and 1.7**.
- The above-listed web-based databases are useful for gathering primary sources allowing the researcher to access all original articles or research papers published on a specific topic in which he is interested. This permits him to work with an eye on gaps in knowledge and practice further or extended research.
- The above-listed electronic evidence-based databases are useful in accessing secondary sources, especially systematic reviews and meta-analyses where all primary source literature is inferred and evaluated.
- Some of the above data bases that are better suited for nursing professionals to access nursing-related research questions and primary and secondary literature accessibility are presented in **Table 1.8**.
- Besides all the above-mentioned electronic databases, Scopus, EMBASE (Excerpta Medica Database), ProQuest, ISI web of knowledge, and Dissertation Abstracts Online can also be used by nursing professionals and nurse researchers to access relevant literature as per the research question.

Formulating a Search Strategy

- Various methods of literature search along with a basic understanding of all available electronic databases assist the reader in understanding ways of formulating search strategies. There are several ways to search for research evidence and plan it well ahead of time to choose a correct database, approach to proceed successfully.

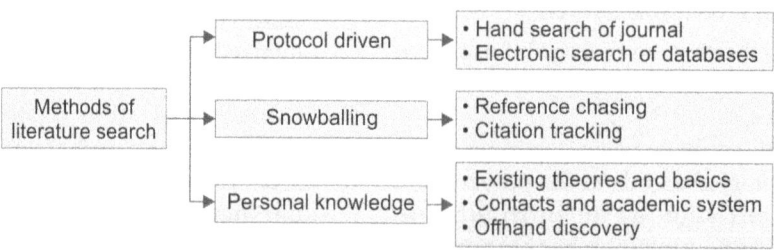

Fig. 1.24: Methods of literature search

Table 1.6: Web-based methods of literature search

Sources	Web address
Search engines	
Google	http://www.google.com
Google Scholar	http://www.scholar.google.com
Yahoo	http://www.yahoo.com
Electronic source of database	
PubMed	https://www.nlm.nih.gov/pubmed
MeSH	http://www.ncbi.nlm.nih.gov/mesh
MEDLINE (Medical Literature Analysis and Retrieval System Online)	https://www.nlm.nih.gov
CINAHL (The Cumulative Index to Nursing and Allied Health Literature)	https://www.cinahl.com
EMBASE (Excerpta Medica Database)	https://store.elsevier.com/embase
SCOPUS	https://www.scopus.com/
Ind Med: Indian Database	https://www.medind.nic.in
ERIC	https://www.eric.ed.gov
ProQuest	http://proquest.com

Table 1.7: Evidence-based databases of literature search

Sources	Web address
The Cochrane Database of Systematic Reviews	http://www.cochranelibrary.com/ or http://www.cochrane.com/
The ACP Journal Club	http://search.ebscohost.com/
Dartmouth EBM Database	http://www.dartmouth.edu/~library/biomed/resources/ejournals.html
Evidence updates	http://plus.mcmaster.ca/evidenceupdates/
e Medicine	http://emedicine.medscape.com/
National Guideline Clearinghouse	http://www.guideline.gov/
Ovid Medline	http://www.dartmouth.edu/~library/biomed/resources/ovid.html
PubMed	http://www.ncbi.nlm.nih.gov/pubmed/
UpToDate	http://www.uptodate.com/online

Table 1.8: Electronic databases relevant to nursing profession/nurse researchers

Sources	Focus area	Web address
CINAHL (The Cumulative Index to Nursing and Allied Health Literature)	It covers all sorts of nursing and allied health-related journals, books, dissertations, and conference proceedings. CINAHL, CINAHL Plus, and various other versions are available. Materials are offered via EBSCOhost. Covers around 3000 journals dating from 1981.	https://www.cinahl.com

Contd...

Contd...

Sources	Focus area	Web address
PubMed/MEDLINE	These were developed by the U.S. National Library of Medicine (NLM) which is recognized as a prime source of bibliographical databases covering biomedical literature published in medical, nursing, and health journals dating from 1966. Available via Ovid search engine but freely available via PubMed website.	http://www.ncbi.nlm.nih.gov/pubmed/
British Nursing Index	The UK-based bibliographical database covers a large number of British nursing and midwifery journals.	www.rcn.org.uk/elibrary (Royal College of Nursing)
The Cochrane Database of Systematic Reviews	Cochrane Library is a house of all secondary sources like systematic reviews of various literature related to nursing, medical and health professions.	http://www.cochranelibrary.com/ or http://www.cochrane.com/
PsycINFO	It belongs to the organization American Psychological Association which covers a wide range of literature related to psychology and other related or relevant disciplines.	http://www.psycinfo.com or https://psycnet.apa.org/

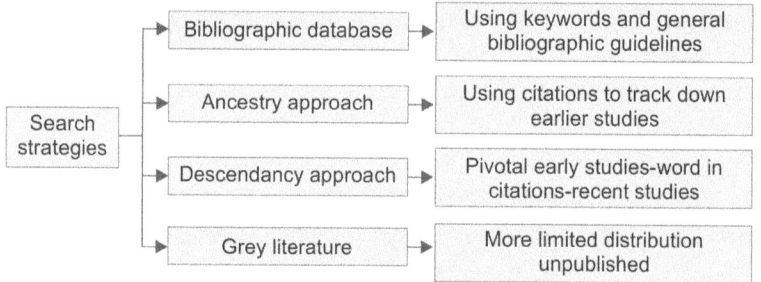

Fig. 1.25: Literature search strategies

- Several other approaches for seeking evidence are: *the bibliographic database, ancestry approach, descendancy approach, and grey literature,* the most common one being *Bibliographic database.* The ancestry approach uses present citations and tracks down similar kind of papers published in the past. The descendancy approach is to find pivotal early/past studies and search forward in citation to find more relevant recent studies on the selected topic that cited the pivotal study. Another strategy that focuses on tracking down named grey literature includes all the unpublished reports and conference proceeding, etc. Various search strategies are depicted in **Figure 1.25**.

Searching Bibliographic Databases

- Literature search usually begins with bibliographic database by many scholars as it contains thousands of journal articles coded as per language, content, or type of journal.
- Several commercial vendors provide software for retrieving information from these bibliographic databases. These can be easily accessed as they are user-friendly and support menu-driven commands.

Unit 1 | Introduction to Computer Applications for Patient Care Delivery System and Nursing Practice

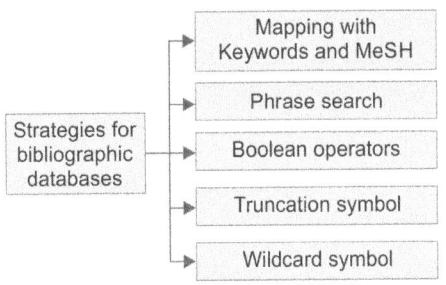

Fig. 1.26: Strategies for Bibliographic databases

Getting started with Bibliographic Database

Various strategies used to retrieve information from bibliographic databases include Keywords, MeSH terms, Phrase search, Boolean operators, Wildcard and Truncation symbols, and filters. These are depicted in **Figure 1.26**.

Mapping with Keywords and MeSH

- One usually begins with Keywords to search for relevant published material matching the research question.
- Keywords are basically any single word or synonyms used to retrieve journal articles or papers published related to that word. Most bibliographic databases support this keyword search as it is the cornerstone of an effective search.
- Keywords can be independent (manipulation) or dependent (effect) variables or their synonyms, and perhaps also the population of the study. Using synonyms or similar words which would yield comparable results need to be chosen carefully as several databases have controlled word stock. Thus looking at database thesaurus is mandatory for choosing correct alternative keywords. For example, if the study is conducted on adolescents' aggression, then keywords can be aggression, anger, rage, violence, adolescents, teenagers, etc.
- Another strategy used while mapping with keywords is using MeSH (Medical Subject Heading) to retrieve better and related results. These are National Library of Medicine's (NLM) controlled hierarchical vocabulary used for indexing articles in PubMed where terms flow like branches, beginning with general terms and continuing with branches of specific terms to proceed further and so on. For example, if the search is about aggression then subheadings will be shown where one can choose and extend the further search, or even restrict the search with major keywords and synonyms which may also be suggested by the database. The example sheet of MeSH terms is depicted in **Figure 1.27**.

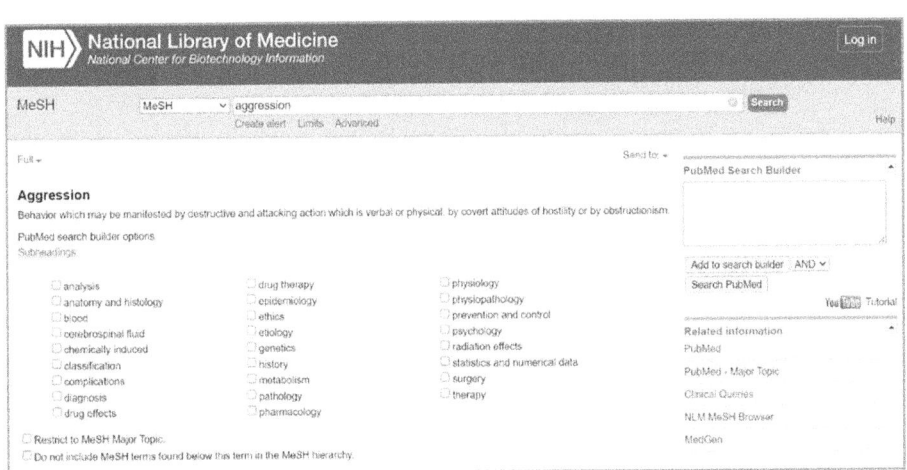

Fig. 1.27: Outlook of MeSH page

Phrase Search

These are any words or phrases used in the database to get the exact result of typed words rather than any consideration of synonyms or associated and relevant words. The results are displayed in the same order of how the phrase was entered without adding any words in between them.

Boolean Operators

- It is a simple strategy of combining keywords to get proper and extended results of literature. These search strategies are supported by most of the available electronic databases.
- AND, OR, and NOT are the three common Boolean operators used in bibliographic databases which are named after the mathematician George Boole.
- Combining two words by using AND between them delimits the search and fetches only published articles that mentioned both the words. For example, typing "Aggression AND Adolescence" in a search box will yield results of only those articles that mentioned both the words in them.
- Combining two words by using OR between them will expand the search and fetch all the published articles that mentioned either of the terms. In a similar example, typing "Aggression OR Adolescence" in a search box will yield results of all the articles that mentioned either aggression or adolescent in them.
- At last, combining two words by using NOT between them narrows the search and will fetch all the published articles that mentioned only the first word but not the second word. In a similar example, typing "Aggression NOT Adolescence" in a search box would retrieve all records with aggression that did not include the term adolescent.
- Further, these Boolean operators can be used to extend the search by adding more terms to get more delimited, expanded and narrowed results as shown in hypothetical **Figure 1.28**.

Truncation and the Wildcard Symbol

- These are other strategies used in a bibliographic database, though the functionality of these strategies varies among available databases.
- Truncation symbol (often an asterisk*) expands the search term to include all forms of a root word that has been entered. For example, a search for *'teen*'* would retrieve all the results that begin with teen such as teen, teens, teenage, and teenagers.
- Wildcard symbol (often a question mark ?) suggests that alternative spelling in a root

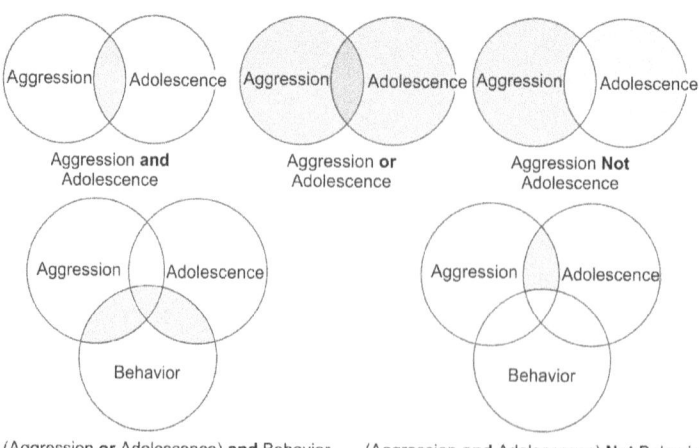

Fig. 1.28: Concept of Boolean operators

word has been entered which yields results of all alternative suggestions. For example, a search for *'wom?n'* would retrieve results with either woman or women.

Filters

- These are simple other strategies used to retrieve articles by just filtering or sorting the search as per need. For example, filtering can be based upon article type, text availability, age, gender, language, and journal categories.
- The above search strategies can be effectively used in databases to retrieve needed literature. The process of literature search can be understood as shown in **Figures 1.29 to 1.31.**

STATISTICAL PACKAGES

- In the field of biostatistics, the collected data was studied and analyzed manually to obtain study results and contribute to evidence-based practice. This required heavy manpower and laborious paper work which could lead to erroneous outcomes.
- This is now taken care of by various software packages which have optimized tasks such as data entry, coding, analysis, easy and fast storage in an errorless manner. These are termed as statistical packages.
- Statistical packages are used to collect, organize, interpret and present numerical information. These are preferred due to the complexity of calculations involved and the need for yielding errorless results among the vast amount of data collected. These make the task of analysis and inference easy in bringing out errorless results and provide comprehensive data with seamless graphical presentation.
- Though software can be errorless and yield results to contribute to evidence-based practice, it needs to be handled only by trained personnel with enough statistical competence.
- Nurses are quite often involved in evidence-based practice to better improve clinical decisions and patient care. This requires the nurses to get familiarized with not only research literature and clinical problems

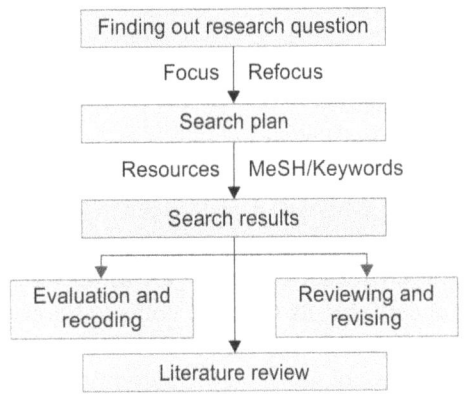

Fig. 1.29: Process of literature search

Nurse staffing and patient care cost in acute inpatient nursing units.

Authors: Li YF; Wong ES; Sales AE; Sharp ND; Needleman J; Maciejewski ML; Lowy E; Alt-White AC; Liu CF

Affiliation: Northwest Center for Outcomes Research in Older Adults, VA Puget Sound Health Care System, Seattle, WA, USA. yugang.li@va.gov

Source: Medical Care (MED CARE), 2011 Aug; 49(8): 708-13

Publication Type: Journal article-research

Language: English

Major Subjects: Health Facility Costs
Hospital Units—Economics
Nursing Service—Economics
Personnel Staffing and Scheduling—Economics

Minor Subjects: Aged; Analysis of Variance; Chi Square Test; Costs and Cost Analysis; Cross Sectional Studies; Female; Health Services Research; Hospitals; Veterans; Length of Stay—Statistics and Numerical Data; Linear Regression; Male; Middle Age; Retrospective Design; United States

Abstract: OBJECTIVE: Studies suggest that a business case for improving **nurse staffing** can be made to increase registered **nurse (RN)** skill mix without changing total licensed nursing hours. It is unclear whether a business case for increasing RN skill mix can be justified equally among patients of varying health needs. This study evaluated whether nursing hours per patient day (HPPD) and skill mix are associated with higher inpatient care costs within acute medical/surgical inpatient units using data from the Veterans Health Administration. METHODS: Retrospective cross-sectional study, including 139, 360 inpatient admissions to 292 acute medical/surgical inpatient units at 125 Veterans Health Administration medical centers between February and June 2003, was conducted. Dependent variables were inpatient costs per admission and costs per patient day. RESULTS: The average costs per surgical and medical admission were $18,624 and $6,636, respectively. Costs per admission were positively associated with total nursing HPPD among medical admission ($164.49 per additional HPPD, P>0.001), but not among surgical admission. Total nursing HPPD and RN skill mix were associated with higher costs per hospital day for both medical admission ($79.02 per additional HPPD and 5.64 per 1% point increase in nursing skill mix, both P<0.001) and surgical admissions ($112.47 per additional HPPD and $13.31 per 1% point increase in nursing skill mix, both P<0.0001). Patients experiencing complications or transferring to an intensive care unit had higher inpatient costs than other patient. CONCLUSION: The association of **nurse staffing** level with costs per admission differed for medical versus surgical admission.

Journal Subset: Biomedical; Peer Reviewed; USA

Fig. 1.30: Example of record from CINAHL search

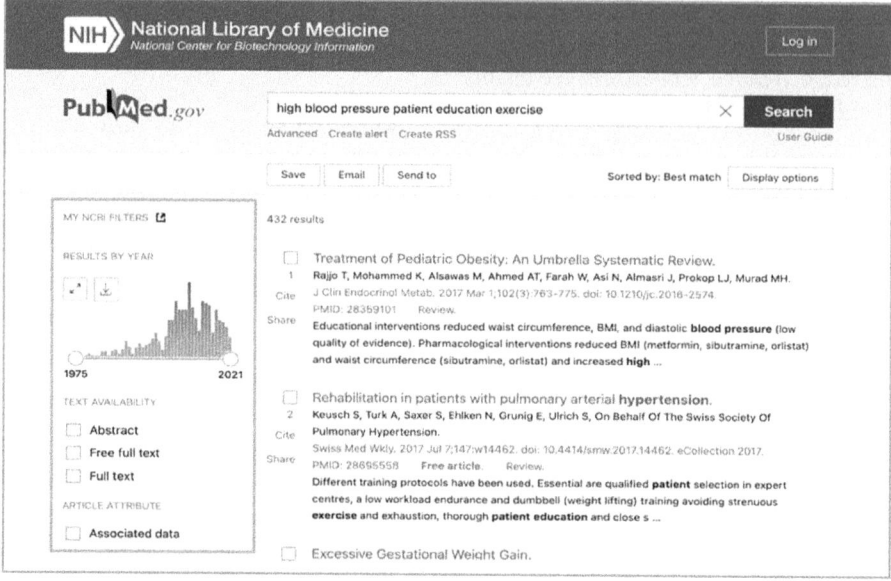

Fig. 1.31: Example of record from PubMed search

but also statistical methods, procedures, and interpretation of data. Hence, the understanding of available statistical packages and the statistics performed becomes part of evidence-based practice among nurses.

Statistics and Software

Various statistical procedures can be performed using statistical packages thereby saving time and effort:
- Descriptive statistics like frequencies, percentages, graphs, central tendencies, and variability.
- Inferential statistics like parametric (t-test, ANOVA) and non-parametric tests, correlation, Chi-square, etc.
- Multivariate statistics like various multiple regressions, analysis of covariance, multivariate analysis of variance, etc.

Uses of Statistical Packages
- All quantitative research studies are analyzed using statistical packages to give a quick and reliable outcome.
- They help in condensing large amount of data and presenting it in the form of tables and graphs for better understanding and outcome.
- They help in drawing conclusions and inferences from the data analyzed based on which statistical decisions are made.
- Most of the data formats like excel, plain text, or SQL database for analysis are acceptable as they are compatible with statistical packages.
- It does not just limit to analyzing the data but also assists in data entry, auto-coding, and transform coding which makes the sheet feasible for easy and quick analysis.
- Statistical packages help in performing all sorts of extensive analyses effortlessly.
- Statistical packages that carry out analysis for qualitative studies are popular among qualitative researchers.

Types of Statistical Software
- As it is cumbersome for many students and researchers to carry out statistical analysis manually due to their poor understanding of mathematics and statistics or lack of being exposed to large amounts of data which is neither condensed nor analyzed,

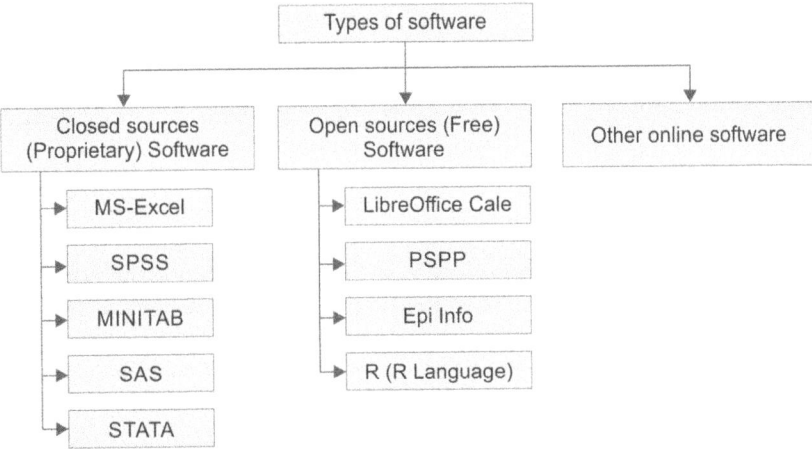

Fig. 1.32: Types of statistical packages

statistical packages come through as a user-friendly, applicable and feasible option.
- It is simple even for a beginner to understand the concepts and navigate through statistical packages and software as many tutorials are freely available on the YouTube. Alternately paid courses and subscriptions to online courses, MOOC courses, biostatistical consultants, and websites are also available.
- All quantitative studies are these days analyzed with the help of statistical softwares. They are available as either closed sources (proprietary) or open sources (free). Various types of statistical packages are depicted in **Figure 1.32**.

Closed Sources (Proprietary) Software

These are statistical softwares available on a proprietary basis to be used only after purchase and installation with proper license code. These are not freely available to the public.

MS-Excel

Excel is a very popular and useful spreadsheet program used for data entry. It is a part of the Microsoft Office suite of programs. These are usually pre-installed in computers and if not require to be purchased from a retail store.

Statistical Uses

- It is a basic tool for data entry that can be analyzed on its page or exported into other statistical software.
- Used for generation of random numbers, basic descriptive statistics like computation of mean, range, percentage, standard deviation, etc.
- While various calculation commands can be entered into Excel, even high-level statistics like ANOVA can be performed. However, statisticians do not recommend the use of Excel for performing complicated statistics as erroneous results might come out due to algorithm related problems in certain versions. It is thereby recommended to export spreadsheets into other softwares for complex data analysis.

Pros

- User friendly and interchanges nicely with various other Microsoft products.
- Excel spreadsheets are easily readable by various other statistical softwares making it possible to get exported and analyzed.
- There is an add-on module that is part of Excel to undertake basic analysis.
- Allows for generating graphs such as bar charts, pie charts, scattered plots, etc.

Cons
- Excel though designed for financial calculations is used for other purposes limitedly.
- Uneconomical as it requires the purchase of Microsoft Office for the system.
- Not preferred for sophisticated statistical analyses though it can be performed with expensive commercial add-ons.

SPSS

SPSS, an acronym for Statistical Package for Social Sciences is a product of IBM with its version 1.0 released way back in 1968, latest version being 23.0. It was originally developed by Stanford University in 1960 itself and labeled as one of the earliest statistical packages available in the market. It mostly resembles Microsoft Excel in its look and is one of the most powerful and widely used statistical packages by academia. It is a proprietary software meaning it needs to be purchased and used with proper license. SPSS can be easily downloaded from the link www.spss.com.

Statistical Uses
- This IBM Product is highly preferred for carrying out all sorts of quantitative analyses.
- Descriptive statistics like frequencies, percentages, graphs, central tendencies, and variability can be performed.
- Inferential statistics like parametric (t-test, ANOVA) and non-parametric tests, correlation, Chi-square, etc can be performed.
- Multivariate statistics like various multiple regressions, analyses of covariance, multivariate analyses of variance, etc., can be performed.
- Other complex and sophisticated analyses such as cluster analysis, time series analysis, power analysis, etc. can also be performed.

Pros
- User-friendly, easy to learn and use.
- Has a command-line (syntax) interface as well as the usual menu-driven interface that makes it a great user interface.
- Resembles Excel, but can handle a large amount of data.
- Excels in descriptive statistics and carries out most of the inferential and multivariate statistics quite easily.
- Has an option for generating fine graphics in SPSS sheet as well as on output documents. Data can be exported into any other document and saved as a Word or Excel file.
- Has its own structural equation modeling named AMOS.

Cons
- By far it is the most expensive package available in the market which needs to be renewed every year.
- Limited functionality: These are highly associated with methods mostly used in social sciences, market research, and psychology.
- Looks similar to Excel.
- Only a few more powerful epidemiological analysis techniques are available.

The outlook of SPSS data and variable views are shown in **Figure 1.33**.

MINITAB

It is a statistical package developed at the Pennsylvania State University in the year 1972 with the recent stable version being 21.1 released in 2021. It helps to predict, visualize, analyze, and harness the power of the data to solve business challenges. These are proprietary software meaning the software needs to be purchased and used with proper license.

Statistical Uses
- Data entry and manipulation
- Identify trends and patterns
- Business statistics

Pros
- Part of introductory statistics
- Easy to learn
- Used in business statistics

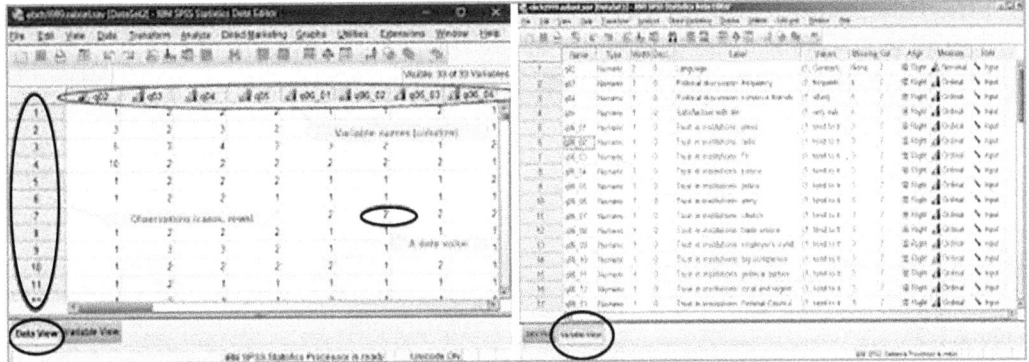

Fig. 1.33: SPSS data and variable views

Cons
- Expensive package
- Not as powerful as other packages for carrying out advanced statistics
- Not preferred for academic research

SAS

SAS, an acronym for Statistical Analysis System was originally developed by North Carolina State University in 1966 and is quite contemporary with SPSS. These are proprietary software requiring purchase and license to use. As the software has many modules, licensing is flexible depending upon the need of the purchaser. SAS can be easily downloaded from the link www.sas.com.

Statistical Uses
- Data entry, retrieval, and management
- All the analyses listed with SPSS are possible with SAS/STAT
- A large variety of statistical methods are available for advanced analysis and numerous other tasks making it popular with the academia and major businesses such as the pharmaceutical industry

Pros
- More powerful than SPSS
- Can be used with both menu-driven as well as syntax file systems
- Highly preferred and commonly used for data management in clinical trials

- Availability of an expansive library of prewritten statistical analysis procedures and robust statistical methods

Cons
- Much harder to learn and use than SPSS
- Expensive and not user-friendly

STATA

STATA is the most recent statistical package available in the market with version 1 being released in 1985. It is user-friendly and more popularly used in the area of epidemiology, economics, and political science. It is a complete, integrated statistical package with the latest version 17 being released in April'21. These are proprietary software that need to be purchased and used with proper license.

Statistical Uses
- Any statistical task including visualization.
- Carry out all types of analyses carried out by SPSS/SAS.
- Meta-analyses are carried out with STATA easily like RevMan software.
- All epidemiological analyses.

Pros
- User friendly and easy to learn.
- Complete, integrated version control.
- Can be used with both menu-driven as well as syntax file systems.
- More powerful than SPSS and equivalent to SAS.

- Effective for performing advanced regression modeling.
- Has its own structural equation modeling.
- Good software for epidemiological procedures.

Cons

- Much harder to learn and use than SPSS
- Very expensive

The outlook of the STATA view is shown in **Figure 1.34**.

Open Sources (Free) Software

The terms 'open-source software' and 'free software' are used interchangeably in most contexts. It is a non-proprietary software where the authors make its source code available to developers who would like to view the code, copy it, learn from it and alter or share it. While the developers are typically encouraged to collaborate and improve upon the open-source software, licenses are still attached to applications with varying requirements.

Advantages of Open-source Software

- Open-source software tends to be more flexible as it offers programmers multiple ways of solving problems thereby encouraging creative solutions.
- Improvements and troubleshooting happens much more quickly as it allows collaboration.
- Is cost-effective as the software allows those unaffiliated with the project access without the authors having to pay for further development.
- It attracts better talent.

Disadvantages of Open-source Software

- Open source software can be difficult to use as they have less user-friendly interfaces or features that many programmers may not be familiar with.
- It may result in both cost and compatibility issues if the hardware used to create the piece of open-source software isn't available with all the programmers working on it.
- These softwares do not come with warranties or indemnification as in the case of proprietary applications.

LibreOffice

LibreOffice is a freely available, fully featured office productivity suite. Its native file format is open document format (ODF), an open standard format. It can open and save documents in many formats, including those used by several versions of Microsoft Office. Its components include a writer (word

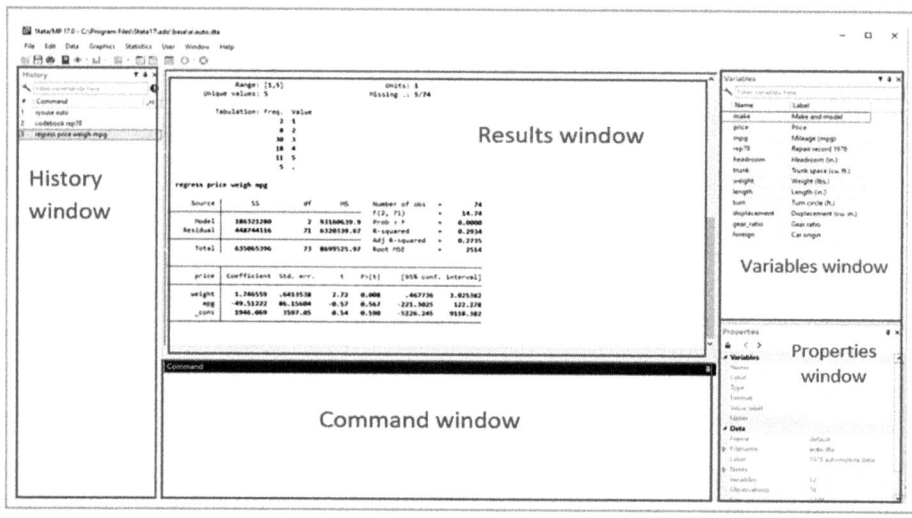

Fig. 1.34: STATA Windows view

processor), calc (spreadsheet), impress (presentations). While new comers prefer this software for its ease, data miners appreciate its comprehensive range of advanced functions.

Statistical Uses
- It is a basic tool for data entry that can be analyzed on its page.
- Used for basic descriptive statistics like computation mean, range, percentage, standard deviation, etc. like Microsoft Excel.

Advantages
- It is an open source with no licensing fees.
- Runs on several hardware architectures and under multiple operating systems.
- The user interface while being consistent provides extensive language support.
- Carries out all descriptive statistics and interoperable with Microsoft Office.
- Extensively used for generating graphs such as bar charts, pie charts, scattered plots, etc.

Disadvantages
Preferred only for basic analyses and not for sophisticated statistical analyses.

PSPP

PSPP is a just free alternative for the proprietary software IBM SPSS. PSPP is a stable and reliable application which carries out all statistics like SPSS with its stable release 1.4.1 in 2020. It is not used as widely as SPSS.

Statistical Uses
- Data entry, retrieval, and management.
- All the analyses listed in SPSS are possible with few exceptions.
- It can perform descriptive statistics, T-tests, ANOVA, regression, association, non-parametric tests, etc.
- Helps in carrying out complex analyses such as cluster analysis, factor analysis, and more.

Advantages
- Available free of cost.
- User-friendly, easy to learn and use.
- Has a command-line (syntax) interface as well as the usual menu-driven interface like SPSS.

Disadvantages
Though similar to a free version of SPSS, not widely used.

Epi Info

Epi Info is a statistical software developed for epidemiology by the Centers for Disease Control and Prevention (CDC) in Atlanta, Georgia for the global community of public health practitioners and researchers. It is in public domain and available free of cost with the recent stable version for windows 7.2.5. It is in existence for more than 20 years.

Statistical Uses
- Data entry, management, customization, and analyses of data.
- Epidemiological analyses such as outbreak investigations, disease surveillance systems, analysis, visualization, and reporting (AVR) components of a larger system.
- All basic analyses performed by other softwares.

Advantages
- Continuing education in the field of epidemiology and public health.
- With multiple modules to complete tasks it goes beyond data entry in questionnaires and customization, and statistical analysis.
- Available freely.

Disadvantages
- Not as powerful as other softwares
- Not a dedicated statistical package
- Not powerful enough to carry out advanced statistics

R (R Language)

Initially, S-Plus statistical programming language was developed and introduced in the year 1988 in Seattle. Later the free version of the same was released as R, a free version of S-Plus in 1996. Being available free for public, it is an open-source software that anyone can access and use from all around the world. R can be easily downloaded from the link http://cran.csiro.au/.

Statistical Uses

- Any statistical tasks that we need it to do including visualization.
- Carries out all types of analyses as carried out by SPSS/SAS including complex analyses such as linear, non-linear, time series, and cluster analysis.

Advantages

- It is free and available to anyone around the globe.
- Has a strong online user community.
- Researchers can program by writing their procedures in R, which are then available to other users.
- Free alternative for SPSS in academia.

Disadvantages

- Much harder to learn and use than SPSS or SAS.
- With only a command-line (syntax) interface available, an expert is required to use it in an errorless manner.

Besides all free version software, there are few other free software available to carry out selective functions with regard to statistics such as Power analysis, Effect size, sample size calculation by G*power software, and many others.

Other Online Software

- These are online platforms where data can be entered directly and output copy-pasted or saved on the document.
- Open-source Epidemiologic Statistics for Public health (OpenEpi) is an example where all epidemiological statistics are performed by data entry online. It also permits performance of power analysis.
- There are various online platforms available for carrying out selected tests and statistics where results are out instantly. However these require data entry everywhere with no option to upload files directly and work on.

Software to Analyze Qualitative Data

Statistical packages are limited to not only analyzing quantitative data but also available for qualitative studies. These help in analyzing narrative data to bring out themes and sub-themes or meaningful units from the descriptive data. This may require greater effort on the part of the users to ensure credibility of the derived data, more clarity and understanding of the package being used. Some examples of qualitative data analysis software are NVivo, ATLAS, Provalis, Quirkos, MAXQDA, Dedoose, Raven's Eye, Qidda and WebQDA, etc.

HOSPITAL MANAGEMENT INFORMATION SYSTEM

Advancement in technology along with an evolving paradigm shift resulting from IT and social changes have recommended significant change and advancement in many fields including health care too. The Healthcare system was expected to take a few innovative steps to evolve into a knowledge-based healthcare system so as to meet global as well as future healthcare demands while adapting to the changing trends. The Hospital Management Information System (HMIS) is needed in every hospital for processing and management of hospital information not only within the hospital areas but also beyond the hospital boundaries such as extending it to meet the purposes of telemedicine and e-healthcare.

Concepts

- HMIS in any hospital is being implemented to manage patient care and administrative functions. It is a process of automation which generates reports for efficient management of the overall system including operations, performance, quality, planning, and decision-making process.
- The digital India movement contributed significantly to the IT sector which in turn brought about a tremendous improvement in every Ministry and its organizations

including Department of Health. This adoption of information technology resulted in providing better care for the people.
- With the meaning of information system in mind it is always easy to define a hospital information management system which is the socio-technical subsystem of a hospital, comprising of all information processing within the hospital as well covering the human and technical sources associated with information processing roles.
- The various HIMS components include hospital functions, business processes, applications, and physical data processing segments.
- Based on this, one can conclude that hospital information system is not a new component and that it was in existence since the invention of hospitals. So, the question is not whether the hospitals need to be equipped with hospital information system, but rather how it could be improved; whether one needs to have all the old traditional information processing tools or need to bring in technology to manage it systematically.
- Every person working in a hospital needs to be considered while framing or structuring the hospital management information system. There is a need for wise integration of various and different information processing tools that are important when looking at information processing systems.

Goals of Hospital Management Information System

- Major goal of the hospital management information system is to adequately enable the better execution of hospital functions for patient care considering the economic hospital management as well as legal and other considerations.
- Legal considerations. For example, data protection of reimbursement aspects, maintenance of patient records, etc.

Tasks of Hospital Management Information System

To support patient care and associated administration, the tasks of hospital management information systems might include various aspects as follows:
- **Patient-related information:** To make patient-related information readily available all the current information must be provided and shared on real time basis to the right person at the right location in an appropriate or usable form for which all the information and data must be carefully and thoroughly collected, stored, processed and systematically documented to ensure that correct, apt, specific and up-to-date patient information can be shared or provided.
- **Knowledge:** Proper hospital management information systems can improve our knowledge on diseases, medications, treatment, side effects, drug interactions, etc.
- **Quality care:** Hospital information management systems assist to make available the information on quality of patient care, and cost-effect situations available within the hospital.

In all, information and knowledge logistics are considered to be a major task of the hospital information system which means making available the right information and knowledge at the right time, at the right place to the right people in the right form will enable the person to make the right decision as shown in **Figure 1.35**.

Importance of HMIS

Importance of hospital management information system can be discussed under various headings as shown in **Figure 1.36**.

Time Saving

- Each part of the hospital along with the people working in it are affected by the quality of the information system. Usually, the data are needed and shared among various personnel working in a hospital

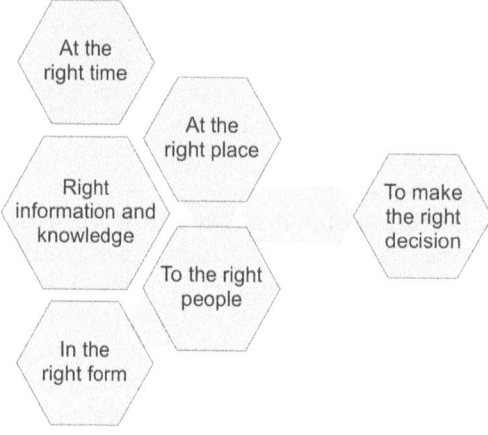

Fig. 1.35: Tasks of HMIS
(Information and knowledge logistics)

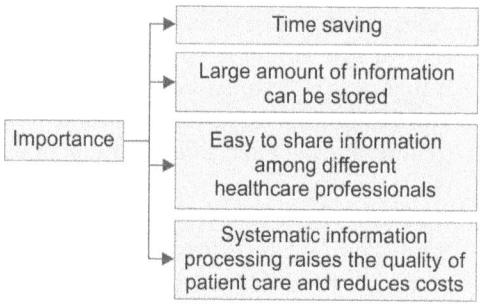

Fig. 1.36: Importance of HMIS

hospital especially if it is a large hospital with multiple departments as the amount of data generated daily about patient care, education, and research is huge.
- For instance, data might cover in-patient and out-patient treatment, operation reports, discharge letters, pathology reports, microbiology reports, radiology reports and clinical chemistry reports. Every year lakhs of new reports and millions of papers are created. To store all this data in a store-room would be difficult as mostly 20–30 years of data would need to be archived consuming huge space. However, if stored digitally 5 terabytes of space would be sufficient to store the entire data including the digital images.

Easy to Share Information Among Different Healthcare Professionals

- Holistic-integrated information processing can be achieved by proper integration of similar and same data as it might be required by various departments within the hospital or between health care personnel or between hospitals and hospital and health insurance team.
- In general, admission data is shared with the departments, treatment reports shared between departments during referrals, and surgical reports considered in discharge letters. Diagnosis and treatment reports are needed for statistics and quality of patient care, discharge data required by the administrative department for census, treatment and diagnostic data required by the billing department and even some administrative data is required to be shared between the hospital and health insurance companies.
- Proper systematic information processing can make the job easier and sharing of data quick and timely thus improving quality of patient care.

with most of them needing various types of data including patient information. If the information processing is systematically managed, it can directly improve the quality of care and reduce costs.
- Hospital personnel like physicians, nurses and administrative personnel are directly affected by the quality of the information system. It is reported that all health care personnel working in hospitals almost spent 25% of their time handling data which requires proper and efficient information processing to benefit them. But it affects them adversely if the information processing is poor and unsystematic.

Large Amount of Information can be Stored

- Considerable amount of data is required to be collected and stored in any given

Systematic Information Processing Raises the Quality of Patient Care and Reduces Costs

- Information processing needs to be done systematically so as to improve quality of patient care and reduce costs.
- An 'unsystematic' information processing system would be chaotic, purposeless, and ineffective leading to low-quality hospital information system. Such a system will not only fail in meeting the information needs of various departments but also result in ending up with poor data quality and higher costs.
- Systematic processing is a purposeful and effective way of handling information and would result in a higher benefit to cost ratio. The health systems need to invest more in systematic information processing as it raises the quality of patient care and reduce cost. These investments include both staff and tools for information processing as it contributes to quality patient care and cost management.

Areas that need to be Supported by an HMIS

Various hospital functions need to be supported by the Hospital management information system to make it practical and easier than carrying it out with most traditional methods. Various functions that need to be supported by HMIS are presented in **Figures 1.37 and 1.38**.

- **Admission of patients:**
  - Patient admission majorly focuses on data related to patient demographics, insurance data and patient safety by ensuring correct patient identification with the unique patient and case identifier. This requires HMIS support.
  - One of the various sub-functions connected with patient admission includes scheduling an appointment. It requires HMIS to make schedules available and support emergency admission.
  - Administrative admission is also a sub-function of patient admission which requires HMIS support in gathering or organizing and recording administrative data such as insurance data, type of admission, patient's relatives, admitting physician, and any referral diagnosis.
  - The hospital management must have adequate data regarding the current occupancy rate of the hospital which the counter clerks can share with relatives

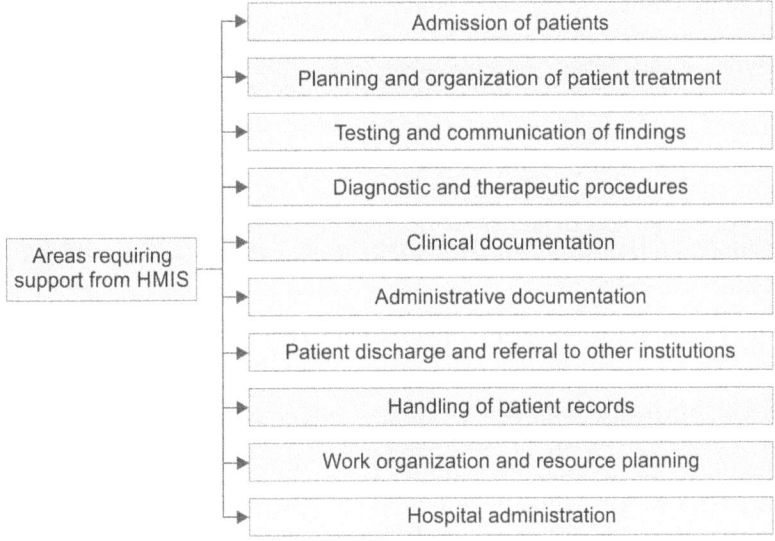

Fig. 1.37: Areas requiring support from HMIS

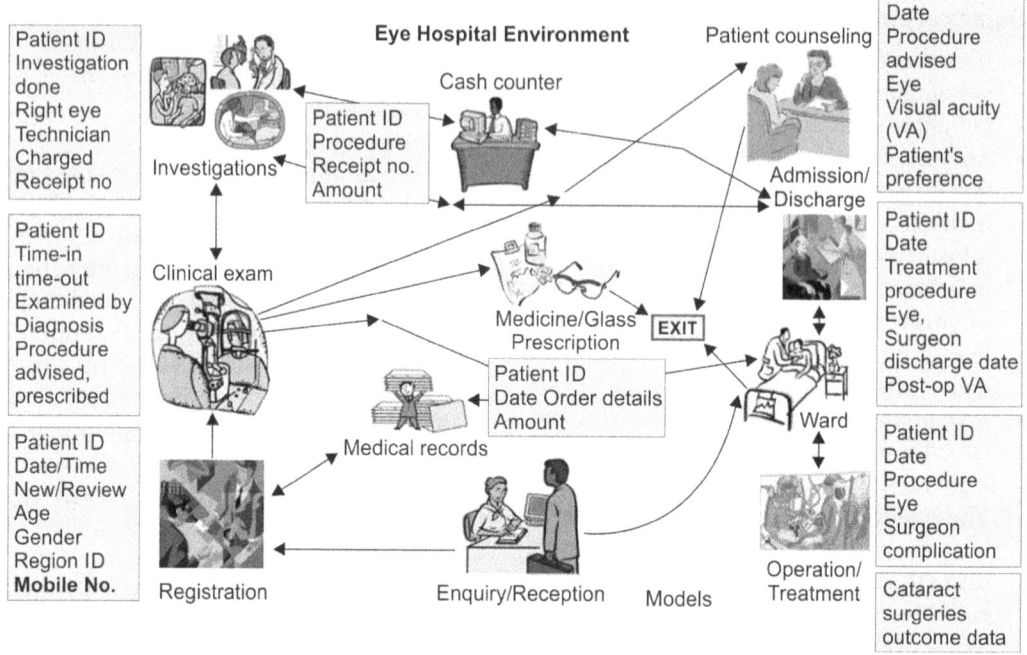

Fig. 1.38: Hospital functions and areas that require support from HMIS

and visitors of patients. It may also assist in generating some general hospital management statistics.
- **Planning and organization of patient treatment:**
  - All clinical procedures and planned care need to be shared, discussed, and agreed upon every time when new information is available. HMIS plays a vital role in making all this data readily available.
  - In addition to having general clinical knowledge about the patients, staff members must be able to access all the available data relevant to patient care specific to the situation.
  - Decision making is required after having gone through all the available data relevant to patient care for diagnosis. For this, the patient needs to be properly diagnosed by having the right consultation with internal or external experts. Data sharing thus becomes mandatory which the HMIS makes it simple.
  - Decisions about clinical procedures and all planned care must be documented in detail which may include type, duration, expert or a responsible person. Also patient consent needs to be well documented.
- **Testing and communication of findings:**
  - All the diagnostic and therapeutic procedures need to be ordered properly by the department to other relevant departments such as laboratory, radiology, or pathology. The test results of these have to be communicated in a proper form as early as possible to the ordering department.
  - HMIS plays a vital role in preparing a proper order with correct entry form systematically, collecting samples, scheduling appointments for procedures, transmitting the order from the department to the testing unit, and reporting findings clearly and correctly in the application format.

- **Diagnostic and therapeutic procedures:**
  - All planned diagnostic, therapeutic and nursing care procedures such as operations, radiotherapies or administration of medications are expected to be executed as planned. However, changes in the planned care need to be communicated among all concerned healthcare workers promptly well within time.
  - HMIS plays a vital role in communicating the changes to all the concerned workers instantly, reschedule it properly or enable all the concerned units and individuals to adapt to the new situation.
- **Clinical documentation:**
  - This includes documentation of all the clinically relevant patient data such as vital signs, orders, results, etc., correctly, completely and making it available quickly among all the concerned healthcare workers. It also refers to recording all the data systematically in a computerized manner so as to enable retrieval of data whenever required, use it for data aggregation and statistics.
  - HMIS plays a vital role in supporting clinical documentation significantly which includes both medical and nursing documentation. Medical documentation includes patient history, diagnosis, therapies and findings, documentation in ICUs, medication orders, and data relevant to clinical trials. Nursing documentation comprises of documentation relevant to nursing care processes like nursing patient history, nursing care and procedure documentation, report writing, vital signs, medications, and other details.
- **Administrative documentation**
  - The hospital must have all the data relevant to patient information and procedures carried out readily available which are the basis for hospital's billing and controlling, cost center and internal budgeting.
  - HMIS plays a vital role in establishing this data and make it available readily so as to improve the administrative functioning of the hospital.
- **Patient discharge and referral to other institutions**
  - When patient treatment is terminated and planned for referral to other treating institutions or rehabilitation centers, HMIS takes the responsibility for communicating patient details and short discharge summary of the patient to the referred hospital quickly.
  - All these treatment data of the patient, procedures carried out, and discharge summary need to be shared between hospitals and treating units while referring the patient to other institutions.
- **Handling of patient records:** All the relevant data of the patient throughout the treatment process must be created, gathered, and stored in such a way that it can be retrieved efficiently. Systematic and computer-based data storage is always easy to retrieve.
- **Work organization and resource planning:** All activities associated with work organization and resource planning such as scheduling and resource allocation, material and pharmaceutical management, maintenance and management of equipment, office communication and basic information processing support require proper data flow and support from HMIS.
- **Hospital administration:** HMIS plays a vital role in establishing data relevant to most of the hospital administration functions. It includes quality management, controlling and budgeting, cost and financial accounting, human resources management, and hospital's general statistical data.

Strategies Used in the Field of HMIS

- There are several strategies that need to be ensured while handling and managing hospital information. Information

management comprises of management of information, management of application components, and management of physical data processing components including computer-based data.
- While planning information management for the hospitals certain tasks such as planning the hospital information system and its architecture, directing its establishment and operation, and monitoring its functions as per the planned objectives need to be considered.
- Simply developing the hospital management information system is not adequate to meet the standards and goals of the information system as it is only proper monitoring that will enable the system to function appropriately. It is also expected that doctors and nurses get recent laboratory findings in shortest possible time and up-to-date therapy and medication interaction information is available all shifts of the day. It is also desirable that sufficient information on economic situation of the hospital is readily available.

Software Used in HMIS

Various Hospital Management Information System softwares used in India besides other Government software are discussed below (Fig. 1.39).

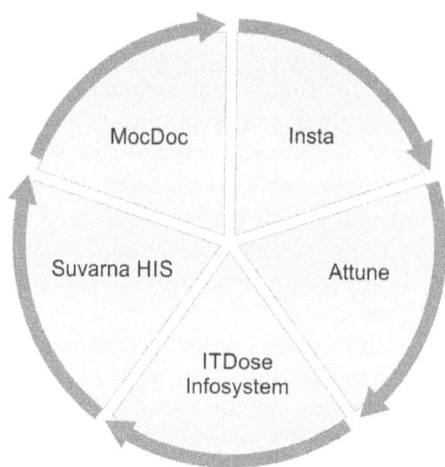

Fig. 1.39: HMIS Softwares in India

- **MocDoc:** It is one of the most popular hospital management information systems available that can be used effectively by incorporating it in out-patient units such as doctor discovery, check-in, mobile apps, prescriptions, appointments, and billing; in inpatient units such as visual bed management, discharge summary, insurance management, ward request, and more. It also covers pharmacy benefits and lab benefits.
- **Insta:** It is known for controlling and monitoring the moving pieces of the hospitals without any difficulty. It manages patients, departments, and staff with ease and enables better decision-making among the patients.
- **Attune:** It is highly preferred for the purpose of increasing revenue, simplifying operations, optimizing productivity, etc. It focuses on billing, insurance, credit tracking, patient referral, in-patient management, radiology information system, CSSD tracking, doctor scheduling, etc.
- **IT Dose Infosystem:** This software has some important features like allocation of duties and staff management, bed allocation, billing, accounting, multi-user accessibilities, doctor scheduling, availability, controlling laboratory and inventory management.
- **Suvarna HIS:** It is cost-effective and the best solution for hospital information management at affordable rates. Important features include hospital module, in-patient services, laboratory system, billing, inventory, online scheduling, diabetes module, nursing module, etc.

REVIEW QUESTIONS

Long Essays (10 Marks)
1. What is a computer? List the components of computer? Write a detailed note on parts of the computer.
2. Explain uses of computer in teaching and learning of nursing students.
3. Write a note on role of computers in nursing practice.
4. Describe impact of computers in scientific research process.
5. Explain in detail the application of computers in nursing administration.
6. What is hospital management information system? Describe tasks and advantages of HMIS.
7. List the important statistical packages. Describe SPSS package in detail.

Short Essays (5 Marks)
1. What are the various components of a computer? Explain any one component in detail.
2. List the parts of a computer. Explain central processing unit.
3. Use of computers in enhancing academic performance of both faculty and nursing students.
4. Forms of computer application in nursing education.
5. Describe modes of internet connection.
6. Purposes of literature search.
7. Methods of literature search.
8. Uses of statistical packages.
9. Features of MS-Excel.
10. What is SPSS package. Explain statistical uses of SPSS.
11. Describe minitab.
12. Explain Epi Info.
13. Importance of hospital management information system.
14. What are the electronic databases relevant to nursing?

Short Answers (2 Marks)
1. Expand ROM and RAM.
2. Expand SPSS and SAS.
3. What is hard disk device.
4. List classification of computers based on power.
5. List types of websites.
6. Types of statistical softwares.
7. List the softwares to analyze qualitative data.
8. List two HMIS softwares in India.
9. List boolean operators.

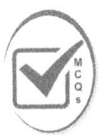

MULTIPLE CHOICE QUESTIONS

1. Which of the following is an input device?
   a. Monitor
   b. Printer
   c. Keyboard
   d. Motherboard

2. Which of the following is an output device?
   a. Monitor
   b. Mouse
   c. Keyboard
   d. Punch cards

3. Which of the following is a memory unit?
   a. Control unit
   b. Logical unit
   c. Central processing unit
   d. Logical processing unit

4. What is mother board?
   a. It is a printed circuit board with various inter-connected electronic components
   b. It is an internal part of the computer which helps to keep components cool
   c. It serves as a primary memory for temporary storing of data
   d. It is a storage device mainly used to store long-term data

5. Which of the following is a word processor?
   a. MS office
   b. MS word
   c. MS excel
   d. MS PowerPoint
6. Ctrl+C short cut key indicates:
   a. Cut selected text
   b. Copy selected text
   c. Paste selected information
   d. Bold highlighted section
7. Which of the following is a spread sheet used to manage large amount of data?
   a. MS office
   b. MS word
   c. MS PowerPoint
   d. MS excel
8. Which of the following is a professional level presentation software?
   a. MS office
   b. MS word
   c. MS PowerPoint
   d. MS excel
9. WWW stands for:
   a. World Wide Web
   b. World Wide Website
   c. World wide Wi-Fi
   d. World Wide Wireless
10. High speed internet connect is called:
    a. Wi-Fi Hotspots
    b. Broadband
    c. Dial-up connection
    d. WWW
11. Following are the Boolean operators, *except*:
    a. AND
    b. OR
    c. BUT
    d. NOT
12. Following are the strategies used to retrieve better review of literature, *except*:
    a. MeSH
    b. Boolean operators
    c. Phrased search
    d. Electronic databases
13. Which of the following software is used to collect, organize, interpret and present numerical data:
    a. SPSS
    b. MS outlook
    c. MS PowerPoint
    d. MS word

ANSWER KEY

| 1. c | 2. a | 3. c | 4. a | 5. b | 6. b | 7. d | 8. c | 9. a | 10. b |
| 11. c | 12. d | 13. a | | | | | | | |

Principles of Health Informatics

INTRODUCTION

Health informatics (HI) also known as healthcare informatics, medical informatics, biomedical informatics or health information system is a relatively new, interdisciplinary field in the healthcare industry.

It encompasses knowledge, skills and tools that enable information to be collected, managed, used and shared to support delivery of healthcare and promote health.

Meaning and Definitions

To understand the meaning of health informatics we first need to define informatics. The term 'informatics' is derived from the French word *'informatique'*. It includes:

- **Science of information:** It studies the analysis, collection, classification, manipulation, storage, retrieval, movement, dissemination, and protection of information. It also deals with acquiring information from raw data systematically.
- **Information processing:** It relates to how the information can be used and what methods are applied to transform healthcare information into useful and usable knowledge.
- **Engineering of information systems:** It refers to engineering of systems that involve input of data and its transformation to information using appropriate methods. It also refers to complementary networks of hardware and software used to collect, filter, process, create and distribute data.

Informatics studies structure, behavior, interactions of natural and artificial systems that store, process and communicate information. Informatics thus does not refer to computer science or computational methods though many of the methods it employs may be related to computer science.

- **Information and communication technology (ICT):** It refers to communication technologies and services used in various applications. It describes these computer, communication and multimedia technologies used to receive, process, store, display and disseminate information. ICT is an umbrella term often used to describe communication within applications in a specific domain. For example, ICT in Health Care.
- **Health informatics:** Health informatics has been defined by the World Health Organization (WHO) as "an umbrella term used to encompass the rapidly evolving discipline of using computing, networking and communications—methodology and technology—to support the health-related fields such as medicine, nursing, pharmacy and dentistry".

'A field that concerns itself with the cognitive, information processing, and communication tools of medical practice, education and research including information science and technology to support these tasks.'
—*Edward H Shortliffe*

'Medical informatics is the application of computer technology to all fields of medicine—medical care, medical teaching and medical research.'
—*Morris F Collen*

'Medical informatics attempts to provide theoretical and scientific basis for the application of computer and automated information systems to biomedicine and health affairs, studies biomedical information and knowledge—their storage, retrieval, and optimal use for problem-solving and decision-making.'
—*Donand AB Lindberg*

ELEMENTS IN HEALTH INFORMATICS

The key elements in health informatics are acquisition, storage and retrieval, communication, manipulation and display (Fig. 2.1).

1. *Acquisition:* It deals with capturing of data generated in the course of providing health care. Various ways to acquire information in clinical environment are as follows (Fig. 2.2):
   - Observation and clinical examination: Healthcare providers collect crucial information from patients using systematic evaluation procedures. They also use their natural senses to collect as much information as possible while examining the patients. For example, inspection, palpation, etc.

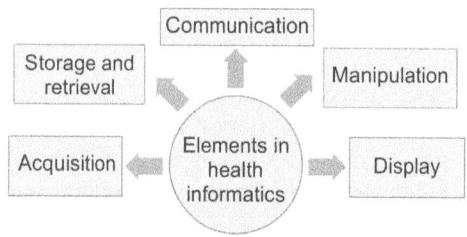

Fig. 2.1: Elements in health informatics

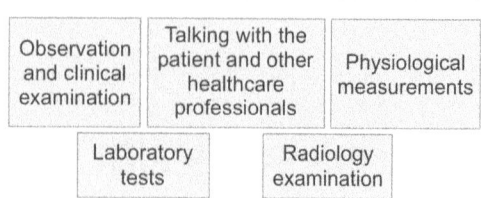

Fig. 2.2: Ways to acquire information in clinical environment

   - *Talking with the patient and other healthcare professionals:* Considering the fact that nurses spend a considerable amount of time with the patient, their observations can serve as a valuable input for the doctor. A nurse is in the best position to observe even small changes or events like loss of appetite, change in skin color or consciousness. Such inputs can be of significant importance as the physician may not be in place to observe it all. Thus, interactions between nurses and doctors can be of great importance.
   - *Physiological measurements:* These may range from simple tests such as measurement of body temperature with a clinical thermometer and measurement of blood pressure to more complicated tests such as measuring the heart function by taking an electrocardiograph (ECG). Majority of such tests are carried out by nurse practitioners.
   - *Laboratory tests:* Laboratory tests involve analysis of samples extracted from patients. For instance, it may involve analysis of blood, urine or tissue samples extracted from patients. These are run both during routine health check-ups (blood, urine, tissue samples) and also during hospitalization to help shape a diagnosis (enzyme concentration, antibody tests).
   - *Radiology exams:* It includes a variety of imaging techniques used to diagnose/treat diseases such as X-ray, ultrasound, computed tomography (CT), positron emission tomography (PET), magnetic resonance imaging (MRI).

2. **Storage and retrieval:** Healthcare related data can be stored by direct entry into electronic medical records (and consequent storage in relational databases in the backend) or using sensors to perform measurements and transmitting the data via a communication module to interoperable systems or scanning handwritten documents and using optical character recognition (OCR) technologies. Healthcare professionals retrieve information using search tools available in graphical user interfaces or electronic medical records.
3. **Communication:** Acquired health information is communicated from the point of data collection to storage for analysis and across subsections of a hospital information system. However, it involves the use of communication protocols and interoperability standards which should not only be technically compatible but also be able to achieve seamless data exchange.
4. **Manipulation:** Data needs to be manipulated, combined and aggregated for statistical and healthcare analytics purposes. It may range from calculating a patient's age to generating prediction models. It may also refer to different forms of data representation depending upon the requirement of the end user.
5. **Display:** It refers to the way data may be displayed for the purpose of easy understanding. It not only includes displaying of information via physical output devices such as monitors, printers, etc., but also via user-friendly interfaces such as human computer interactions and functional dialogue systems.

HEALTH INFORMATION SYSTEM

Health information system management is the primary function of any health informatics professional. The term health information system is used to describe any system that employs computer hardware and software

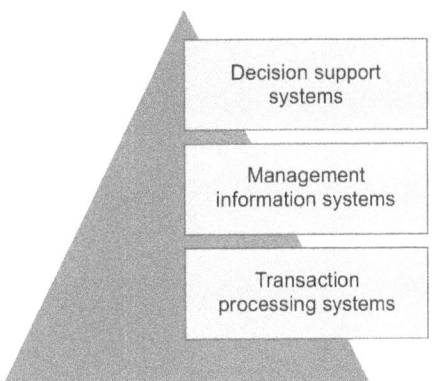

Fig. 2.3: Basic types of information system

to capture, store, manage and transmit information associated with the health of individuals. Basic types of information systems are (**Fig. 2.3**):

- **Transaction processing systems:** It is a type of information system that collects, stores, modifies and retrieves the data transactions of an organization. Examples, patient billing system, hospital admission and discharge system.
- **Management information systems:** It is a set of systems and procedures that gather data from a range of sources, compile it and present it in a readable format. These software systems provide management tools for organizing and evaluating departments and their staff. Examples, emergency department, laboratory information system.
- **Decision support systems:** It is a computerized program used to support determinations, judgments and courses of action in an organization. These computer systems in addition to gathering data, use analytical models and tools to improve the outcome of decision-making tasks. Example, clinical decision support system.

Types of Health Information Systems

Healthcare organizations have various systems working together within a broader information technology environment. The various health information systems are presented in **Figure 2.4**.

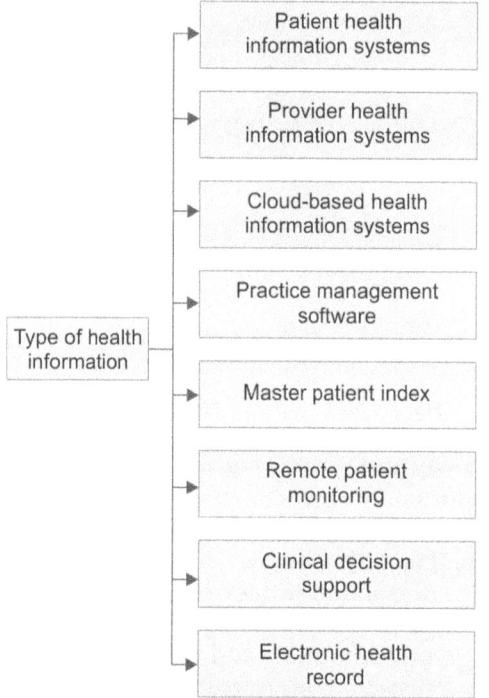

Fig. 2.4: Types of health information systems

- **Patient health information system/patient portals:** These are primarily web portals (websites or apps) wherein patients can log into their personal accounts to access medical history which may include details of their previous doctor visits. These portals help the patients to view lab test results, physician orders, nurse's notes, recommended medicines and follow-ups. It allows the patients to be a part of their own treatment and know the status of payments or insurance benefits. These portals often enable doctors and nurses to transmit confidential messages to patients, be it sharing of lab reports or simply recap the discussion had during the previous visit. There is also an option to message their provider securely and confidentially and pose follow-up questions.
- **Provider health information systems:** These systems contain information on population health, trends in the hospital or any other data relating to treatment decisions.
- **Cloud-based health information systems:** These systems make available common records across various departments and facilities thereby allowing each provider in the chain to access the same information. They also play an important role in collaborative care. It thus provides a clear picture of the patient's treatment history, minimizes redundant treatments and keeps all providers on the same page.
- **Practice management software:** These are mostly used by the front office managers of hospital set-up to automate administrative work such as keeping track of appointments, generating and dispatching bills, etc.
- **Master patient Index:** This system provides an entry for every registered patient whose individual files are linked across various databases thereby consolidating all the information connected to the patient treatment history.
- **Remote patient monitoring or telehealth:** It helps in keeping a track of patient's vital signs, blood pressure and other biometrics even when the patient has returned home. This is made possible with the help of sensors which the patients may wear inconspicuously and unobtrusively at home, school or work. The sensors transmit information back to the provider automatically. It allows the providers to monitor patients with conditions even such as diabetes remotely. It also permits the providers to determine when a patient may require further clinical intervention.
- **Clinical decision support (CDS):** It enables the providers to access and evaluate data from clinical and administrative subsystems. Information thus collected helps the providers to make prudent decisions about the likely clinical treatment. For example, the CDS information can help a provider prepare a diagnosis or predict on how different medications will interact. While CDS system relies on trends from

an entire patient population, the providers can use the filtered information to take the best possible decision for each individual patient.
- **Electronic health record:** The electronic medical record is essentially a digitalized version of the paper chart that provides a long-term holistic view of the patient's health. It includes the following information:
  - Patient testing and treatment history
  - Demographic data
  - List of medications administered
  - History of present illness

Essentials of Health Information Systems and Technology

Health information systems can benefit a healthcare organization in numerous ways. The essentials of health information system includes both hardware and software requirements.
- Effective implementation of health information systems requires a secure wireless network connecting all associated devices and enabling the access and sharing of information from anywhere within the organization.
- It requires workstations for the healthcare providers such as doctors, nurses, technicians and administrators to access records from. These may include desktops, laptops and tablets.
- It requires employee training, best practices for maintaining network security and ensuring patient privacy, data encryption and backup to safeguard data from cyberattacks, hackers or system failures. It also requires cyber insurance to protect the organization from legal liability in the event that patient data is compromised.

Most of the larger hospital settings are likely to have an information technology team led by a chief information officer. Health information system provides an option for the decision makers to make the best possible use of resources to achieve optimal patient outcomes as efficiently as possible.

APPLICATIONS OF HEALTH INFORMATICS

Following are the applications of health informatics (**Fig. 2.5**):
- **Translational bioinformatics:** It includes research on the development of novel techniques for the integration of biological and clinical data and the evolution of clinical informatics methodology to encompass biological observations.
- **Clinical research informatics:** It includes use of informatics in the discovery and management of new knowledge relating to health and disease. It manages the information related to clinical trials and also involves informatics related to secondary research use of clinical data.
- **Clinical informatics:** It is the application of informatics and information technology to deliver healthcare services. It is concerned with information use in health care by clinicians.
- **Consumer health informatics:** It analyzes consumer's needs for information, studies and implements methods for making information accessible to consumers and integrates consumer's preferences into health information systems.

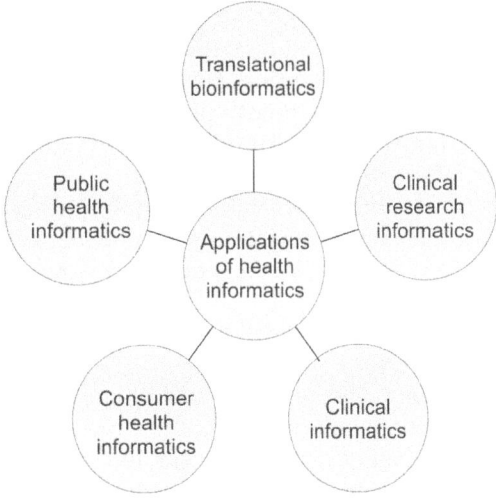

Fig. 2.5: Applications of health informatics

- **Public health informatics:** It is the application of informatics in the area of public health including surveillance, reporting and health promotion.

OBJECTIVES OF HEALTH INFORMATICS

Health informatics is the intersection of information science, computer science, and health care. It studies resources, devices and methods required to optimize acquisition, storage, retrieval and use of information in health. The main objectives of health informatics are:
- To provide solutions for problems related to data, information and knowledge processing.
- To study the general principles of processing data, information and knowledge in medical and health care.
- To provide a structure for pooling, communicating and applying clinical evidence.

NEED FOR HEALTH INFORMATICS

- To organize, store and manage health data while using electronic health records.
- To have easy access to patient information so as to help physicians and nurses arrive at quick solutions.
- To make an appropriate healthcare decision. Better information leads to better decisions.
- To communicate with policymakers for policy planning. Healthcare, health management, health policy and health planning all depend on having good information to make decisions.
- To enable better collaboration and co-ordination among healthcare providers.
- To streamline medical quality assurance processes.
- To improve cost-efficiency in healthcare delivery.
- To increase accuracy and efficiency in practice management.
- To advance patient care and life sciences research, health professions education and public health.

PRINCIPLES OF HEALTH INFORMATICS

According to the American Medical Informatics Association (AMIA), health informatics applies principles of computer and information sciences to the advancement of patient care and life sciences research, health professions education and public health. The main principles of health informatics are:
- The health information system should be developed in a coordinated manner to facilitate interconnectivity.
- Recognize the needs of primary health care.
- Guarantee all privacy and confidentiality requirements.
- Serve the needs of both the individual patient and healthcare professional needs.
- Improve effectiveness and efficiency of healthcare services/delivery.
- Enable quality assessment and quality improvement.

BENEFITS OF HEALTH INFORMATICS

Health informatics applies information technology to healthcare delivery in a systematic manner. It deals with resources, devices and methods required to optimize the collection, storage, retrieval and communication of health-related data. It focuses on problem-solving, decision-making and assuring highest quality care in all basic and applied areas of biomedical sciences. The benefits of health informatics are depicted in Box 2.1.
- **Reduces healthcare cost and time:** Health care costs are expensive and also wasteful as half of all the medical expenditures are related to repeated procedures, expenses associated with traditional methods of sharing information, delays in care and errors in care or delivery. With an electronic and connected system in place much of misuse can be restricted with timely care being delivered to reduce malpractice claims and errors. Earlier incompetence and obstruction can be replaced with better communication and efficiency.

> **Box 2.1: Benefits of health informatics**
>
> - Reduces health care cost and time
> - Provides ease in decision-making
> - Improves health care quality, outcome and safety
> - Shares knowledge
> - Improves access to information
> - Reduces error rates
> - Improves diagnoses and treatment
> - Reduces the length of hospital stays
> - Reduces mortality
> - Improves delivery of care
> - Empowers patients
> - Increases coordination
> - Improves communication
> - Maintains data confidentiality and patient privacy
> - Improves compliance of accreditation standards
> - Improves education
> - Accelerates research

Application of computer science and information technology to the many different facets of healthcare creates great efficiencies by minimizing and automating labor-intensive or time-consuming tasks and lowering healthcare costs.

- **Ease in decision-making:** Electronic record system enables physicians and nurses to make better and quicker decisions through on-line access to evidence-based results, assists in placing orders and receives alerts for significantly abnormal test results. This results in fewer errors being made and fewer resources being consumed. Having information at the right time supports clinical decision-making.

- **Improves healthcare quality, outcome and safety:** Quality of care delivered and access to knowledge and information are two important factors that can reduce errors and improve positive outcomes. Technology improves quality and safety in key areas. Nurses can receive alerts regarding patient care to prevent orders from being missed. Sharing of data can aid in decision-making with the patients. The most significant achievement of health informatics is the way it promotes improved outcomes. Electronic medical records result in quality care as the medical team is able to provide better diagnoses with little chance for errors. With manual jobs getting automated, doctors and nurses are able to spend more time with the patients thereby improving efficiency. This results in saving of time and money for hospitals, clinics and providers, so also for patients, insurance companies and the Government. Electronically generated reminders for screening and follow-up improve patient treatment adherence by 10 to 15%.

- **Shares knowledge:** Medicine is referred to as a "practice" as the healthcare providers are always learning and honing their skills. Health informatics provides an easier way to share knowledge on patients, diseases, therapies and medicines. As the knowledge is passed back and forth between providers and patients, the practice of medicine gets better thus aiding everyone with the chain of care.

- **Improves access to information:** Access to information for patients and providers can improve the quality of decision-making besides reducing errors resulting from missing documentation. Health informatics makes it possible for multiple users to share information concurrently within and outside the hospital for various purposes. Through Electronic Health Records (EHR) information can be shared between providers caring for the patients, third party payers and reporting agencies such as public health. Patients have real-time access to their health information. With mobile applications available, patients can carry all the information they need in the palm of their hands. Some even allow messaging services directly to their clinicians, offering a convenient way to access their doctor without scheduling an appointment. The use of communication technology based on the Internet makes it possible to provide health and social care to a patient directly even from a remote location.

- **Reduces error rates:** Health informatics reduces medication errors to ensure patients receive accurate prescriptions based on the information found in patient records. Having these processes automated through quality information systems managed by informaticists reduces errors, making care more effective and efficient.
- **Improves diagnoses and treatments:** Automated data sorting can help drive preventive care enabling clinicians to more readily identify patients with higher risks. This provides proper assessment and treatment even before a more severe health concern occurs.
- **Reduces the length of hospital stays:** Having the necessary tools to detect early patient risks can help the clinician provide treatment without requiring extended hospital stays. Informatics systems maintain data that equip healthcare providers with access to real-time patient records and medical information in an attempt to drive critical decision-making so as to provide the best patient care.
- **Reduces mortality:** Studies have suggested that introduction of information technology in hospitals reduces mortality and complications.
- **Improves delivery of care:** Delivery of care for various conditions can be improved as there is lesser trial and error on combining team-based practice with EHR.
- **Empowers patients:** Telehealth services allow patients to hold non-emergency appointments with their health care providers facilitating easier and more convenient healthcare delivery to more patients. This option will continue to benefit patients with limited mobility and those with limited access to transportation and nearby healthcare facilities. Patients are able to access their EHRs and review prescriptions and laboratory results to improve self-care. This access to one's own health history allows the patient to play an important role in personal health care and get empowered. Patients with access to healthcare portals are able to educate themselves about the diagnoses and prognoses while keeping a track of medications and symptoms. They are able to better interact with doctors and nurses resulting in better outcomes. It makes the patient feel that they are a precious part of their own healthcare team.
- **Increases co-ordination:** With patients receiving care from many different people in one hospital stay, health care is getting increasingly specialized. Patients are involved in many different conversations regarding care which may include medical tests, therapies, medication, discharge instructions, etc. Unless these conversations are held in a combination with one another newer problems may arise affecting care adversely. This requires increased co-ordination for which health informatics is the only way forward.
- **Improves communication:** It facilitates enhanced communication between providers and between providers and patients.
- **Maintains data confidentiality and patient privacy:** Health informatics professionals are using block chain technology to find new methods for data encryption. This ensures that patients and doctors do not have to worry about data breaches and compromised data and that the records are completely safe. They can also see which health providers have viewed their files allowing them to monitor privacy.
- **Improves administrative functions:** For a leader to be able to shape the policy of an organization he has to be equipped with up to date and relevant data. Being able to understand the activities taking place in the organization, the authorities can determine education needs, improve quality programs and create a culture

of safety and accountability for the staff. Health informatics helps streamline administrative tasks that healthcare professionals usually handle such as filling paper work, processing billing codes and verifying insurance information. Electronic health records make it easy to not only create backup in digital format but also access it from anywhere and anytime with proper permission.

- **Improved compliance of accreditation standards**: Most electronic health record related software packages come with preset documentation standards for providers and staff.
- **Improves education**: Healthcare technology has many facets of patient and staff education incorporated in the patient record. Educative tools as regards procedures, medications and disease processes are available in electronic health records.
- **Accelerates research**: Health informatics also aids in accelerating research and solving public health challenges.

LIMITATIONS OR DISADVANTAGES

Despite the growing benefits of health informatics, some of the identified potential limitations or disadvantages with technology are presented below (**Fig. 2.6**).

- **Impersonalization of care**: One of the main criticisms of approaching patient care through information and technology is that it results in lesser personal care and lack of empathy. Knowing the patient becomes a function of the data available and algorithms rather than the interaction in real time and space thereby enhancing the risk of miscommunication.
- **Cyber security risks**: As technology has a major role to play, the risk related to breach of protected health information is very high. Patient data and other private information is susceptible to network hackers. The additional risk of alteration in data leading to wrong healthcare decisions

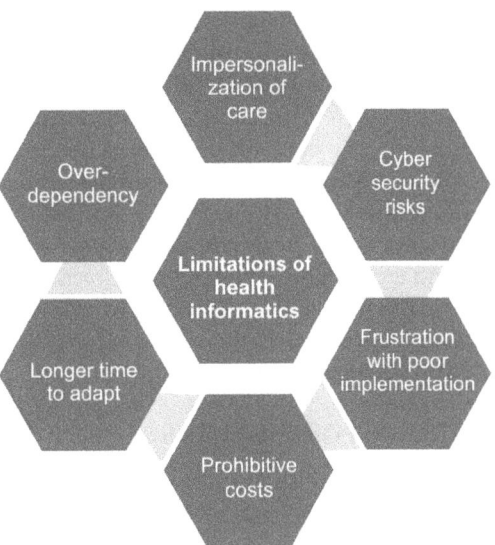

Fig. 2.6: Limitations of health informatics

also cannot be ruled out. Alteration of device functionality can lead to adverse events.
- **Frustration with poor implementation**: Too much reliance on technology may not result in desired outcomes and at times also be counterproductive especially if the Artificial Intelligence (AI) implementation is poor. Clinicians may end up spending more time struggling with technology rather than providing the needed patient care.
- **Prohibitive costs**: Costs associated with sophisticated health technology, upgrades, maintenance and support, changes in workflow, lower revenues associated with temporary loss of productivity and ongoing training and support for end users can serve as a disincentive for hospitals to adopt and implement EHR. Higher input costs may make quality health care inaccessible to a sizeable population which is living below the poverty line.
- **Longer time to adapt**: As technology is constantly evolving, there can be new softwares, upgrades and ways of doing things. In order to keep up with it and maintain the competitive edge, the healthcare staff will be required to continually evolve and

change the way they work. This can be a real struggle for the older staff.
- **Over-dependency:** With increasing dependence on data and technology and no way to revert to manual methods the cost and impact of system downtime (accumulated time during which the system is not performing in accordance with the required standard of performance) can rise rapidly. Such failures can erode the confidence and damage the reputation of the healthcare unit.

TRENDS FOR THE FUTURE

The field of health informatics expanded significantly in the decades following its first practical use in the 1950s when dental data was collected by the National Bureau of Standards. In 2009, the Health Information Technology for Economic and Clinical Health (HITECH) Act was created to promote and expand the adoption of health information technology—focusing mainly on the use of electronic health records (EHRs) by healthcare providers. Today, the International Medical Informatics Association (IMIA) oversees member organizations involved in health informatics worldwide.

Healthcare though for ages has been employing the paper-based system, it is now fast becoming obsolete due to its limited functionality and emergence of various data-capturing techniques. The challenge however comes from managing and streamlining large volumes of data. Some of the emerging trends include:
- Health data experts can utilize the health informatics data to track and draw insights for drawing public health management programs.
- Health informaticians can use newer technologies to perform predictive analysis about the likelihood of individual patients and larger patient population getting certain diseases.
- Digitization of healthcare in clinical settings will help in revolutionizing approaches at all levels of care with emphasis on precision medicine and person-centered care.
- Health informatics will provide greater interoperability, i.e., an ability to access, exchange, integrate and cooperatively use data in a coordinated manner both within and across organizational, regional and national boundaries enabling better care coordination, patient outcomes and reduced costs.
- The newer trends will empower the patients by providing them access to their health information.
- Existing and developing technologies can be used to support open, proactive, two-way communication between hospitals, clinicians, patients, vendors and other healthcare stakeholders.
- Focus is on offering a robust heath data infrastructure by providing faster, more interoperable and accessible patient records, reduction in errors, reduction in redundant testing, production of more complete and accurate healthcare records.
- Newer technologies which are at the core of successful health informatics are able to distinguish between large amounts of data and meaningful data at breakneck speeds enabling its seamless integration within an organization.

The rapid evolution of healthcare informatics has made it a critical component of the modern concept of public health and national healthcare policy.

USE OF DATA, INFORMATION AND KNOWLEDGE FOR MORE EFFECTIVE HEALTHCARE AND BETTER HEALTH

Health informatics is a scientific discipline that deals with the collection, storage, retrieval, communication and optimal use of health-related data, information and knowledge. This discipline utilizes methods and technologies of information science for the purpose of problem-solving, decision-making and assuring quality health care in all areas of biomedical sciences. Data, information and

Use of Data, Information and Knowledge for Effective Health Care

Data is the basic element of cognition on which all constructs are based and stored in information systems. Information and knowledge are derived from data. Attaching meaning to data transforms them into semantic data or information. Knowledge at the next level implies contextualized information (adding related information to something to make it more useful). This can mean including background information, patterns, trends, outliers, and more to help a reader make sense of what the data is really saying.

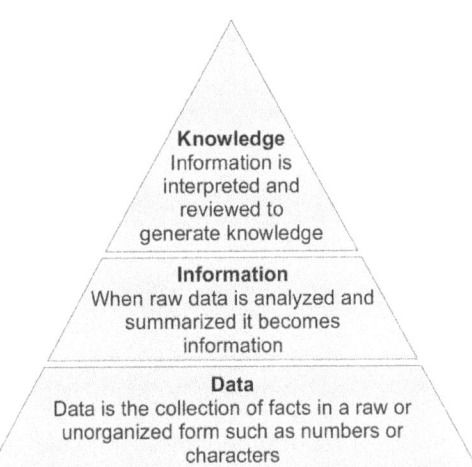

Fig. 2.7: Central concepts in health informatics

knowledge are central concepts in health informatics (**Fig. 2.7**).

- **Data:** Data is the collection of facts in a raw or unorganized form such as numbers or characters acquired from many sources. It requires cleaning and processing. Without context and analysis, data has little meaning. Data in its simplest form consists of raw alphanumeric values.
- **Information:** When raw data is analyzed and summarized it transforms to information. Information can be defined as either data organized into meaningful unions or data placed in context with relevance, purpose and meaning. Unlike data, information has various purposes in creating knowledge, decision-making and guiding further actions. Information is useful data that has been processed in a way to improve the knowledge of the person using the data. Information is essentially processed data.
- **Knowledge:** Information is interpreted and reviewed to generate knowledge. It is combined with intelligence, evidence and qualitative data and presented to form decision-making. Knowledge is the justifiable belief based on data and information. Knowledge itself may be processed to generate decisions. Knowledge is needed to produce actionable information that can lead to impact.

Types of Data in Healthcare Sector

Healthcare organization collects, processes and analyzes different types of data. Various types of data in healthcare sector are presented in **Figure 2.8**.

- **Clinical data:** It refers to information about patient care. It is collected from the patient during care or observed or obtained from electronic medical records, hospital information system, image centers, laboratories, pharmacies, physician's notes, physiological monitoring, etc. Examples are medical history, surgical interventions, investigation reports, etc. Clinical data can further be classified into narrative (recorded by clinician), numerical measurements (blood pressure and temperature), coded data (selected from a controlled terminology system), recorded

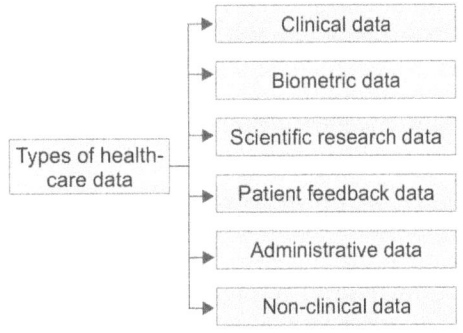

Fig. 2.8: Types of healthcare data

signals (EKG, EEG), pictures (radiographs, photographs and other images).
- **Biometric data:** Data provided from various devices that monitor weight, pressure, heart rate, oxygen saturation, glucose level, etc.
- **Scientific research data:** Data from scientific research activities and results of research, drug trials, new inventions, etc.
- **Patient feedback data:** Data provided by patients may include description of preferences, level of satisfaction, information from systems for self-monitoring of their activity, exercises, sleep, meals consumed, etc.
- **Administrative data:** It refers to information that is collected, processed and stored in automated information systems. This data includes admission details, claims information, physician office visits, etc.
- **Non-clinical data:** It refers to information not directly related to patient treatment but still influencing the way professionals use healthcare facilities and resources.

The above generated data is stored in paper and digital form. It is also difficult to apply traditional tools and methods for management of unstructured data. Advanced analytical tools and technologies are needed to manage healthcare data.

Information and Knowledge Process in Health Care

Healthcare organizations are constantly generating health-related data. The primary purpose of health information systems is to help organizations capture this data, interpret it and put it to practical use. After the data is collected, it must be analyzed for making necessary decisions and changes in the organizations.

Information and knowledge process refers to organizational processes that ensure the availability of information and knowledge for professionals within an organization through the following four elements (**Fig. 2.9**):
- **Information collection:** Information is collected from the patient during care or observed or obtained from electronic

Fig. 2.9: Elements in information and knowledge process

medical records, hospital information system, image centers, laboratories, pharmacies, physician's notes, physiological monitoring, etc. Examples are medical history, surgical interventions, investigation reports, etc.
- **Information transfer and storage:** Patient information in health care is mediated through information technology in electronic patient records. Electronic patient records enable easy storage and retrieval of patient information. Through this process information is integrated for knowledge creation and sharing.
- **Knowledge creation and sharing:** Knowledge is created through the collection of experience, the generation of new understanding by combining research findings. Knowledge sharing is an activity in which people make knowledge available to another or others. It can result in the construction of common meanings and the creation of new knowledge.
- **Information and knowledge use:** It refers to meaningful and purposive actions of knowledge use in practice and decision-making by various professionals in a health organization with expected positive organizational and patient outcomes.

Healthcare Big Data Analytics Applications

Medical facilities use both structured and unstructured data in their practice. While the structured data has a predetermined schema that is extensive, free form and comes in a

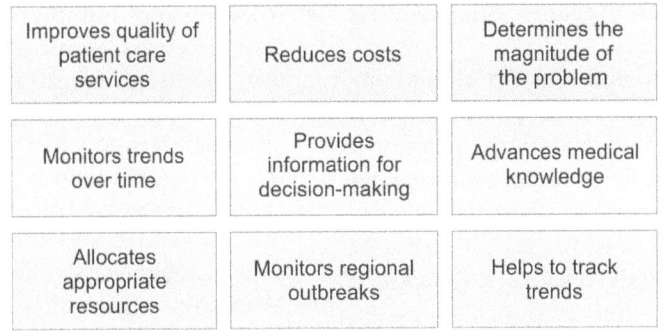

Fig. 2.10: Benefits of healthcare data management

variety of forms, the unstructured data referred to as Big data does not fit into the typical data processing format. Big data refers to massive amount of data sets that cannot be stored, processed or analyzed using traditional tools. It remains stored but is not analyzed. It requires a specific technology and method to transform it into value. Integrating data stored in both structured and unstructured formats can add significant value to an organization. Applications of big healthcare data analysis are as follows:

- **Diagnosis:** Identification of disease causes
- **Patient treatment:** Selecting treatment options
- **Precision medicine:** Treatment adjusted to a specific patient-personalized medicine
- **Preventive medicine:** Predictive analytics for disease prevention
- **Telemedicine:** Patient health monitoring
- **Health population support:** Big data monitoring to capture disease trends, outbreaks, etc.
- **Medical research:** Data-driven medical research
- **Cost reduction:** Greater insight into medical data translating into better patient care resulting in long-term savings

Benefits of Healthcare Data Management

A healthcare knowledge management system can create a more efficient flow of information between all healthcare providers, which can ultimately lead to increased efficiency and productivity. Various benefits of healthcare data management are presented in **Figure 2.10**.

- **Improves quality of patient care services:** Better data leads to better care. Immediate access to information allows for faster response and more effective treatment. Healthcare data management provides convenience to both the patient and the provider. With more complete documentation available for healthcare professionals patient can benefit from lower wait times, faster diagnoses, more efficient treatment, easier billing and insurance claims and better communication.

- **Reduces costs:** With more data available and the use of predictive modeling, healthcare professionals are equipped to be more proactive. This data not only helps in identification of unnecessary medical activities and procedures but also provides actionable insights making it easier to prevent readmissions, diagnose chronic conditions early, optimize treatments and improve care co-ordination. All these reduce healthcare costs.

- **Determines the magnitude of the problem:** Data describes what is known about the problem, place the problem in context, describe what already exists and identify gaps and population at high risk. It also helps in estimating disease prevalence and incidence.

- **Monitors trends over time:** Data provides a source of baseline information. Progress can be measured against this baseline information.

- **Provides information for decision-making:** Analysis of large volumes of data provides information on needs and resources. This helps in decision-making process of diagnosis and detection of more effective interventions for patients. By utilizing data in the health sector, medical providers and administrators can identify areas of risk or improvement within current pathways. With this information they can work to correct areas where patient care is lacking and increase the quality of overall patient experience. This can help improve patient care, promote strategic planning and utilize resources in a more efficient manner.
- **Advancement of medical knowledge:** Data helps in diagnosing rare illnesses, make connections between diseases and lifestyle choices, study the effects of treatment, etc. Through this data, healthcare professionals can analyze patient histories and similar case studies so as to hone their treatment decisions.
- **Allocates appropriate resources:** Through data analysis administrators can not only monitor patient footfalls in various departments but also allocate staffing and resources to where they are needed the most. This data is used to develop comprehensive care plans, improve patient outcomes and allocate organizational resources judiciously.
- **Monitors regional outbreaks:** Basic analysis of this data can reveal incidence and prevalence of diseases, track cases and monitor regional outbreaks. It also helps in prediction of occurrence of specific diseases or worsening of patient's condition.
- **Helps to track trends:** Collected data is stored and utilized to make a diagnosis and track trends following patient health condition.

The process of data analysis, patterns and trends allows health service providers to offer a more accurate and insightful diagnoses of patients and personalized treatment. It also helps to monitor patients, support medical research and health population, provide better quality of medical services and patient care, and reduce costs.

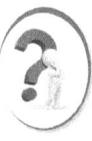

REVIEW QUESTIONS

Long Essays (10 Marks)
1. Write the meaning of data, information and knowledge. Explain their uses in effective health care.
2. What is the meaning of health informatics? Explain applications of health informatics.
3. Describe benefits of health informatics.

Short Essays (5 Marks)
1. Describe types of health information systems.
2. What are the essentials of health information system?
3. Narrate the need for health informatics in India.
4. Write the meaning of data, information and knowledge.
5. What is healthcare bigdata?

Short Answers (2 Marks)
1. What is information processing?
2. Meaning of information and communication technology.
3. Meaning of health informatics.
4. List the elements of health informatics.
5. What are the basic types of information systems?

MULTIPLE CHOICE QUESTIONS

1. What is the meaning of information processing?
   a. It is related to methods applied to transform healthcare information into useable knowledge
   b. It is related to input of data and its transformation to information
   c. It is related to study of analysis, collection, classification and manipulation of information
   d. It is related to communication technologies that are used in various applications

2. Following are the key elements of health informatics, except:
   a. Acquisition
   b. Display
   c. Process
   d. Manipulation

3. Which of the following deals with capturing of data generated in the course of providing health care?
   a. Acquisition
   b. Display
   c. Process
   d. Manipulation

4. Which of the computer programs is used to support determinations, judgments and courses of action in an organization?
   a. Transaction processing system
   b. Management information system
   c. Decision support system
   d. Manipulation support system

5. Which of the following is a web portal where the patient can log into his personal account to access his healthcare data?
   a. Patient health information system
   b. Provider health information system
   c. Cloud-based health information system
   d. Master patient index

6. Which of the following links individual files across various databases?
   a. Telehealth
   b. Master patient index
   c. Electronic health record
   d. Remote patient monitoring

7. Which of the following is a limitation of health informatics?
   a. Maintains data confidentiality
   b. Empowers patients
   c. Cyber security risks
   d. Maintains data privacy

8. Which of the following is a raw or unorganized form of facts?
   a. Data
   b. Information
   c. Knowledge
   d. Characteristics

9. Which of the following information can be categorized as non-clinical data?
   a. Admission details of a patient
   b. Geographical reach to health organization
   c. Patient feedback about organization
   d. Laboratory results of a patient

10. Which of the following refers to massive amount of data sets that cannot be stored, processed or analyzed using traditional tools?
    a. Big data
    b. Electronic data
    c. Biometric data
    d. Clinical data

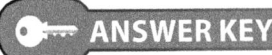

ANSWER KEY

| 1. a | 2. c | 3. a | 4. c | 5. a | 6. b | 7. c | 8. a | 9. b | 10. a |

Information System in Health Care

UNIT 3

INTRODUCTION

Information has today revolutionized every sector, making the management process swift and seamless. The healthcare sector is no exception. The field of healthcare informatics combined with healthcare data, information technology and business has gained an enormous push from technology. Health information system has been a technological boon for the health industry, making the management of healthcare data more efficient. Its implementation has helped in improving the efficiency and quality of patient care, reducing operational cost, making administration data error-free, step-up patient involvement in healthcare decision-making and provide timely access to complete and accurate information.

Hospital information system is one of the information technology tools covering all functions and operations carried out in the process of care in various wards of a hospital.

Historical Development of Health Information System

- The concept of health information system was introduced way back in the 1920s, when healthcare professionals realized that documenting patient care is important in treating patients with complete and accurate medical history. Health records were soon recognized as being critical to the safety and quality of the patient experience.
- In the 1960s, hospital information system was first introduced by some pioneering institutions most of which were academic teaching hospitals. These developed their own hospital information systems (HISs). Large hospital systems acquired mainframe computers primarily for business and administrative functions. The staff used them for managing billing and hospital inventory.
- In 1970s, lower cost and minicomputers enabled the placement of smaller, special purpose clinical application systems in various hospital departments.
- The advancing technology of the 1960s and 70s introduced the beginning of a new system. The development of computers encouraged the use of computers in maintenance of medical records.
- In 1980s, widespread availability of local area networks fostered the development of large Health Information Systems (HISs) with advanced database management capabilities and large mini- and microcomputers being linked to a number of clinical workstations and bedside terminals. During this period there was a shift from paper-based recording system to computer-based recording system.
- The 1980s saw massive developments in healthcare software development.

Introduction of computerized registration suggested that the patients were now benefitted from a more efficient electronic check-in process for the first time ever. These breakthroughs encouraged the software developers to focus on individual hospital departments. With the laboratories being well adapted to the new software, computer healthcare applications began finding a place in the market.

- During 1990s, commercial vendors increased their system development efforts. Interoperability became the main design requirement for HISs and electronic patient record (EPR) systems.
- 1990s–2000s—With medical Informatics becoming mandatory in most medical schools, it consolidated its position as an independent discipline. However, hospital information system continued to be implemented in some hospitals mostly for administration purposes. Notable progress was made in e-health and telemedicine research, databases, medical imaging, electronic health record (EHR) including confidentiality, data protection, standards, etc.
- A wave of medical errors and patient deaths caused by healthcare providers renewed the search for a viable EHR system in 2000. Electronic health records would allow providers to make better decisions and provide better care while reducing the incidence of medical error by improving the accuracy and clarity of medical records.
- 2000–2010—Notable progress in e-health, finding the hidden gaps and difficulties in real implementation, integration and interoperability, modest rate of user acceptance, quality assessment, clear contour of subdisciplines: bioinformatics, neuroinformatics, etc.
- Beyond 2010, open system architectures and interconnection standards hold promise for full interchange of information between multivendor HISs and Electronic Personal Record (EPR) systems and their related subsystems.

Traditionally information systems have addressed issues relating to admissions and discharge, payroll, billing, insurance, and related tasks in healthcare organizations. These systems helped healthcare organizations improve efficiency in their operations and achieve cost reduction. The role of healthcare information systems has metamorphosed with the emphasis turning to information and knowledge management. Information systems that have resulted from this shift include clinical decision support systems, knowledge management systems, communication systems, and simulation systems for use in teaching and surgery.

Health information systems have blended into medical practice mostly in the form of a laptop computer, personalized digital assistant (PDA) or any other portable device that moves with physicians or other healthcare workers. Knowledge management systems have allowed healthcare workers to incorporate evidence-based medicine into their practice of medicine.

Meaning and Definitions of Health Information System

Healthcare information system is a process whereby health data is recorded, stored, retrieved and processed for decision-making.

Health information system refers to any system that captures, stores, manages or transmits information related to the health of individual or the activities of organization that work within the health sector.

Health information systems refer to the interaction between people, process and technology to support operations, management in delivering essential information so as to improve the quality of healthcare services.

Health information system is the intersection between healthcare's business process and information systems to deliver better healthcare services.

Health information systems are interdisciplinary in nature and can be defined as acquiring, storing, distributing, and using information in a healthcare environment, and usually involving the use of information technology.

A health information system is broadly defined as a system that integrates data collection, processing, reporting, and use of information necessary for improving the effectiveness and efficiency of health services through better management at all levels of health services.
—*United Nations Development Program*

Health information system as integrated efforts to collect, process, report and use health information and knowledge to influence policy making, program action and research, are essential to the effective functioning of health systems worldwide.   —*WHO*

Human resource management information system refers to any system that captures, stores, manages or transmits information related to the health of individuals or the activities of organizations that work within the health sector. This definition besides incorporating district level routine information system and disease surveillance system also includes laboratory information system, hospital patient administration system and human resource management information system.

Key Elements of a Health Information System

- Used synonymously, the terms healthcare information systems, health information systems and hospital information systems are often used to refer to the same concept. The two main types of Health Information Systems are: 1. Electronic Medical Records (EMR) and 2. Clinical Decision Support (CDS).
  - Electronic medical records allow healthcare providers to track patient's health over time, scan through inputs from other consulting physicians or recall their own clinical assessment from a previous hospital visit.
  - Clinical decision support provides timely reminders and suggestions to medical practitioners. It may recommend screening tests based on patient's age and medical conditions and drug allergy information.
- Electronic medical records and clinical decision support systems together form the backbone of the hospital information system.
- A well-functioning HIS is an integrated effort to collect, process, report and use health information to influence policy and program decision-making.
- At a policy level, decisions informed by evidence contribute to more efficient use of resources while at the delivery level they provide information about the quality and effectiveness of services.

Components of a Health Information System

Following are the components of health information system (**Fig. 3.1**):
- **Resources:** HIS resources include financial and human resources, infrastructure, policies and coordination.
- **Indicators:** A core set of indicators are needed to assess changes in three major

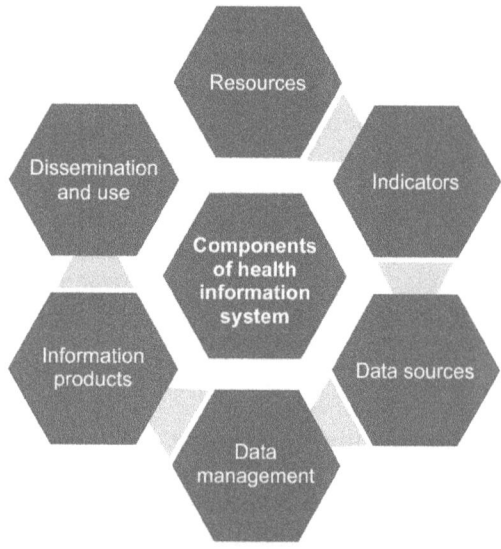

Fig. 3.1: Components of health information system

domains: determinants of health, health system and health status.
- **Data sources:** It includes health information data sources which can either be population-based or institutional-based.
- **Data management:** It refers to data storage, safeguarding data quality and data processing.
- **Information products:** Involves transforming data into information.
- **Dissemination and use:** Refers to use of information for decision-making, institutionalizing information use and demand.

A well-functioning HIS should
- Generate and compile information from service delivery points to district level routine information systems, disease surveillance systems, laboratory/procurement information systems, hospital patient administration systems and human resource management information systems.
- Detects events that threaten public health security.
- Analyzes, synthesizes and communicates information for use in planning and implementation.

Application Fields of HIS
- Patient management (patient record, scheduling of appointments, emergency care, inpatient and outpatient care information);
- Clinical management (medical reports, electronic prescription, surgery appointments)
- Diagnostics and treatment (lab reports)
- Supplies management (storeroom, ordering of supplies, pharmacy, current assets)
- Financial management (accounts payable and receivable, banking control)
- Support services (hospital infection control, asset maintenance, vaccine control)
- Research and education (library, convention center scheduling, recruiting and personnel)

Need for HIS
- Sharing information about health gives a clear picture of health and illness across populations. This knowledge can help in the prevention of spread of disease and improve health outcomes.
- Information is essential for health system policy development and implementation, governance and regulation, health research, human resources development, health education and training, service delivery and financing.
- Good governance of a health system requires reliable and timely information. For example, decision makers need to know where the resources are being deployed and whether people are getting the desired services.
- An effective and integrated health information system is the foundation for a strong health system and the key to making effective evidence-based health policy decision.
- Without health information systems sound decisions cannot be made.
- Information is used in a wide range of situations which may range from developing national strategies and plans to monitoring progress against national priorities and ensuring accountability for results.
- The role of Health Information System is to ensure the production, analysis, dissemination and use of reliable and timely data by decision-makers at all levels of the health system. The HIS is therefore reliant on the quality of data collected. Having quality and up-to-date data is necessary for agencies to respond quickly to public health crises.
- Information is important to understand the progress pertaining to health of populations, performance and quality of healthcare systems.

Benefits of Health Information System
A health information system enables healthcare organizations to collect, store, manage,

analyze and optimize patient treatment histories and other important data. Healthcare administrators, doctors and nurses who access patient and population health data can make crucial decisions about patient care. Some of the benefits of health information system are presented in **Figure 3.2**:

- **Organized and coordinated treatment process:** Health information system shares protected health information between organizations in a hassle-free manner. This process enables the patient to get continuous and coordinated treatment from healthcare providers. This form of treatment is more required for patients whose diagnoses need cross-specialty treatment. It improves the delivery of care and patient outcome. It also provides meaningful information on the health status of the community and ensures accountability.
- **Improved patient safety:** Through HIS, patient data can be saved and shared across multiple databases to improve patient safety. HIS provides alert notification every time an issue relating to patient health arises. For example, healthcare providers receive a program alert about the harmful effects the patient may experience due to the intake of an unprescribed medicine. This allows healthcare providers to avoid committing serious mistakes.
- **Better patient care:** Healthcare information promotes excellence in care. Patient care can be improved by collecting and saving patient information which may include diagnosis reports, medical history, allergy reactions, vaccinations, treatment plans, medications, lab investigation reports, etc. HIS provides a complete and orderly framework to healthcare providers thereby helping them to communicate effectively with their patients and provide quality care.
- **Hassle-free process of performance analysis:** HIS allows administrators to access staff performance, analyze patient care and monitor the efficiency of the organization. HIS computerizes every record thereby limiting paper work. It also allows patients to review the level of care being received from healthcare providers and in doing so analyze the effectiveness of the organization.
- **Transfiguration in clinical procedures:** With HIS, administrators can view patient flow and each patient experience. Careful attention to this helps administrators to describe the type of people using a service and the type of services being mostly utilized. It also identifies the areas where change is required for improving quality care.

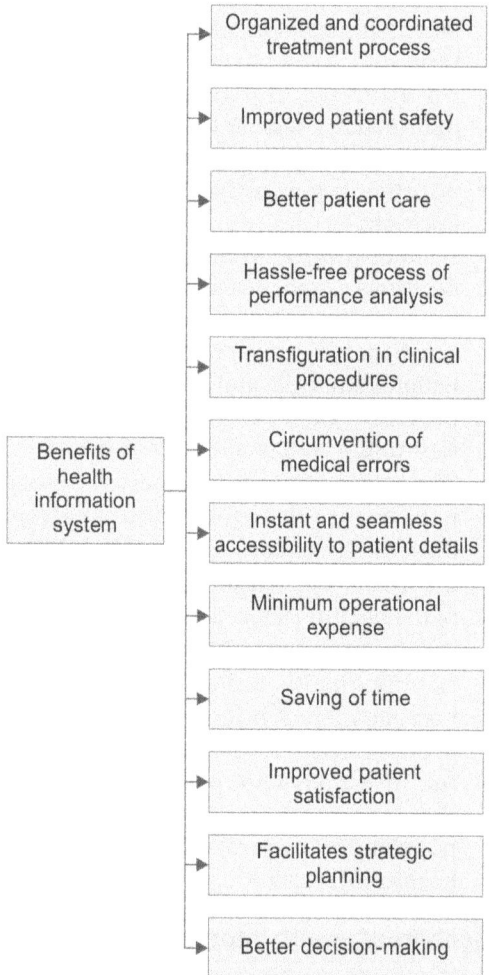

Fig. 3.2: Benefits of health information system

- **Circumvention of medical errors:** HIS computerizes and automates all data thereby ensuring error-free reports and sharing of information with the patient. This reduces medication errors and ensures patient safety.
- **Instant and seamless accessibility to patient details:** HIS collects patient data from various sources, analyses and ensures quality. It also converts data into information for health-related decision-making. The more reliable the information is, better is the chance to make any decision, implement any policy, execute any regulation, conduct health research, training and development programs and have a check on service delivery.
- **Minimized operational expense:** HIS enables health organizations to assign resources in a planned manner and save potentially huge expenses and resources.
- **Saving of time:** By computerizing and automating all patient information, HIS saves a significant amount of time thus making patient care coordinated and hospital management seamless.
- **Improved patient satisfaction:** HIS improves the satisfaction level of the patients thereby making them rely on the service.
- **Facilitates strategic planning:** HIS is the core building block of a health system. Healthcare information is used in strategic planning and priority setting as well as within clinical diagnosis and management, quality assurance and improvement.
- **Better decision-making:** A core value of the health information system is that better health information will lead to better decision-making and as such better health. Through HIS, problems can be identified, progress tracked and impact of interventions evaluated. This helps in implementing evidence-based decisions.

Essentials of Health Information Systems

To realize the benefits of information system, the organization must have proper technological infrastructure in place. It includes both fundamental software and hardware requirements.

Effective implementation of health information system requires:
- All associated devices to be connected over a secure wireless network enabling information to be accessed and shared from anywhere within the organization.
- Convenient workstations from which providers, nurses, technicians and administrators can access records. These may include desktops, laptops and tablets.
- Comprehensive employee training for best practices to maintain network security and ensuring patient privacy.
- Data encryption and backup, both of which can help safeguard data from cyber attacks, hackers or system failures.
- Cyber insurance, which can protect the organization from legal liability in the event that patient data is compromised.

ARCHITECTURE OF INFORMATION SYSTEM IN MODERN HEALTHCARE ENVIRONMENT

The success of an information system depends on a clear strategy, proper design and implementation of the system. For this purpose, the health system in addition to having a technological structure and hardware software support must meet the needs and expectations of the system users. Successful implementation of information system leads to efficient and effective organizational processes and work procedures at the individual level.

Meaning of Information System Architecture (ISA)

ISA refers to the business processes and policies, system structure, technical structure and product technologies required for an information system.

The architecture comprises a detailed description of design, content, list of current hardware, software and network capabilities of the computerized system.

Architecture is a blueprint depicting how the data processing system, telecommunication networks and data are incorporated.

Components of Information System

There are five components of an information system **(Fig. 3.3)**:
1. **Hardware resources:** It refers to the physical aspects of a computer used in processing of information. These include:
   a. *Computer peripherals:* These devices are used to input the data, store the data and provide the output in a computer. It includes keyboard (for data input), printer (for output information) and magnetic tapes (for storing information).
   b. *Computer systems:* It comprises a central processing unit containing microprocessors and numerous interconnected peripheral devices.
2. **People resources:** People play a crucial role in effective operation of all information systems. They range from information system specialists to end users or clients, data resources, software resources, network resources.
3. **Data resources:** These are valuable resources that must be managed effectively to benefit an organization. These are organized, stored and accessed by data resource management technologies in the form of knowledge base and database. Knowledge base comprises knowledge in various forms such as facts and rules. Database contains processed and organized data.
4. **Software resources:** Software is a generic term used to refer to applications, scripts and programs that run on a device. It is a set of instructions, programs or procedures for operating a computer and executing specific tasks. Instructions used to direct and control the computer hardware are known as programs and the instructions used to process data are known as procedures.
5. **Network resources:** E-business operations of an organization will succeed only if telecommunication technologies and network are in place. These include network infrastructure and communication media. Network infrastructure refers to the hardware, software and data technologies used to support and control the organization network. Example, modems, Internet work processors and communication control software. Communication media are used to deliver and receive information or data. Example, twisted pair wire, coaxial and fibre-optic cable, microwave cellular and satellite wireless technologies.

Classification of Information System Architecture

- **Client-server architecture:** The client server software architecture is a flexible, message based and modular infrastructure. It aims to improve usability, interoperability, flexibility and scalability. Components of this architecture include: client, requesting machine and server. These are connected to each other by a local area network (LAN) or a wide area network (WAN). The server notes the client query, processes the query and returns the result to the client. The client decodes the user request into specific protocols to enable processing, tackle the user interface, present the result to the user, wait for the server to respond, send the request to the server and convert the response into a readable format **(Fig. 3.4)**.

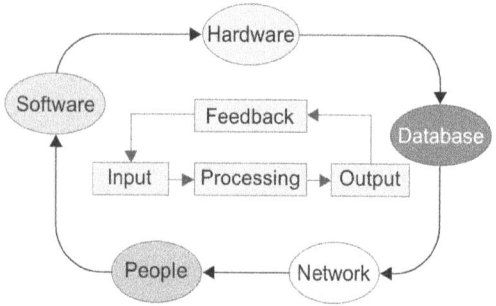

Fig. 3.3: Components of information system

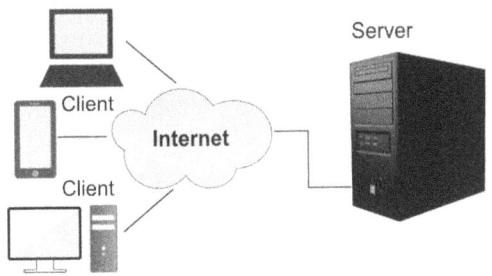

Fig. 3.4: Client server architecture

- **Mainframe architecture:** In a mainframe, the terminal accepts the query from its users but does not validate it. This type of architecture is not in vogue now.
- **Distributed system:** A distributed system comprises a collection of independent computers which are connected by a network and distributed by operation system software. This enables the computers to co-ordinate their activities and share the system resources.
- **Web-based architecture:** It is an extension of the client/server architecture. In the web-based application, the client machines have web browsers which are networked to a web browser by LAN or WAN.
- **Cloud architecture:** The cloud computing architecture refers to the structure of the system which includes on premise and cloud resources, services, middle ware and software components with their geo-location externally visible properties and their inter-relationships. In cloud computing, the right protection is dependent on the correct architecture of the corresponding application.
- **Grid architecture:** Grid architecture refers to sharing of resources in a distributed environment in a particular design. The resource layers comprise computers, storage system, electronic data catalogues, sensors and telescopes connected to the network. Each layer has a specific function with higher layer being user-centric and lower layers being hardware centric. Network is the lowest layer which connects the grid resources. The middle ware layer supplies the tools that facilitate participation of different elements in a grid-like server, storage, network, etc. It is referred to as the brain of the computing grid. The application layer is the highest layer of a grid comprising application in science, engineering, business, finance, etc., and also portals and development tool-kits to support applications.

Hospital Information Systems

The term hospital information system refers to that component of health informatics which focuses largely on administrative, financial and clinical needs of hospitals. It is designed to manage patients and their related information in a centralized way via electronic data processing and predict health status within the hospital environment.

Meaning of Hospital Information System

This is a centralized system that digitally manages the administrative, financial and clinical data of a hospital.

HIS is a comprehensive, integrated information system intended to manage all the aspects of hospital operations such as medical, administrative, financial and legal issues.

The term hospital information system (HIS) encompasses both patient care and patient management systems which support healthcare delivery and financial and resource management systems. It also supports the business and strategic operations of a hospital.

Mode of Functioning

The hospital information system plays an important role in simplifying the workflow of hospitals by digitizing the entire operations of a hospital. The two main parts are: clinical modules and administrative modules (Fig. 3.5).

The clinical module of this system is patient-centric. It deals with patient appointments, registrations, billing, medicines, treatments and surgeries. The clinical part relieves tasks

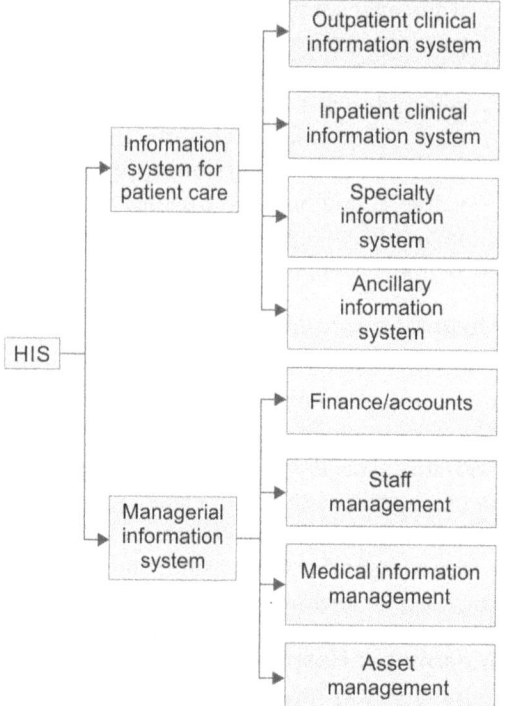

Fig. 3.5: Parts of hospital information system

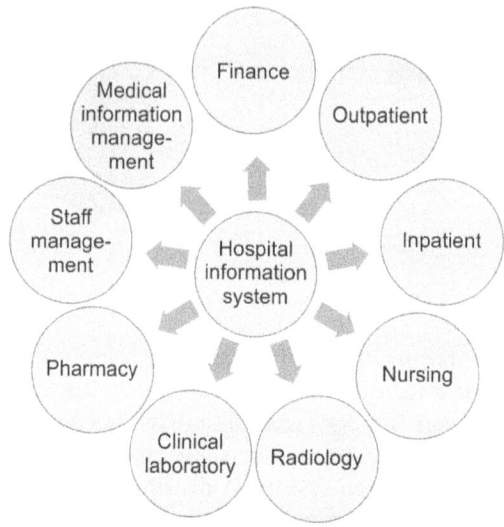

Fig. 3.6: Hospital information system

of a consultant thereby allowing him to spend more time with the patients and consult more patients as well.

The administrative module of a hospital information system handles the back office information which includes accounts, stores, asset management, human resource management, corporate billing, insurance billing and so on. It allows the hospital management to keep track of the revenue, outstanding payments, purchases and stocks.

The hospital information system software helps in controlling financial, inpatient, nursing, radiology, clinical laboratory, outpatient, pharmaceuticals and pathology data (**Fig. 3.6**).

The hospital information system operates online and covers the relevant hospital network through the intranet.

The success of a hospital information system lies mainly on it being user-friendly. It is possible only if the system development team consists of healthcare professionals, a company in the healthcare domain, has close connection with every type of staff in a hospital so that they can understand their ability.

A hospital information system is successful only if it is user-friendly and has a team of healthcare professionals having good rapport with the hospital staff. It enables them to realize the abilities and strengths of each hospital staff.

Elements of Hospital Information System

The primary use of hospital information management system is to manage and take care of healthcare management. The following elements enable it to function perfectly (**Fig. 3.7**).

- **Core systems:** This is concerned with the operational requirements for the running of day-to-day tasks.
- **Financial systems:** This addresses information system for patient care, managerial information system to include hardware and software requirements.
- **Communication/networking systems:** This is concerned with decisions regarding hospital management, short- and long-term decisions about patient care and disaster recovery.

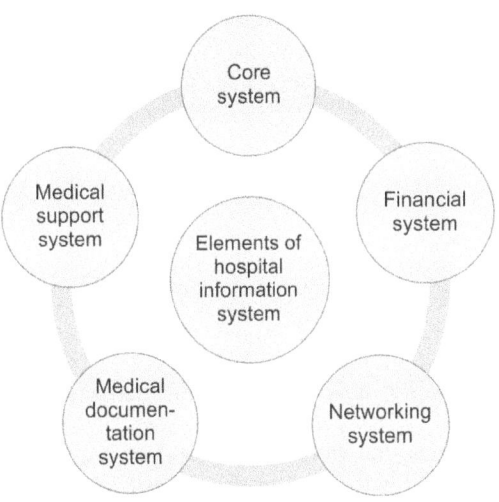

Fig. 3.7: Elements of HIS

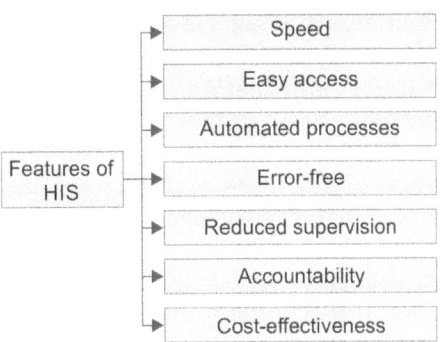

Fig. 3.8: Features of HIS

- **Medical documentation systems:** This addresses the maintenance of records, accreditation and legal records.
- **Medical support systems:** This addresses clinical and medical patient care activities in the hospital.

Features of HIS

The key features of HIS are presented in **Figure 3.8**.

- **Speed:** It is one of the important features of HIS. Communication between various interlinked departments, reporting of laboratory tests, emergency and non-emergency communications are speeded up because of the HIS.
- **Easy access:** Hospitals generate a lot of data which needs to be stored and managed. It is necessary to share it among various departments for taking crucial decisions. The quick and easy access feature of HIS enables correct decision-making and better quality of care.
- **Automated processes:** Once coded and implemented the HIS is practically automated. Picking the name of the service, test or drug will automatically fetch the rate and bill it to the selected patient ID. Also it does not face fatigue issues as in humans.
- **Error free:** After the initial implementation of HIS, the processes run on their own with minimum mandatory inputs from employees. This ensures minimum errors that too owing to human errors.
- **Reduced supervision:** Minimum supervision is required as each task is coded to be performed in a certain manner based on the employee input.
- **Accountability:** As every employee working on HIS is provided an individual login with access controls, accountability is automatically fixed which otherwise is not possible in a manual process.
- **Cost-effective:** HIS implementation requires minimum stationary and storage space thereby freeing up manpower for other important activities. This makes HIS cost-effective and operationally efficient thereby improving hospital revenues.

CLINICAL INFORMATION SYSTEMS

Medical care is nowadays being provided in multiple settings and at multiple locations, thus creating a need for clinicians to combine the available clinical data and share it so as to provide a holistic picture of the individual patient.

Meaning of Clinical Information System

A clinical information system (CIS) is one that is designed specifically for use in a critical care environment. It can network with other computer systems in a hospital and draw information from them into an electronic patient record, which clinicians can view at patient bedside.

Clinical information system (CIS) is a computer-based system meant to gather, store and alter clinical data on patients. These systems may be used at single locations or across the entire healthcare system.

Clinical information systems (CISs) are part of hospital information systems that provide instant access to current patient data as regards medical history, clinical notes, treatment, laboratory reports and images either directly or via data networks facilitating direct patient care.

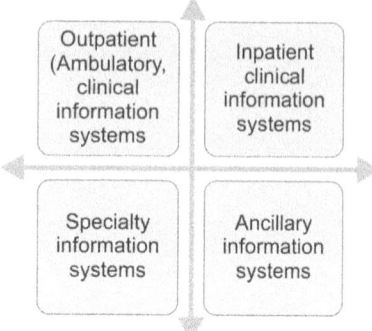

Fig. 3.9: Areas of clinical information system

Infrastructure and Information Flows of Clinical Information System

A CIS consists of a wide range of networking technology, clinical databases, electronic medical records, clinical informatics research evidence systems. Major role of CISs is to capture, store, process, and transfer information to clinical decision-makers on time for arriving at a correct and rapid decision. For example, a CIS can import data from instruments such as vital signs monitors, ventilators, and infusion devices, store them safely, and display them in specific tables and formats easily.

Information from various CISs is entered into an electronic health record which is then networked to different databases as per requirement. Clinical information from EHRs and other systems is then exchanged for effective treatment and decision-making. CIS interconnects with other subsystems in the hospital such as pharmacy, laboratories, radiology, and image processing storage solutions.

Major Areas of Clinical Information System

Clinical information systems provide a clinical data repository that stores patient clinical data and their interactions with care providers. The repository encodes information capable of helping physicians decide about the patient's condition, treatment options and wellness activities besides the status of decisions, actions undertaken and other relevant information that could be helpful in performing those actions. Major areas of clinical information system are presented in Figure 3.9.

- **Outpatient clinical information system:** It has two components: clinical administration and OPD healthcare delivery. Clinical administration includes registration, follow-up visits and billing functions. OPD healthcare delivery system includes OPD electronic medical record which is tailored for OPD visits. OPD starts with initial registration, goes through physician visit, lab investigations and ends up with minor procedures or medication prescription.
- **Inpatient clinical information system:** Inpatient clinical information system is much more complex and intense and a combination of various workflows. Inpatient visit begins with admission, goes through treatment and procedures and ends up with discharge. Once the patient is admitted, an initial assessment is carried out by the doctors and nurses, the physician advises lab investigations and medications or referred to specialists. After the results and referrals, a reassessment is done which may result in new medication or additional tests being ordered. The inpatient clinical workflows are:
  - *Clinical documentation:* It includes progress notes, nurses' notes, TPR charts, medication charts, laboratory

reports, diet sheets and other support staff documentation.
- *Computerized provider order entry (CPOE):* They allow a physician to communicate electronically with various departments. It also handles other orders like IV drips with rate of administration, dietary orders, physiotherapy orders, etc. This system alerts the physicians on potential drug-drug or drug allergy interactions. It reduces prescribing errors and significant toxicities at clinically prescribed doses.
- *Electronic medication administration record:* It helps to reconcile administration of medication.
- *Care plan:* Nursing care plan functions for planning of patient care, communicating patient care needs among the nursing and support teams, document changes in patient's condition and his response to treatment.
- *Work lists:* These are a list of tasks and interventions for each patient generated to provide suitable instructions for nursing and supporting staff.
- *Order sets, clinical protocols and templates:* Setting up of templates and order sets for standardized clinical protocols in the inpatient area. For example, protocol for myocardial infarction. This facilitates implementing of standard evidence-based guidelines for best practice across the healthcare organization.
- *Alerts and clinical decision supports:* These help in checking for errors and making correct clinical decisions like dose adjustments for renal insufficiency. These features are very important for the inpatient EMR as they lead to significant reduction in medication and other errors thereby improving patient safety.
- **Specialty information systems:** These are clinical information systems that cater to specialty departments with unique workflows that cannot be configured into a general EMR system. Example, emergency department information systems, ICU information systems, OT information systems.
  - *Emergency department information systems (EDIS):* It is a highly dynamic, high movement and quick turnover area. The visiting patients may include those with minor ailments to those who are critically sick. The EDIS allows registration of patients with minimal data entry mostly using quick fill templates on a touch screen for the purpose of clinical documentation and ordering of investigations and medications which is simultaneously integrated with inpatient systems.
  - *Intensive care unit information system (ICUISs):* It is a high care arena with critically ill patients requiring intensive level of care. Vital signs and other critical parameters are monitored constantly with the help of bedside monitors and devices. An ICUIS should thus be able to provide protocol templates and flow sheets, have automatic capture of physiologic parameters from monitors, graphically display trends to help in decision-making, automatically calculated dose adjustments in accordance with fast-changing parameters, etc. By providing protocol templates and flow sheets, CISs in ICU reduces the time spent on documentation. This allows the physician to spend the available time on direct patient care. They support the continuous assessment and adjustment of medication, automatic capture of physiological parameters from patient monitors, and display of patients' vital conditions.
  - *Cardiovascular information system (CVIS):* It plays a vital role in monitoring, managing, evaluating, and policy development issues related to cardiac diseases. It integrates all cardiology requests, procedures, images, and reports with other clinical information

systems allowing physicians to extract images and reports from any computer inside and outside of the hospital through a portal.

A CVIS can offer structured templates for echo, pediatrics, peripheral vascular, Cath lab, and other systems. The demand for CISs has gone up with cardiovascular picture archiving and communication systems (CPACS) that provide effective data analysis and accurate therapeutic decisions in a short period of time. Additionally, hospital information systems are integrated with CVISs for exchanging 4D echocardiography, nuclear medicine, computed tomography (CT), angiography, and pediatric echocardiography reports.

- *Oncology information system (OISs):* These systems combine radiation, medical and surgical oncology information into a complete oncology specific EMR which helps physicians to manage their patients' complete information from diagnosis through follow-up.

- **Ancillary information system:** This includes laboratory information system, pharmacy information system and radiology information system.
  - *Laboratory information system:* Through CISs, accuracy and accessibility can be fostered in lab samples at clinical laboratories. The physician can follow each step of the testing process (from administration of tests to the receipt of test results) supporting timely decision-making and diagnosis. These systems are rich sources of data that can be used for policy-making, quality projects and research.
  - *Pharmacy information system (PIS):* It supports the distribution and management of drugs, and maintaining drug and medical device inventory. PIS manages inpatient and outpatient dispensing of order entry drugs. It allows the pharmacist to identify the physician's order; validate the medication based on drug-to-drug interactions and timing of medications and then dispense the drug for administration. It plays a vital role in preventing dosage errors by providing an individual dosage limit according to patient's age, gender and other factors. The integration of CPOE and PIS has virtually eliminated the need for pharmacy staff to re-enter medication orders from the CPOE system.

Benefits of CIS

The main function of CIS is to collect, store, manage and integrate data from various sources. A good CIS contributes positively to patient safety, workflow efficiency, point-of-care decision support and management of patient data. The key benefits of CIS are presented in **Figure 3.10**.

- **Easy access to patient data:** CIS captures the data electronically and makes it potentially available to a large number of systems. Besides providing convenient and direct access to instant updates of a patient's medical records, it also provides remote access to complete information at all points of care. It is highly beneficial in OPD settings as it enhances

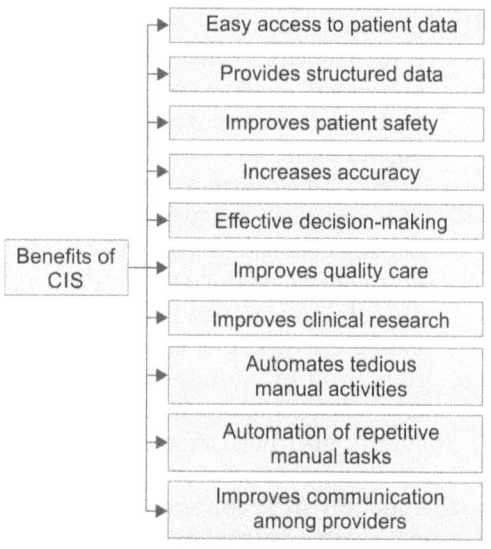

Fig. 3.10: Benefits of CIS

continuity of care. Internet-based access improves the ability to remotely access patient data in real-time and provides clinicians with x-ray and scans in a timely manner. The patient record can be accessed from geographically distant workstations in the ICU, hospital and even from other remote sites. As long as the system is live, the record is easy to locate and always available.

- **Provides structured data:** The clinical information captured in CISs is well organized, making it easier to maintain and explore for relevant information. The information is also legible making it less likely for mistakes to happen due to illegible writing. CIS improves data quality and the analysis of patient's data by combining it with the physician's own knowledge.
- **Improves patient safety:** The built-in error checking and knowledge-based methods result in improved patient safety. CIS alerts physicians on potential drug–drug or drug–allergy interactions. It reduces prescribing errors and significant toxicities at clinically prescribed doses. It plays a vital role in preventing dosage errors by providing an individual dosage limit according to patient's age, gender and other factors leading to reduction of adverse drug interactions while promoting more appropriate pharmaceutical utilization. Development of better and more effective security protocols can lead to reduced human error and increased patient safety.
- **Increases accuracy:** Greater precision is achieved due to reduction in human errors, availability of traceable records from multiple sites simultaneously and connection with other bedside equipment and information systems. The CIS automates the process of electronic data collection from monitors, ventilators, infusion pumps, dialysis/filtration equipment, cardiac-assist devices and other bedside devices and provides a real-time spreadsheet with arithmetic accuracy.
- **Provides information for effective decision-making:** Healthcare providers can have access to all information and services at a single point of contact. CIS provides users with the tools to acquire, manipulate, apply and display appropriate information to aid in the making of correct, timely and evidence-based clinical decisions. It improves clinical decision-making during patient encounters and provides universal access to patient information in real time.
- **Improves quality care:** Errors in prescription and administration are a leading cause of adverse events with associated morbidity. A major contribution of CIS to clinical safety and quality is through the provision of an electronic prescription and administration record for drugs and fluids. Incorporation of clinical documentation and progress notes provides a legible and attributable record of events thus contributing to clinical safety and quality. An effective CIS warrants cost reduction, workflow improvement and standardization of procedures. It has a huge potential to reduce medical errors, increase legibility, cut unnecessary healthcare costs and boost the quality of healthcare. Test turnaround times are faster for providing quicker diagnosis.
- **Improves clinical research:** Patient information can be made available to physicians for the purpose of training and research. Data mining of the information stored in databases could provide insights into disease states and help to manage patient problems.
- **Automates of tedious manual activities:** CIS captures the data electronically and makes it available to a wide range of systems. This practically eliminates the need for manual data input or transcription.
- **Automation of repetitive manual tasks:** CIS improves accuracy through reduction in human error, availability of attributable records simultaneously from multiple points of care and integration with other

bedside equipment and information systems. This obviates the need for repetitive manual data entry or transcription while making the data accessible for a range of purposes that may include clinical, business and research reporting.
- **Improves communication among providers:** In intensive care units, CIS can communicate with the computer systems across the hospital. It consolidates data from all the available systems into an electronic patient record that physicians may access at the patient's bedside. It therefore improves communication among various healthcare providers.

Barriers of CIS

Despite its benefits, CIS can present the following barriers **(Fig. 3.11)**:
- **High cost of acquisition:** High basic infrastructure costs of clinical information technology vis-à-vis low perceived return on investment can be a stumbling block for many healthcare organizations.
- **Privacy and security concerns:** There are still great many concerns in the healthcare industry about the privacy of patient data on a computer system and how to keep such information secure.
- **Clinician resistance:** Clinicians normally have very limited time to interact with their patients. If their interactions with a CIS during these sessions prove to be more time-consuming than necessary, there is bound to be some resistance for its use.
- **Integration of legacy system:** It poses a stiff challenge to many organizations.
- **Lack of technology:** Most of the healthcare institutions lack the basic technology.

An efficient, cost-effective and reliable system is therefore needed to strengthen the hospital information system.

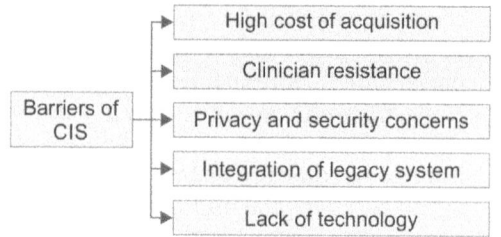

Fig. 3.11: Barriers of CIS

REVIEW QUESTIONS

Long Essays   (10 Marks)
1. Write the meaning of health information system. List the elements and components of health information system.
2. Describe in detail on application fields and benefits of health information system.
3. Describe in detail on major areas of clinical information system.
4. Explain benefits and barriers of clinical information system.
5. Explain parts of hospital information system.
6. Explain elements of hospital information system.
7. Describe features of hospital information system.

Short Essays   (5 Marks)
1. Essentials of Health Information System.
2. Components of information system.
3. Classification of information system architecture.

Short Answers   (2 Marks)
1. Meaning of hospital information system.
2. Meaning of information system architecture.
3. Meaning of clinical information system.

MULTIPLE CHOICE QUESTIONS

1. Which of the following information systems provides timely reminders and suggestions to medical practitioners?
   a. Electronic medical record system
   b. Clinical decision support system
   c. Information system architecture
   d. Client server architecture

2. Which of the following HIS improves patient safety?
   a. Alert notification
   b. Hassle-free process
   c. Circumvention of medical errors
   d. All of the above

3. Which of the following is an essential of the health information system?
   a. Collection of patient information
   b. A secure wireless network
   c. Legal issues
   d. Cyber attacks

4. A detailed description of design, contents, list of current hardware and software network capabilities of a computer system is called as
   a. Hospital information system
   b. Information system architecture
   c. Information system network
   d. Information system components

5. Which of the following is a hardware resource?
   a. Central processing unit
   b. Network infrastructure
   c. Communication media
   d. Data resources

6. In which of the following areas is a clinical information system widely used?
   a. Intensive care units
   b. Rehabilitation units
   c. Community health units
   d. Hospital reception units

7. Which of the following is a major barrier in implementing CIS in India?
   a. Legal issues
   b. Lack of trained technicians
   c. High cost of acquisition
   d. Less number of hospitals

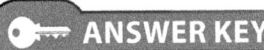

ANSWER KEY

1. b   2. d   3. b   4. b   5. a   6. a   7. c

Shared Care and Electronic Health Records

UNIT 4

INTRODUCTION

Worldwide focus is recently on improving quality health care, cost containment and enhanced patient experience. This has ushered the way to development of improved tools and methods for maintaining patient data in digital form. The Electronic Health Record (EHR) is one such solution to support the healthcare facility. It would not only reduce medical errors but also reduce clinician workload significantly and serve as a major cost cutting measure for the organization.

Meaning and Definition of Electronic Medical Record and Electronic Health Record

The EHR is an electronic version of a patient's wellness history. It is a digital record of health information. It contains past medical history, vital signs, progress notes, diagnoses, medications, immunization dates, allergies, lab data and imaging reports. It also contains other relevant information, such as insurance information, demographic data and data from personal wellness devices. It includes information from all the clinicians involved in patient's care. All authorized clinicians involved in a patient's care can access the information to provide care to that patient and share information with other healthcare providers such as laboratories and specialists. EHRs follow patients to their specialist, hospital, nursing home or even across the country. It automates access to information and has the potential to streamline the clinician's workflow with an ability to support other care-related activities directly or indirectly through various interfaces including evidence-based decision support, quality management and outcome reporting.

An electronic medical record (EMR) is a digital version of a patient's chart in clinician offices or hospital. These are online medical records of the standard medical and clinical data from one provider's office. It contains patient's medical history, diagnoses and treatment by a particular physician, nurse practitioner, specialist, dentist or surgeon. It works well within a practice as they don't have to travel outside the practice. These are used by providers for diagnosis and treatment. Comprehensive and accurate documentation of patient's medical history, tests, diagnosis and treatment in EMRs ensures appropriate care throughout the hospital or clinic. It allows effective communication and coordination among healthcare members for comprehensive care.

- **Departmental EMR:** It contains patient medical information recorded by a single hospital department (e.g. radiology, pathology, pharmacy).
- **Inter-departmental EMR:** It contains patient medical information recorded by two or more hospital departments.

- **Hospital EMR:** It contains patient clinical information from a single hospital.
- **Inter-hospital EMR:** It contains patient medical information recorded by two or more hospitals.

Electronic Health Record refers to information in electronic form containing the past, present and future health status or healthcare provided to subject of care.
—*Katehakis and Tsiknakis, 2006*

Electronic Health Record is a warehouse of information containing health information of a subject in computer readable form, stored, transmitted securely and accessed by authorized users. —*International Organization for Standardization, 2005*

Electronic Health Record is a central database used by various individuals and organizations to record patient information. It contains clinical data and wellness data as well.
—*Knaup et al, 2007*

Electronic medical record is an electronic record of health-related information on an individual that can be created, gathered, managed and consulted by authorized clinicians and staff within one health care organization.

Difference between Electronic Medical Record and Electronic Health Record

The terms 'electronic medical record' and 'electronic health record' though used interchangeably, the difference between the two terms is quite significant. The term EMR came along first and was mostly used to refer to 'medical'. They were used by clinicians mostly for diagnosis and treatment. Alternately, 'health' refers to 'the condition of being sound in body, mind or spirit; freedom from physical disease or pain'. As the word 'health' has a more extensive meaning than the word 'medical', EHRs also go a lot further than EMRs.

An EMR is a digital record of medical information while an EHR is a digital record of health information. Both are shared care records. Shared care record is a collection of patient information stored in one area that care providers both contribute to and have access to thereby giving a full picture of those in their care. Differences between EHR and EMR are presented in **Table 4.1**.

Trends in EHRs

Having evolved during the past several years, medical records are an essential feature of

Table 4.1: Differences between electronic medical record and electronic health record

Electronic medical record (EMR)	Electronic health record (EHR)
It is a digital version of patient medical and treatment history	It is a digital record of patient health information regarding wellness, health and health care of an individual
It is a narrower view of a patient's medical history	It is a broader view of a patient's overall health
It is generated and maintained within an institution such as a hospital, integrated delivery network, clinic, or physician office	It is a longitudinal collection of health information from all sources
Designed to be shared outside individual practice	Designed to be shared with other providers and labs for updating information
Patient record does not easily travel outside the practice	Allows a patient's medical information to move outside the practice with other healthcare providers and specialists
Mainly used by providers for diagnosis and treatment	Accessed by a number of providers for decision-making, diagnosis and care beyond one provider's office
Primary purpose is to improve the quality of patient care and patient safety	Primary purpose is to support an effective and life-long, high-quality safe integrated health care

any hospital care organization. The recent innovations in healthcare information technology have transformed the way health information is recorded. In 1920s, all medical records were kept manually using a paper-based system. Patient visit details, their history, diagnosis, lab results, medication, etc., were recorded on paper and stored in a medical record room. The last decade of healthcare reform led by advancement in technology and use of computers has revolutionalized the way patient medical information is recorded and organized electronically. The electronic way of recording patient health information has developed progressively in recent years. The trends in electronic health records are described below.

From paper-based system to computer-based system: In the past, medical records were stored in a paper-based format, allowed to be viewed only by limited personnel in the health organization. This paper-based record had limitations in terms of accessibility and availability as its movement was restricted by locked doors, access cards and sign-in and sign-out procedures and allowed to be used only by one user at a time. Record completion was delayed as it was updated manually. The physician was in control of care and documentation processes and authorized the release of information. Patients rarely viewed their medical records. Neither did unauthorized access to patient information trigger any alerts nor was it known if any information was viewed by unauthorized personnel. The electronic system has today replaced the paper-based records. It has the ability to process more data and store it through the use of modern information technologies to yield better knowledge. The future of healthcare information system looks towards a near 'paperless' era.

From local to global information systems: While earlier healthcare information systems were limited to departmental units (e.g., radiology or laboratory) or just within a healthcare practice system (e.g. a hospital or a clinic) modern healthcare systems target regional, national and even a global reach.

From healthcare professionals to patients and consumers: Originally, healthcare information systems were designed to be used mainly by physicians and administrative staff but were later passed on to be used by nurses. Since then, the trend has shifted to involve more patient input.

From using data for patient care to research: Over the years, patient data has been used beyond patient care management to a more general use involving research in healthcare and even education.

From technical to strategic information management orientation: Previously, computer-supported information systems focused on problems resulting from the technical aspects of the systems, concerns about the organizational problems and social issues. However, at the turn of the millennium, the management aspects have become more relevant.

From numeric data to more complex forms of data: Not only has the technology that supports health information systems advanced in technological complexity, the data that is being received and processed has also become complex, from numeric data through alphanumeric data to imaging and even molecular data.

Trends of the decade: The main trends of 2010–2020 include Big data approach; cloud computing; social networks on health; certification of educational programs in medical informatics; full interoperability—communication, semantic interoperability; integration of molecular and genetic Health Information Systems, deployment of home monitoring systems and tele-assistance; deeper penetration of IT tools in medical research (modeling and simulation, digital patient, etc); advanced decision support systems.

Key Factors to Support Electronic Medical Records

In 2003, the institute of medicine issued 8 key functions to support EMRs:
1. Physician access to patient information such as diagnoses, allergies, lab results and medications
2. Access to new and past test results among providers in multiple care settings
3. Computerized provider order entry
4. Computerized decision-support systems to prevent drug interactions and improve compliance with best practices
5. Secure electronic communication among providers and patients
6. Patient access to health records, disease management tools and health information resources
7. Computerized administration processes, such as scheduling systems
8. Standards-based electronic data storage and reporting for patient safety and disease surveillance efforts.

Benefits of Using Electronic Records in Health Care

Both EHRs and EMRs offer benefits to patients and healthcare providers. Electronic records are expected to make healthcare more efficient and affordable, making a good investment for nation's health care. The benefits of electronic health records can be categorized into patient benefits, practitioner benefits and organizational benefits **(Fig. 4.1)**.

Patient Benefits

From a patient's perspective, benefits of electronic records include: improved quality of care, safe and more reliable treatment, improved diagnosis and treatment, significant reduction in medical errors and patient empowerment.

- **Improved quality of care:**
  - Computerized records being easy to read, the risk of misinterpretations or errors in diagnosis and treatment are minimized.
  - It provides faster access to most recent health history and medical best practices for the purpose of reference. It provides greater support in making point of care decision.
  - It can integrate evidence-based clinical guidelines with clinical practice easily and effectively so as to improve patient safety and quality care.
  - It improves accuracy of documentation making diagnosis and claims submission easier and quicker.
  - Through automated alerts potential risks can be detected and immediate treatment initiated.
  - Timely reminders help in patient screening and preventive checkups.
- **Safe and more reliable treatment:** Improved information access makes prescribing medication safer and more reliable. More complete information means more accurate diagnoses.
- **Reduction in medical errors:** With fast, accurate and updated information medical errors are minimized and healthcare improved.
- **Patient empowerment:** EHRs improve access to patient medical information thereby promoting patient participation and healthier lifestyles with more frequent use of preventive care. It also facilitates care coordination.
- **Easy access to information:** EHR systems contain a portal which the patients can use to access their own medical records. This prevents the need for unnecessary calls or appointments to obtain information from the physician. The patient can access data electronically on his own with utmost ease.
- **Improves satisfaction:** Patient satisfaction is also enhanced with EHRs in several other ways such as easy accessibility, improvement in continuity of care and patient education material delivery.

Practitioner Benefits

Implementation of electronic records serves many benefits for both doctors and

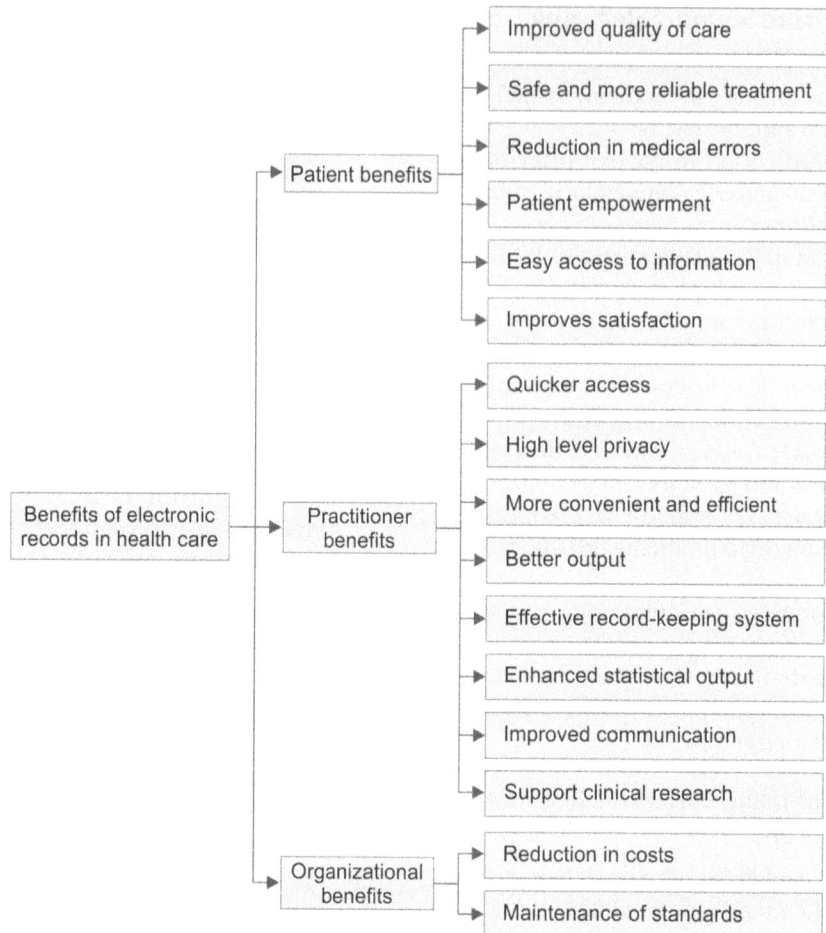

Fig. 4.1: Benefits of electronic records in health care

health practitioners: quick access, high level privacy, better output, superior record-keeping system, improved statistical output, enhanced communication and clinical research support.

- **Quicker access:** Electronic medical records software converts the information in hard copies into digital data. Computerized records can be accessed instantly with a few keystrokes. Data can also be accumulated from different sources and quickly referred to. The importance of electronic health records is that they facilitate sharing of patient data such as medical records, charts, medications and test results across multiple healthcare environments. The ability to transfer patient data at shortest possible notice between departments is a huge advantage. Through EHRs updated information can be shared real time among the healthcare team thereby resulting in faster diagnosis.
- **High-level privacy:** EMR software provides better security to patient data during the entire transaction than paper records. It converts the data into an encrypted format which can be accessed only by authorized users.
- **More convenient and efficient:** Health care and other staff no longer have to waste time sorting through cumbersome paper records. Users can access electronic health

records quickly and efficiently with just a few strokes on the keyboard.
- **Better output:** Improved access and data tracking system helps doctors to serve a greater number of patients. Workflow is smooth with lesser interruptions enabling the doctors to manage multiple patients in a single day. This results in improved workflow and productivity, better patient outcomes due to reduction in errors within medical practice.
- **Effective record-keeping system:**
  - EHR systems provide the flexibility to connect with other medical records for the purpose of reference. This allows the patients to fix appointments and locate the records easily even while switching between doctors, hospitals or even locations.
  - Instances of patient files getting misplaced or lost are eliminated. This is a positive development so far as health-related safety of patients and patient welfare are concerned.
  - Patient charts are more complete and clearer with no more decoding of illegible scribbles. Other benefits include effective reports collection, quick recording, immediate response from radiology images, etc.
  - A patient may be transferred from one hospital to another within a city or a country. The use of EHRs facilitates moving of patient records across nations or even the globe thereby allowing health professionals to take good care of the new patient.
- **Enhanced statistical output:** It provides benefits to doctors and other medical professionals by enabling compilation of data in chronological order. It authenticates the information immediately and accepts only trusted sources with doctors' approval which is not quite possible with paper charts and reports. Information can be extracted in different forms such as graphs, pie chart, tables, etc. It allows the doctors to monitor the difference in readings and patient progress during each visit. Management can assess the performance of each individual and department and use the unbiased data for internal audits.
- **Improved communication:** Electronic records improve communication of information among healthcare professionals. This helps in improved care coordination, reduction in medical errors and greater safety for patients.
- **Support clinical research:** Advanced e-prescribing, clinical documentation capabilities and an improved bottom line in healthcare practice enhance support for clinical research.

Organizational Benefits

From an organizational point of view electronic health records help in saving overhead costs, increase revenue and record positive return on investment. Hospital standards can be better maintained using electronic health records.

- **Reduction in costs:**
  - Overhead costs may be reduced by lowering administrative costs (such as chart filing, transcriptions, phone calls, photocopying charts, faxing medical information), optimum use of space and paper.
  - As patient's medical records are kept at a single location, duplicated diagnosis and testing is avoided saving both time and cost. It results in practice efficiencies and healthcare planning.
  - EHRs give strong protection and a simple interface for long hour usage.
  - Organizations can do away with costly file cabinets, folders and printing and paper costs.
  - All office medical records can be stored in an individual computer hard drive and backed up in the cloud.
  - Resource consumption can be cut down by reducing the number of paper forms and duplicate or needless lab orders.
  - Transcription services and overtime labor expenses can be reduced.

- EHRs solve logistical problems associated with the paper system and also optimize documentation of patient encounters.
- Employing coding applications facilitates easier billing besides improving reimbursement services.
- **Maintenance of standards**
  - Electronic records support health policy decisions.
  - Collect and analyze data more easily, create reports faster, explore data trends more thoroughly and effectively thereby controlling inventory.
  - Can play a crucial role in implementing telemedicine projects.

Disadvantages of EHR

Though electronic records offer many valuable benefits to patients, practitioners and organizations they are also a source for certain inconveniences and inefficiencies. Some of the disadvantages of electronic records are presented in **Figure 4.2**.

- **Potential privacy and cyber security issues:** EHRs are vulnerable to attacks by hackers. There is always a possibility of sensitive patient data falling into wrong hands.
- **Regular updation:** The instantaneous nature of electronic health records requires immediate updation after each patient visit or every time there is a modification in information. Failure to do so will make the records lose their merit and utility and also result in inaccurate data being shared among the healthcare team members.
- **Alarming patients pointlessly:** When a patient has access to his own medical information at will, it can expose him to information that he may not completely understand. The ability to access information one does not thoroughly understand could lead to a host of misunderstandings thereby creating panic and taking inappropriate actions.
- **Malpractice liability concerns:** There are several potential liability issues associated with EHR implementation. For example, medical data could get lost or destroyed during transition from a paper-based to a computerized EHR system which could lead to treatment errors. Physicians can be held liable for their inability to access medical data at their disposal.
- **Expensive and time-consuming:** Costs involved in setting up of EHRs are high. Even if new EHRs are running smoothly, it still requires a lot of time and effort to train the personnel.
- **Power outages and computer breakdown:** Power outages and computer failure can make the information inaccessible. An essential part of EHRs is the ability to have an information technology team available 24/7 to solve technical problems real time. Failure to do so will escalate patient care interruptions.

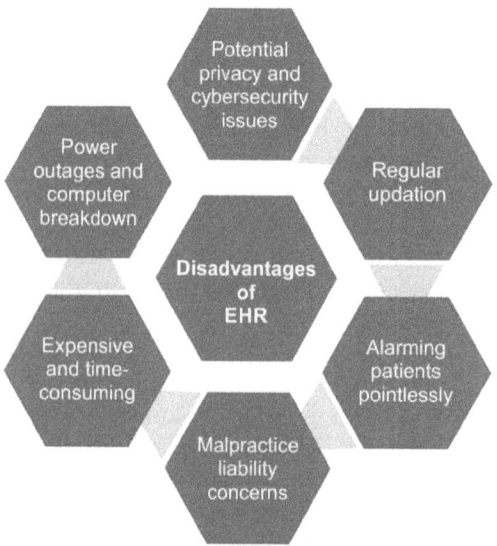

Fig. 4.2: Disadvantages of EHR

Barriers in Implementation of Electronic Records

Common barriers in implementation of electronic records are presented in **Figure 4.3**.

- **Cost constraints:** EHR implementation requires high capital costs. Many EHR systems require specific hardware and

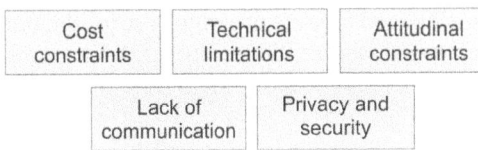

Fig. 4.3: Barriers in implementation of EHRs

networks or interfaces. It also includes staff training costs.
- **Technical limitations:** One hurdle often faced by organizations to implement EHRs is the technical limitations. Integrating present clinical system with EHR often requires pairing specific devices which are compatible with one another.
- **Attitudinal constraints and behavior of individuals:** Attitude of staff members can affect the successful implementation of EHRs. Many might be resistant to change or learning the use the EHRs. A negative mindset affects the individual's ability to gain the knowledge of a new system. Concern regarding unintended consequences of technology use can also be a barrier.
- **Lack of communication:** Effective communication is the key to successful adaptation of EHR. Lack of preparedness and improper communication with staff hinders the switch from paper to electronic records.
- **Privacy and security:** Safety and privacy concerns of protected health data are the biggest barriers in implementing electronic health records.
- **Other barriers** include lack of proper planning, unavailability of skilled resources for implementation of EHRs.

ETHICAL ISSUES IN ELECTRONIC HEALTH RECORDS

EHRs are being implemented increasingly in many developing countries to improve the quality of health care and make them cost effective. Common issues that need to be addressed in electronic medical record system are privacy, security and confidentiality.

Privacy, Security and Confidentiality

Adequate medical documentation assures patient confidentiality and ensures that standards of care are being met.

Privacy refers to the right of someone to determine for themselves when, how and the level at which accessing personal information is transferred or shared by others. It is the right of an individual to keep information about themselves from being disclosed to others. Privacy can be violated through employers, health or life insurance coverage or participation in government benefit programs.

Security is defined as the level at which accessing someone's personal information is restricted and allowed for those authorized only. Increased use of smart phone devices, exchange of data between and among organizations, clinicians, government organizations and patients may lead to unforeseen or unintentional instances of data breach. Another security thereat could be data getting hacked, manipulated or destroyed by internal or external users. Transferring or sharing sensitive health data when not authorized can also result in a data breach.

Security breaches threaten patient privacy when confidential health information is made available to others without the individual's consent or authorization.

Three basic information technology security requirements are: confidentiality, integrity and availability.
- **Confidentiality:** Information shared as a result of clinical interaction is considered confidential and must be protected. Confidentiality simply means restricting the access of information to unauthorized persons either during storage, transmitting or while being treated. It guarantees protection of information from being modified or deleted by unauthorized users or undesired modifications done by authorized users.
- **Integrity:** Integrity assures that the data is accurate and not been manipulated.

Data is collected and used across systems in the organization and the continuum of care in outpatient setting, in-patient setting, rehabilitation centers and so forth. This data can be manipulated intentionally or unintentionally as it moves between and among the system. Poor data integrity results mostly due to documentation errors, improper use of options such as cut and paste. This practice is unacceptable because it increases the risk for patients and liability for clinicians and organizations. Another feature that can effect data integrity is the drop-down menu and dispositions of relevant information in the trash. Such menus limit the choices available to the clinicians who in a hurry may choose the wrong option leading to major errors.

- **Availability:** If the system is hacked or overloaded with requests, information therein may become unusable. To ensure continuing availability, electronic health record systems often have redundant components known as fault-tolerance systems. If a component fails or experiences trouble, the system switches to the backup component automatically.

Need for Safety of Electronic Medical Records

Patient information includes identification data, diagnosis, treatment and progress notes, and laboratory results. Information can be stored on paper, video or even electronic files. Information can be released for treatment, payment or administrative purposes without patient's authorization. The patient has a legal right to view, obtain a copy of and amend information in his or her health record. Patient-related information should be released to others only with the patient's permission or be allowed by law. When a patient is unable to do so because of his underage or mental incapacity, decisions about information sharing should be made by the legal representative or legal guardian of the patient. Healthcare units have switched from paper-based records to a much more efficient electronic system. Electronic health records are interactive with many users, reviewers and stakeholders for documentation. In the current scenario safety of information is paramount as technology can introduce certain hazards into the system.

- The growth of information technology has resulted into a scenario whereby the health data of patients are affected by security and privacy threats.
- With considerable rise in both government and private transactions along with the inappropriate intrusions in the present 'Digital Age', privacy protection has entered a new dimension.
- Information present in EHRs is very sensitive and related to patient's medical history, diagnoses, treatment and follow-ups.
- Compromising health-related data of a patient may not only lead to loss of job, insurance, housing, etc., but also invite hatred and embarrassment in the society. It is thus essential to keep the information secured from being manipulated or misused.
- Patient's medical records are usually shared by several departments in the hospital like anesthesia, medicine, orthopedic, etc. This can be a major threat to patient's privacy as the data is accessed by multiple users in the system.
- The need for confidentiality in health sector is in response to privacy concerns due to the sensitive nature of patient and client data. Hence there is a need for health organizations to devise a strategy for securing electronic records.
- For the patient to trust the clinician, hospital records must be kept well protected.
- Patients wish to control the access to their medical information in EHRs just like they do in net banking transactions, property or investment portals, etc.
- Mechanism of safety for electronic medical records in terms of both patient diagnosis and security of health records is one of the main elements that electronic medical record companies design into their software systems.

- Common privacy protection tools include HTTPS, paid VPN like Air VPN, Cryptostorm, Hide Me, Express VPN, Earth VPN, etc. and DNS.

Solutions/Safeguards to Protect Private Patient Information

Managing an electronic health record system effectively requires a multidisciplinary team approach including the use of telecommunication, instrumentation and computer science to enable exchange of medical data across departments and wider regions. Medical professionals must be well aware of the security measures required to protect their patient data and other in-house data. There are five ways in which electronic health record entities can provide superior security and privacy solutions once the EHR is implemented (**Table 4.2**).

- Enhance administrative controls
- Create physical inaccessible systems for unauthorized individuals and monitor their access
- Install technical safeguards
- Update policies and procedures
- Identify security weaknesses and threats and address them

Table 4.2: Safeguards to protect private patient information

Security components	Security strategies
Administrative safeguards	• Privacy protection refers to patient data not being disclosed to third parties as an enforced obligation and without their explicit consent. • Health data should not be publicly available. • Patient information should be shared only with patient's prior permission or as permitted by law. • During the transition phase, the EHR vendor must work closely with the healthcare provider for a smooth and secure transition. • The company should provide comprehensive guide for users in provider's practice. • Every organization must hire an information security officer to co-ordinate with the health information technology experts involving in creating an inventory of system users and technologies. • Security measures and ongoing educational programs must include all users. • Workforce training should be conducted on a regular and frequent basis.
Physical safeguards	• Building alarm systems should be installed. • Offices to be kept locked when not in use. • Screens should be shielded from secondary viewers.
Technical safeguards	• Confidentiality should be maintained by ensuring that information access is provided to authorized personnel only. • Access control tools like passwords and PIN numbers to help limit access to information to authorized individuals should be in place. • Secure user IDs, passwords and appropriate role-based access are used. • Basic standards for password maintenance should include: changing them at regular intervals, setting minimum number of characters and prohibiting reuse of passwords. Many organizations adopt a two-tier approach to authentication by adding a biometric identifier scan such as palm, finger, retina or face recognition. • Provide identification and verification requirements to all system users. • Have exigencies in place for data recovery or restoration. • Access the list of authorized users. • Provide automatic software shutdown routines. • Ensure routine audit of access and changes to EHR are conducted. • End users should be sensitive to the fact that unlike paper record activity, all EHR activity can be traced based on their login credentials.

Contd...

Contd...

Security components	Security strategies
	• Anti-hacking and anti-malware software is installed and working. • Contingency plans and data backup plans are in place. • Confidentiality through technological means such as data encryption or regulating the physical access to the system. It is also achieved through working on moral dispositions such as professional silence. • Data encryption means health information cannot be read or understood except by those using a system that can decrypt it with a key. • Employing data protection security measures such as firewalls, antivirus softwares and intrusion detection softwares. • Security program to ensure integrity of the data along with a fully operational system of audit trails.
Organizational safeguards	• Conduct regular reviews of agreements and make updates accordingly. • Identify security weaknesses and threats and address the concerns by risk rating them. • Monitor logs to patient information through audit trail programs to track unauthorized and unethical activity.
Policies and procedures	• Guide employees through the stringent privacy and security training process. • Designate user access and pre-established role-based privileges based on roles and responsibilities of the hospital staff as it is a critical component of medical record security. • Set alerts to flag suspicious or unusual activity such as reviewing or attempting to access information pertaining to an alternate patient. Administrators have the facility to pull out reports on specific users or user groups to review and chronicle their activity. • Security team should conduct monthly review of user activities. • Routine updates are made to document security measures. • Security risk analysis is performed periodically and every time a change occurs in practice or technology.

CHALLENGES OF CAPTURING RICH PATIENT DATA IN A COMPUTABLE FORM

EHRs are used to capture and manage information collected during patient appointments. As use of electronic health record systems becomes more widespread internationally, there is considerable international policy interest in increasing the proportion of the patient record that is captured in structured and/or coded format as opposed to the more traditional free-text representation of clinical data. However, finding an optimal balance between the more clinically intuitive free-text record and the more computable structured and/or coded record is very challenging.

- **Structuring** is the process of organizing information according to a logical model that is meaningful for humans (i.e., rendering it possible to navigate and locate information easily) and/or computers (information is processable by computers).
- **Coding** is the translation of clinical terms and concepts into a computer interpretable format to support automated processing and reasoning. A well written patient history may be a narrative or structured document. A patient history captured using a form or template will be structured, but not necessarily coded. Several arguments have been advanced in favor of increasing the structure and/or coding of the patient history.

Challenges in Capturing Rich Patient Histories

An electronic health record is a software used to securely capture, store, share and mobilize data about an individual patient.

Capture data: The main aim of capturing data is to record accurate, current, trusted data

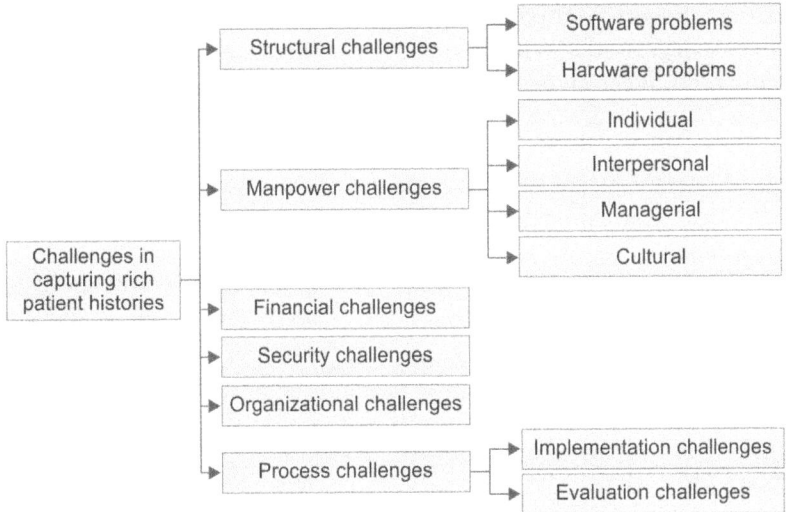

Fig. 4.4: Challenges in capturing rich patient data

at the source—irrespective of whether that source is analog or digital. This could be health data or health relevant data entered by health providers and administrators or that entered by patients themselves.

Retain data: The main aim of retaining data is to ingest and store data in a way that is secure and yet also accessible to health providers. To ensure maximizing its value, data needs to be presented in a way that can be understood and analyzed easily.

Share data: The value of data can be multiplied when it is shared or integrated with other health providers. Furthermore, if data is accessible to patients themselves, this can empower them to self-regulate their behavior and be proactive about their treatment and prevention.

Mobilize data: Most importantly, viewing the above three steps (capture, retention and sharing) is the launch pad to translate data into meaningful information and insights that can be gained to improve health services and patient outcomes.

To capture, retain, share and mobilize data effectively, health providers need a comprehensive strategy that encompasses standards, governance and interoperability; privacy and security; monitoring and evaluating outcomes. Various challenges involved in capturing patient data are discussed below (**Fig. 4.4**):

- **Structural challenges in capturing rich patient histories:** Structural challenges are usually software or hardware related such as the system type, system version, system quality, technical issues, inadequate technical support, usability of system, lack of computers, possibility of data loss and documentation.
  - *Software problems*
    - Possibility of information loss
    - Mismatch between software response speed to user speed
    - Outdated software
    - Limitations due to quality aspects of the system
    - Repetitive and time-consuming documentation
    - Usability problems
  - *Hardware problems*
    - Old and elementary systems
    - Lack of computers in hospitals
    - Technical issues
    - Poor technical support system
    - Technical resource constraints
    - System hanging

- **Manpower challenges:** Manpower challenges can be categorized into individual, interpersonal, managerial, and cultural issues. These challenges are listed below:
  - *Individual*
    - Lack of incentive to use system
    - Unrealistic user expectations and satisfaction
    - Lack of required skills
    - Lack in understanding usefulness and ease of use
    - Inappropriateness for individualization
    - Longer time for the new user to adjust to the system
    - Inattention to users' needs
    - Lack of technicians
    - Documentation errors
  - *Interpersonal*
    - Communication
    - Poor dissemination of knowledge
  - *Managerial*
    - Lack of computer systems and IS program in hospitals
    - Training of new personnel by unspecialized staff
    - Limitation in access to training
    - Employing staff without basic computer skills
    - Project management
    - Lack of significant approach to risk identification and risk management
    - Lack of desire in utilizing information while decision-making
  - *Cultural:*
    - Not adept with the use of computer system
- **Financial challenges:**
  - Lack of resources and harmonized tools as barriers to information access
  - High costs
  - Increased workload
  - Vulnerable structure
  - Decrease in financial efficiency
  - Failure in providing quality data
  - Threats to data quality
- **Security challenges:**
  - Inadequate IT-security for the protection of data
  - Legal challenges
  - Privacy concerns
  - Safeguards of information security
  - Incompatible views towards privacy protection and support
- **Organizational challenges:**
  - Inadequate training about systems
  - Lack of user participation at system designing stage
  - Cost involvement
  - Lack of interoperability between various systems
- **Process challenges:** It includes issues related to implementation and evaluation. These are human, managerial, organizational and technical factors.
  - Human factors include resistance to application of new technologies and lack of acceptance
  - Managerial factors include lack of recovery plan, disaster management and instability of leadership
  - Organizational factors include lack of a perfect implementation plan and well-defined strategy
  - Technological factors include lack of sufficient guides in the system, lack of functionality and usability, and unsuitable flexibility

Overcoming Challenges

- Some challenges are beyond the control of the hospital management, e.g., financial challenges in a government hospital. However, leadership of the hospital can influence policy and push for budgetary allocation.
- Technical and time challenges are more user related and can be addressed by training the staff and involving them in the whole change process thereby ensuring a positive buy-in.
- To realize the benefits of EMR adoption, tremendous effort needs to be put in

by the top management and other key stakeholders.
- The governing body of the institution should in collaboration with the public health department come up with policies on how to overcome the challenges and have strategies in place to actualize their goals.
- Public-private partnerships and donor funds can be utilized to raise funds necessary for putting the IT infrastructure in place. This will address the economic challenges to EMR adoption.
- The entire user group needs to undergo induction training on EMR systems. The new staff should be sensitized at the entry level itself to enhance user acceptance.
- Training addresses the technical and technological challenges. Selecting an experienced person to champion the process is advisable.
- The ease with which electronic records can be transferred or shared provides a considerable likelihood for breaches in confidentiality.
- Additionally, technology provides a means to enhance the security and privacy settings by requiring providers to use passwords to access the EMR. It also limits the accessibility to data based on individual's role. Added tracking and auditing features exist with electronic record-keeping systems that allow monitoring of persons entering medical records.

ELECTRONIC HEALTH RECORDS STANDARDS FOR INDIA

Pre-defined standards for data capture, storage, view, presentation and transmission are required so as to have a greater longevity for any medical record. The Ministry of Health and Family Welfare (MoHFW), GoI, notified Electronic Health Record (EHR) Standards in September 2013.

These standards were chosen from the best available standards from around the world keeping in view their applicability and suitability to the Indian context. The notified standards were supported by professional and regulatory bodies. Revised EHR standards for India were notified in December 2016.

The aim is to provide a set of internationally proven standards with focus on accomplishing syntactic and semantic interoperability of health records, meaning any person in India can approach any health service provider/practitioner, diagnostic center or pharmacy and yet be able to access a fully integrated and ever ready health record in an electronic format. This is not only empowering but also the vision for an efficient 21st century healthcare delivery.

The Goals of EHR Standards

- Promote interoperability
- Support the evolution and timely maintenance of adopted standards
- Promote technical innovation using adopted standards
- Encourage participation and adoption by all vendors and stakeholders
- Keep implementation costs as low and reasonable as possible
- Consider best practices, experiences, policies and frameworks

Health Record IT Standards

- **Identification and demographics:** Patient unique identifiers are necessary to identify a patient in a health record system. For example, a patient UIDAI Aadhar number or any central or state government issued photo identity card number can link all artifacts and records of the patient. Recommended standards are:
  - ISO/TS 22220:2011 Health informatics- identification of subjects of health care.
  - MDDS-Demographic version 1.1 from E-Governance standards, Govt. of India
- **Architecture and functional requirements:** A health record system must meet architectural requirements and functional specifications. To meet the needs of service delivery the health record system must

be clinically valid, meet legal and ethical requirements, support good medical practices. Recommended standards are:
- ISO 18308:2011 health informatics—requirements for an electronic health record architecture
- ISO/HL7 10781:2015 health informatics-HL7 electronic health records system functional model release 2 (EHR-FM)

- **Information model:** A health record system must accumulate observable data and information for all clinically relevant events and encounters. Captured artefacts should have common semantic and syntactic logical information model and structural composition. Standardized data capture makes it possible to communicate and exchange data across systems. Recommended standards are:
  - ISO 13940 Health informatics—system of concepts to support continuity of care
  - ISO 13606 Health informatics—electronic health record communication
  - Open EHR foundation models release 1.0.2

- **Medical terminology and coding:** Common terminology standards are essential to maintain semantic interoperability between various health record systems and express unambiguous meaning of data captured, stored, transmitted and analyzed. Coding terminology standards are used for storing clinically relevant terms and observations. Classification and aggregation of infoRecommended standards are:
  - *Primary terminology:* SNOMED CT
  - *Test, measurement and observation codes:* Logical observation identifiers names and codes
  - *Classification codes:* WHO Family of International Classification (WHO-FIC) and Logical Observation Identifiers Names and Codes (LOINC)
    - WHO ICD-10: International Classification of Diseases (ICD)
    - WHO ICF: International Classification of Functioning Disability and Health (ICF)
    - International Classification of Health Interventions (ICHI)
    - International Classification of Diseases for Oncology (ICD-O)

- **Image, multimedia, waveform and document:** Cater to the need of data records and files of various types such as documentary records of various diagnostic, prescriptive data or information generated, images, waveforms (ECG/EEG), audio (Such as digital stethoscope), video such as endoscope/USG. Recommended standards are:
  - NEMA digital imaging and communication in medicine PS3.0 2015
  - Image: JPEG lossy with size and resolution not less than 1024 px × 768 px at 300 dpi
  - Audio/video: ISO/IEC 14496-coding of audiovisual objects
  - Scanned documents: ISO 19005-2 document management-Electronic document file format for long-term preservation part-2: use of ISO 32000-1

- **Data exchange:** So as to be able to enable data exchange across healthcare systems, it is desirable to capture and provide as comprehensible medical information as possible. To capture and retain information in standardized format the recommended standards are:
  - Event/message exchange: ANS/HL7 V2.8.2-2015 HL7 standard version 2.8.2 – An application protocol for electronic data exchange in healthcare environments
  - Summary records exchange: ASTM/HL7 CCD release 1
  - EHR archetypes: ISO 13606-5:2010 Health Informatics-Electronic Health record Communication
  - Imaging/waveform exchange: NEMA DICOM PS3.0-2015 using DIMSE services

- **Discharge summary:** Logical information model which includes data elements for discharge/treatment summary has to be in line with the format as specified by Medical Council of India (MCI) notification. The printed reports should meet MCI prescribed formats whenever any discharge or treatment summary is prepared.
- **E-prescription:** Pharmacy practice regulations, 2015 notification No. 14-148/2012-PCI by Pharmacy Council of India (PCI). E-prescription has to satisfy requirements of the format for medical prescription as specified by the pharmacy council of India. Electronic version should be digitally signed by a registered medical practitioner. The pharmacists shall be able to print a copy of e-prescription in the required format along with other relevant digital authentication details.
- **Personal healthcare and medical devices interfacing:** Required for clinical data exchange, retrieval, storage, etc. for medical devices. Recommended standards are:
  - IEEE11073 health informatics standards and related ISO standards
- **Principles of data change:** The data once entered into a health record system must become immutable. However, there should be a provision for updation/appending. A complete audit trail of such change is maintained by the system.
- **Other relevant standards:** Bureau of Indian standards and its MHD-17 committee
  - ISO TC 215 set of standards
  - IEEE/NEMA/CE standards for physical systems and interfaces
- **Data privacy and security:** Basis security and privacy requirements
- **Information security management:** Overall information security management
  - ISO/DIS 27799 Health informatics—information
  - Security management in health using ISO/IEC 27002
- **Privilege management and access control:** Access control standards
  - ISO 22600:2014 Health informatics—privilege management and access control
- **Audit trail and logs:** Audit trail standards
  - ISO 27789:2013 Health informatics- Audit trails for electronic health records
- **Data integrity:** Secure Hash algorithm (SHA) used must be SHR-256 or higher
- **Data encryption:** Minimum 256-bits key length; HTTPS, SSL v3.0 and TLS v1.2
- **Digital certificate:** ISO 17090 Health Informatics- Public Key Infrastructure

Interoperability and Standards

- Interoperability is the ability of different subsystems to access and use the data reliably and quickly from various sources without the occurrence of errors. Interoperability among healthcare information systems facilitates communication in the form of information sharing and improving high availability.
- The primary aim of interoperability standards is to ensure syntactic (structural) and semantic (inherent meaning) interoperability of data amongst systems at all times. The need for it within a healthcare information system is to deliver life-long clinical care to the person being cared for and be able to maintain his/her health at optimal levels.
- To achieve interoperability, information models would need to be harmonized into a consistent representation. In other cases, organizations may use the same information model but use different vocabularies or code sets (for example, SNOMED CT or ICD10) within those information models.
- To achieve interoperability at this level, standardizing vocabularies or mapping between different vocabularies may be necessary. For some levels such as the network transport protocol, a widely used industry standard (e.g., TCP/IP–Transmission Control Protocol and Internet

Protocol) will likely be the most appropriate.
- To achieve true interoperability it is anticipated that multiple layers—network transportation protocols, data and services descriptions, information models, and vocabularies and code sets will need to be standardized and/or harmonized to produce an inclusive, consistent representation of the interoperability requirements.

International Standards for EHR

The spotlight is now on digitization of healthcare sector across the world. The focus is on improving healthcare of citizens, integration of medical information across all hospitals, automating patient data, adoption of IT services for clinical services and health management. Governments are facing difficulties due to economic resources and lack of skilled manpower. While the developed countries are utilizing commercial EHR systems, the developing countries are using open-source softwares like HOSxp, OpenEMR and OpenVistA.

IMPLEMENTING ELECTRONIC HEALTH RECORDS IN INDIA

With India slated to become the most populous country in the world very soon, there is an ever-growing need for ramping up quality health care. Accordingly, the Government is engaged in digitizing its health care using EHRs to provide better patient data management. The key objective is to provide equal access to treatment at a reasonable cost. Electronic Health Records are at the core of India's goal for digitalizing the healthcare system and moving towards universal health coverage (UHC).

India is taking cognizance of the benefits of EHR systems in terms of improved patient coordination, increased patient participation, improved medical research, and reduction in healthcare costs. On 23rd September 2018, Government of India (GoI) launched the UHC scheme known as the 'Ayushman Bharat Yojana'. This national health insurance scheme has two main components:

1. The Pradhan Mantri Jan Arogya Yojana (PM-JAY) aims to provide a ₹ 5.00 lakhs insurance cover to the bottom 40 percent of the population for secondary and tertiary care, and
2. Establishment of around 1,50,000 health and wellness centers across the country for primary care, especially in rural areas.

Health data of the scheme beneficiaries is being collected regularly and their records digitized thereby taking steps towards implementing EHR systems. Several national-level policies such as National Digital Health Blueprint (2019) are being formulated to create a pan-India digital health record system. At the provider-level, large health systems like Tata Memorial Hospital and Max Hospitals Private Limited have implemented electronic medical record (EMR) systems and are moving towards EHR.

Policies to Enable EHR Adoption in India

India follows a quasi-federal structure of governance wherein health is treated as a state subject in the Constitution of India. It is therefore up to the discretion of the state governments to implement policies formulated by the central government.

Healthcare policies are largely formulated and implemented by the Ministry of Health and Family Welfare (MoHFW). The government's policy think-tank, NITI Aayog (National Institution for Transforming India) supports the MoHFW in its endeavors. A number of schemes like the 'Ayushman Bharat Yojana' are jointly managed by the MoHFW and NITI Aayog. Some key policy and strategy documents supporting the move towards EHR include MoHFW', National Digital Health Blueprint (NDHB) of 2019 and the NITI Aayog's Health System for New India, Building Blocks (NITI Aayog, 2019) released in 2019.

The NDHB (2019) provides an action plan for realizing digital health. It recognizes the need to establish a specialized organization, the National Digital Health Mission (NDHM) to drive the implementation of NDHB and facilitate the evolution of a national digital health ecosystem.

Key features of the blueprint include:
- Federated architecture
- Set of architectural principles
- Five-layered system of architectural building blocks
- Unique Health ID (UHID)
- Privacy and consent management
- National portability
- Electronic health record
- Application of standards and regulations
- Health analytics
- MyHealth App for increased patient participation
- Multiple access channels like call centers for support, and
- Digital Health India portal for increased data sharing between healthcare providers and patients

While the NDHB (2019) lays out the blueprint to create a National Health Exchange (NHE) accessible to all citizens, the NITI Aayog (2019) discusses the key issues being faced as well as the components and standards required for the success of digital health in India.

NDHB Outlines Six 'Pillars' of Digital Health in India

1. Selection of a governance entity
2. Registries for health data
3. Strategy for the development of a unified health information system
4. Design for health insurance information systems
5. EHRs for patients and healthcare providers, and
6. Creation of a health information infrastructure for the integration of all the mentioned components

Status of EHR Adoption in India

EMR adoption gained popularity in the last decade as most of the private hospitals adopted the EMR system in some form of the other. However, public healthcare centers in villages and remote areas with digital access issues still continue to maintain paper records.

EMRs allow for enhanced patient data tracking though they are not designed to be shared outside a particular practice. This makes it hard to share them across medical facilities like labs, pharmacies, and specialists.

Components in Electronic Health Record Adoption

There are four broad components of an electronic health record adoption, the activities of which are presented in **Table 4.3**:
1. ICT infrastructure
2. Policy and regulations
3. Standards and interoperability
4. Research, development and education

Barriers to Implementing EHR Systems in India

Barriers to implementation of EHRs are presented in **Figure 4.5**.

- **Low public health expenditure:** The Indian government spends a meager 1.13 percent of its gross domestic product (GDP) on health care (NITI Aayog, 2019). Data from the Organization for Economic Co-operation and Development (OECD) shows that India's average spending on health care is lower than that of both developed and developing countries.
- **Infrastructure issues:** Government hospitals lack computers and data storage facilities. Given that a large number of rural hospitals are public hospitals, uniform EHR implementation is difficult without addressing this issue.
- **Issues with data sharing and data security:** EHR systems across the globe are maintained through the effective use of a unique identifier. In the USA, the social security number and in the UK, the national insurance or NHS number is used for this purpose. Additionally, stringent laws like the Health Insurance Portability and

Table 4.3: Components in electronic health record adoption

Component	Activities
ICT infrastructure	• Creation of basic ICT infrastructure • Creation of national secure health net • Creation of storage and exchange infrastructure • Use of free and open-source software • Use of personal health record system
Policy and regulations	• National health IT policy protection of privacy • Regulations related to sharing of health information • Use of health information liability for technical failures
Standards and interoperability	• Use of unique patient identity • Conformation testing facility • Support for adoption of standards • Guidelines for health IT solutions
Research, development and education	• Research development in health IT • Human resource development • Development of online courseware • Dissemination of best practices • International collaboration

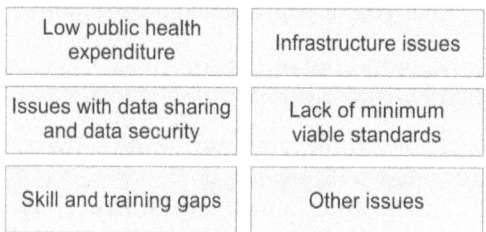

Fig. 4.5: Barriers to implementing EHR systems in India

Accountability Act (HIPAA) of 1996 in the US and the General Data Protection Regulation GDPR in the European Union (EU) ensure that health data remains secure. India does not have a comprehensive or sector specific (for health care) data security Act. India has a unique identifier called Aadhar. However, the lack of regulatory framework and policy with respect to the security of Aadhar makes it difficult for use in handling sensitive patient information.

- **Lack of minimum viable standards:** The EHR Standards 2016 mention a list of ISO standards that hospitals may comply with. However, hospitals can voluntarily choose the standards they want to comply with. In countries such as Australia and the USA, there are minimum standard requirements that entities must abide by for effective record management and interoperability.
- **Skill and training gaps:** Doctors, nurses and other medical staff are ill equipped to enter the data online. Also hospitals have to spend time and money on training and sensitizing their staff in technology related matters. In certain cases, the staff themselves are unwilling to enter patient data online as the doctor to patient ratio is very high in India making data entry cumbersome and time-consuming.
- **Other issues:** Apart from poor IT infrastructure and broadband connectivity, which is core to an efficient digitalization process, other issues include low spending on information technology (IT) for implementation of EHR in the hospitals. While the private hospitals in India spend just about 2.5 percent of the total hospital budgets on IT, the share is much lower when it comes to the government hospitals. Major chunk of the hospital budget is spent on revenue-generating apparatus such as hospital beds and wards.

Recommendations

India may have to actively redress the above issues by examining EHR models adopted by

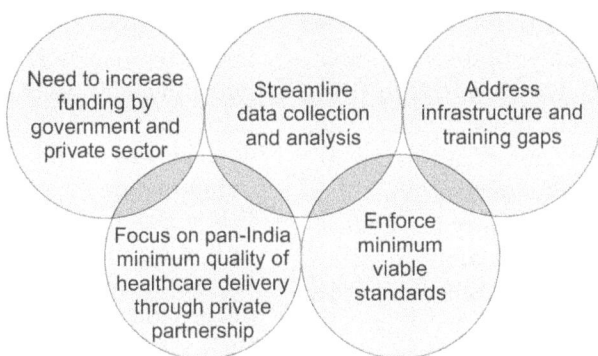

Fig. 4.6: Recommendations to address issues related to implementation of EHR

developed countries and customize them to meet the requirements of the country. Some recommendations to address these issues are discussed below (**Fig. 4.6**):

- **Increased funding by the Government and private sector:** As per National Health Policy 2017, the government is desirous of increasing public health expenditure from 1.5 percent in 2017 to 2.5 percent of GDP by 2025. This should include the cost of training medical professionals with EHR systems, rules, and standards. Also digitalization of district-level hospitals and primary healthcare centers should be completed in a time-bound manner.
- **Focus on minimum level of healthcare delivery through public–private partnership:** While Government hospitals have a larger presence in rural areas, private hospitals which account for nearly 60 percent of the healthcare system in India are mostly concentrated in urban areas. There is an urgent need to equip all hospitals with basic technology, infrastructure, and training.
- **Streamline the data collection and analysis:** A robust data collection system is an integral part of EHR. It is important to define the data required, prioritize fields, and divide data fields across various user roles and stakeholders.

A suitable mechanism should be developed for capturing structured and unstructured data and converting it into formats suitable for securing it in a repository thereby making it easier to maintain the health data. UHID along with Aadhar card can be used for both identification and security purposes. For regions with poor infrastructure, a mechanism needs to be evolved to assist in the securitizing of digitized data.

- **Enforce minimum viable standards:** The National Health Policy 2017 recommended the creation of National Electronic(e) Health Authority (NeHA) or National Digital Health Authority (NDHA) as a regulatory body for the deployment of digital health interventions in the healthcare sector through a Parliament Act called "Digital Information Security in Healthcare Act (DISHA). Though it served as a nodal authority to streamline all the efforts needed to develop integrated national health information architecture and address the growing concerns for EHR standards, the standards were not enforced thereby raising multiple concerns by the stakeholders. To ensure secure interoperability, the MoHFW should specify appropriate global EHR standards such as the Fast Healthcare Interoperability Resources (FHIR) standards in line with the global best practices. This will ensure that the patient records are readily "available, discoverable, and understandable".
- **Addressing infrastructure and training gaps:** Modern EHR systems require computers, high-speed seamless

broadband connectivity along with quality power supply. Before boosting the health-tech, it is essential to first set up the required infrastructure. For effective implementation of health record systems, government directive should be passed making it mandatory for clinical establishments across the country to set up basic computer infrastructure along with Internet connectivity.

Further, practitioners at primary healthcare centers should be provided with smart phones/tablets to allow real-time data collection under the Ayushman Bharat Yojana. Training in use of technology should be introduced for students of healthcare as a part of their course curriculum. The National Skill Development Council can partner with medical schools and hospitals on digital training too.

Development of Standardized Electronic Health Record

- Patient data present in digital format is stored in the standalone machines in individual care delivery setting.
- These discrete pieces of information could hamper critical sharing of data between various levels of healthcare facility.
- Standards play a major role in improving interoperability of HIS. Thus, standard coding provides easy sharing of health information, reduces uncertainty, improves workflow and enables accurate analysis of healthcare data.
- The primary aim of healthcare information system is to ensure delivery of lifetime clinical care. To meet this requirement, syntactic and semantic interoperability of data should be maintained at all times.
- With the data not being interoperable or semantic it is difficult to make the patient data accessible at all levels of healthcare providers.
- To meet the consistent representation of interoperability requirements, standardizing vocabularies or mapping between different vocabularies is necessary. It is necessary to include standard terminologies and codes (in computer processable form) into a HIS support automation so as to ensure the data is analyzable at all points of time.
- EHR makes it possible to not only capture and store distinct patient health data but also make it accessible at the point of care including primary health center (PHC), sub-health center (SHC) and taluk health center (THC). EHR holds health-related information such as patient history, laboratory test reports, and images of the diagnosis stored in a digital format made available to healthcare providers through a computer network.
- Compared to EMR, the EHR provides a more comprehensive report of the patient's overall health. The record may or may not be significant depending upon the current problem the patient is suffering from.
- Thus, an EHR record provides information on various clinical encounters in a chronological order thereby assisting healthcare professionals in providing quality healthcare.
- In the area of health care, cloud computing has played an increasingly important role in providing storage and computing power for the massive volumes of data. It can improve the delivery of diagnosis and treatment by utilizing medical resources through technologies such as cloud computing and Internet of Things (IoT). This could be an excellent solution for the country's needs to have improved healthcare at all levels in the healthcare system.

Proposed EHR Model

- The proposed EHR model connects all the users of the health information system into one single point to record and share the patient health information through EHR network **(Fig. 4.7)**.
- The primary purpose is to enable efficient and continuous care of the patient. It is a cloud-based framework which enables

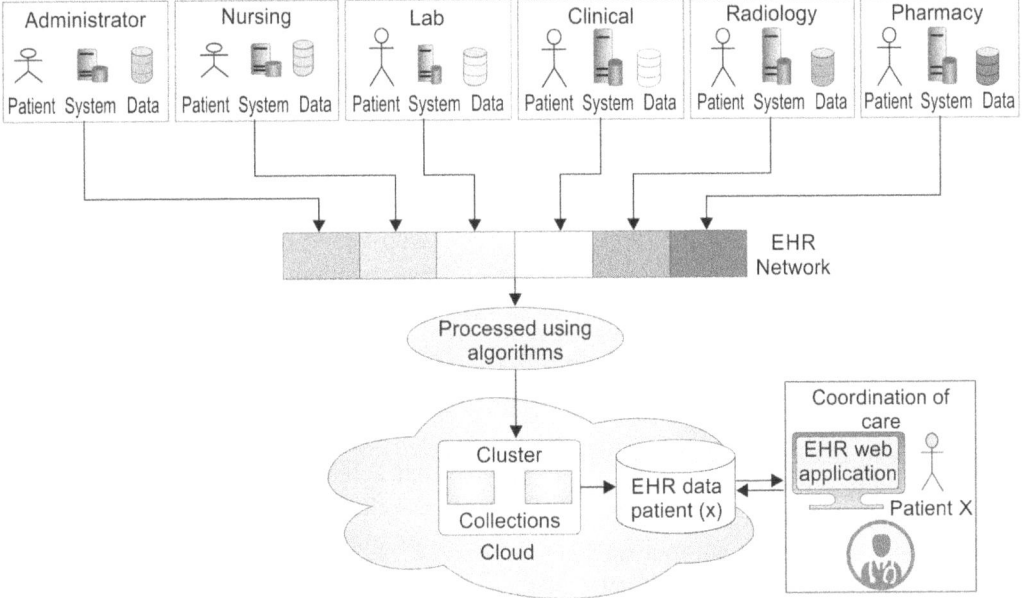

Fig. 4.7: Proposed EHR model

- all levels of healthcare professionals to contribute to the EHR content.
- The cloud resources are shared with primary, secondary and tertiary care levels of health care.
- Data captured from each healthcare setting is processed and stored in a global cloud data base called the EHR universal health service provider database.
- At the point of care, healthcare professionals are allowed to access patient data securely with EHR web application for the coordination of care.
- To develop an integrated system there is a need to collate health data from all the administrative, physician, nursing, laboratory, radiology and pharmacy modules.

Components of EHR System

- The first component of an EHR system is the administrative system module where data such as patient registration details (patient demographic data), admission, discharge, and transfer of record from one hospital to other is maintained.
- The second component of the system is the nursing module, where apparent information of the patient such as height, weight, blood pressure and BMI values are recorded.
- The third component of the EHR includes laboratory data such as microbiology, biochemistry, etc., which plays an essential part in clinical process by furnishing relevant data to healthcare service provider. Approximately 60% to 70% of the quality decisions are decided based on the lab results.
- The fourth module includes radiology-related data and images such as X-ray, CT scan, MRI. Medical imaging system called Picture Archiving Communication System (PACS) is an imaging technology for managing digital images. The key component of the EHR system is the clinical documentation module used to capture patient's clinical data such as diagnosis, procedure, complication and medication. A clinical document in the electronic form helps the healthcare provider to validate and provide quality care to the patient.

- An EHR serves the purpose by providing a comprehensive, concise and accurate information of the patient thereby helping the subsequent healthcare service provider to take appropriate decision.
- Another important module in the EHR system is the pharmacy which holds comprehensive medication history including medication name, drug code, drug name, dosage, quantity, and allergic reaction, etc. This results in administering safe and effective medication to the patient.
- The proposed model uses Aadhar ID or any other valid document the patient is carrying during the first visit to the hospital. This number is used to generate unique ID of the patient. Once the National Digital Health Mission (NDHM) is implemented all over the state, same ID can be used in place of the system generated unique ID to access the patient details.
- The developed model uses MongoDB Atlas Cloud Cluster which stores a variety of health data and has multiple collections to form a cluster in the cloud. For retrieval operations, information extracted from the collections in the cluster are processed and then displayed to the end-user.
- For storing, data which is generated from user inputs is retrieved from the web application and processed to attain certain standard formats before storing in the collections. This way a systematic data flow is established and sanctity of the model maintained. The established web-based EHR system is a platform independent application which runs on any computer, laptop or mobile phone connected to the Internet.
- An EHR application usually performs two major functions: Read and Write. For Read operations information is extracted from specific collections in the cluster, processed using algorithms mentioned ahead and then displayed to the end-user. However, for Write operation information generated from user inputs is retrieved from the website and then processed to attain certain standard formats before storing in the collections. This way a systematic data flow is established and sanctity of the model maintained. Cloud storage helps our work to attain a global platform accessible from any part of the world independent of date and time. These few factors guide the model in attaining EHR fluidity by making patient records globally available to verified users.

REVIEW QUESTIONS

Long Essays (10 Marks)
1. Write the meaning of electronic health records. What are the advantages and disadvantages of EHR?
2. Describe ethical issues in EHRs.
3. Describe electronic health records standards for India.
4. Narrate solutions to protect private patient information.
5. Privacy, security and confidentiality issues in electronic health records.
6. Explain challenges in capturing rich patient data in a computable form.
7. Explain policies to enable EHR adoption in India.
8. Components of EHR system.

3. Explain benefits of using electronic records in health care.
4. Explain barriers in implementation of electronic records in India.

Short Essays (5 Marks)
1. Differences between electronic medical record and electronic health record.
2. Describe key factors to support electronic medical records.

Short Answers (2 Marks)
1. Define electronic health records.
2. Meaning of privacy and security.
3. List the organizational challenges in capturing rich patient data.

MULTIPLE CHOICE QUESTIONS

1. Which of the following is a digital version of patient medical information in clinician offices?
   a. Electronic health record
   b. Electronic medical record
   c. Computer-based record
   d. Computerized record

2. What is privacy?
   a. It is the right that someone's personal information is restricted and allowed for those authorized only
   b. It is the level at which accessing someone's personal information is restricted and allowed for those authorized only
   c. It is the restriction of information to persons that are not authorized to access data during treatment process
   d. It is the right of an individual to keep information about themselves from being disclosed to others

3. What is security?
   a. It is the right that someone has to determine for themselves when and at what level accessing personal information is shared to others
   b. It is the level at which accessing someone's personal information is restricted and allowed for those authorized only
   c. It is the restriction of information to persons that are not authorized to access data during treatment process
   d. It is the right of an individual to keep information about themselves from being disclosed to others

4. What is confidentiality?
   a. It is the right that someone's personal information is restricted and allowed for those authorized only
   b. It is the level at which accessing someone's personal information is restricted and allowed for those authorized only

c. It is the restriction of information to persons that are not authorized to access data during treatment process
d. It is the right of an individual to keep information about themselves from being disclosed to others

5. What is data integrity?
   a. It assures accuracy of data
   b. It assures availability of data
   c. It assures confidentiality of data
   d. It assures authorized sharing of data

6. Which of the following is a key to preserving confidentiality?
   a. Using passwords
   b. Using personal IDs
   c. Use of Aadhar ID
   d. All of the above

7. What is data encryption?
   a. It is a security measure that includes firewalls and antivirus softwares
   b. It is a security measure whereby health information can be read using key to decrypt
   c. It is a security measure achieved through working on moral dispositions
   d. It is a security measure achieved through controlling system access

8. What is coding of data?
   a. It is the process of organizing information according to a logical model
   b. It is the process of translation of clinical terms and concepts into computer interpretable format
   c. It is the process of capturing and managing information collected during patient appointment
   d. It is the process of capturing, retaining, sharing and mobilizing the data

9. What is interoperability?
   a. It is the ability of different subsystems to access and use the data reliably and quickly from various sources
   b. It is the ability of a record system to accumulate observable data and information for all clinically relevant events
   c. It is the ability to meet the needs of service delivery
   d. It is the ability to link all artifacts and records of a patient

10. What is structuring of data?
    a. It is the process of organizing information according to a logical model
    b. It is the process of translation of clinical terms and concepts into a computer interpretable format
    c. It is the process of capturing and managing information collected during patient appointment
    d. It is the process of capturing, retaining, sharing and mobilizing the data

ANSWER KEY

| 1. b | 2. d | 3. b | 4. c | 5. a | 6. d | 7. b | 8. b | 9. a | 10. a |

Patient Safety and Clinical Risk

UNIT 5

INTRODUCTION

Health information technology offers a number of opportunities for reforming healthcare by reducing human errors, improving practice efficiencies and clinical outcomes, facilitating care coordination and strengthening tracking data over time. However, successful implementation of patient safety strategies requires clear policies, effective leadership skills, safety improvements, skilled health care professionals, and effective involvement of patients.

PATIENT SAFETY

Patient safety is a primary component in delivery of quality essential health services. There is a clear consensus that health services across the world should be safe, effective and people-centric. Prevention of errors and adverse effects associated with healthcare are important to ensure patient safety. Further, to realize the benefits of quality health care it must be ensured that health services are timely, equitable, integrated, and efficient.

Meaning and Definitions

Patient safety is a discipline that emphasizes safety in health care through the prevention, reduction, reporting, and analysis of errors and other type of potential harms that often lead to adverse patient events.

Patient safety is a fundamental element of health care defined as the freedom of a patient from unnecessary harm or potential harm associated with the provision of health care.

"Patient Safety is a health care discipline that emerged with an aim to prevent and reduce risks, errors, and harm that occur to patients during the provision of health care."

(World Health Organization, 2019)

"Patient safety is a discipline in the healthcare sector that applies safety science methods toward the goal of achieving a trustworthy system of healthcare delivery. Patient safety is also an attribute of health care systems; it minimizes the incidence and impact of, and maximizes recovery from, adverse events."

(Emanuel et al., 2008)

Nature of Patient Safety

- Patient safety being a relatively new discipline among health care professions, it is being introduced in the undergraduate curriculum in recognition of patient safety as a discipline.
- Though it is a subject within heath care quality, its methods predominantly come from disciplines outside medicine, mostly cognitive psychology, human factors engineering (HFE), and organizational management science.
- Their methods came from biology, chemistry, physics, and mathematics.

- Applying safety sciences to health care requires hiring of experts from new source disciplines like engineering, but without any deviation from the objectives or inherent nature of medical profession.
- The goal of patient safety is to minimize adverse events and eliminate preventable harm in health care.

ADVERSE EVENTS IN HEALTH CARE

Patient harms, collectively referred to as adverse events are events wherein care resulted in an undesirable clinical outcome not caused by underlying disease that prolonged patient stay or caused permanent patient harm or required life-saving intervention or contributed to death.

Instances of adverse events indicate or may indicate that a patient has received poor-quality care. Every year many patients suffer injuries or even die due to unsafe or poor health care. As many medical practices and health care associated risks are emerging as major challenges for patient safety, it is essential to support the management of clinical risks to ensure safety of care. Some of the important patient safety issues as recognized by the World Health Organization are (**Fig. 5.1**):

1. **Medication errors:** It is a failure in the treatment process that leads to or has the potential to lead to patient harm. A medication error may include faulty prescription of medicine and dosage regimen, administering or taking the medication with wrong drug, formulation, label, dose, route, frequency or duration and monitoring therapy. Medication errors result in significant morbidity and mortality.
2. **Healthcare-associated infections (HAIs):** These are infections that people contract while receiving health care for an alternate condition. It can occur in hospitals, ambulatory services and even in long-term facilities. HAIs can have serious emotional, financial and medical consequences besides being a major cause for illness and death.
3. **Unsafe surgical care procedures:** Common errors in surgeries include unnecessary or inappropriate surgeries, anesthesia mistakes, wrongly cutting an organ or another part of the body, leaving instruments or foreign objects within the patient body, infections etc. Unsafe surgical care causes substantial harm.
4. **Unsafe injections practices:** While unsafe injection practices in health care settings can transmit HIV and hepatitis B and C infections, they can also be a direct hazard to patients and health care workers.
5. **Diagnostic errors:** Diagnostic errors refer to failure in providing an accurate and timely explanation for a patient's health problems. Considered as missed opportunities to make a proper diagnosis based on available evidence, these errors occur when the diagnosis is delayed, wrong or missed altogether.
6. **Unsafe transfusion practices:** Unsafe transfusion practices expose patients to risk of adverse transfusion reactions and transmission of infections.
7. **Radiation errors:** Radiation errors include overexposure to radiation and cases of wrong-patient and wrong-site identification.
8. **Sepsis:** Delayed diagnosis of sepsis puts patient's life to risk as it is resistant to antibiotics and can lead to rapid deterioration in clinical condition.
9. **Venous thromboembolism (blood clots):** Venous thromboembolism is a

1. Medication errors	2. Healthcare-associated infections	3. Unsafe surgical care procedures
4. Unsafe injections practices	5. Diagnostic errors	6. Unsafe transfusion practices
7. Radiation errors	8. Sepsis	9. Venous thromboembolism

Fig. 5.1: Patient safety issues

commonly prevalent and preventable cause of patient harm contributing to one-third of the complications attributed to hospitalization.

10. **Other patient safety issues:**
    - Infections as a consequence of medical procedures
    - Resistance to antibiotics on account of overmedication
    - Slip-and-fall accidents in hospitals and long-term care facilities
    - Non-usage of personal protective equipment
    - Failure to ensure proper sanitization in patient rooms and clinical facilities
    - Care transition and discharge problems stemming from poor communication

IMPORTANCE OF PATIENT SAFETY INITIATIVE

Patient safety is a fundamental component of universal health coverage. It is now recognized as an issue of global importance and priority with global awareness fostered by the World Health Organization. The World Health Assembly (WHA) adopted a resolution on patient safety which endorsed the establishment of world patient safety day to be observed annually by member states on 17th September every year. The purpose of World Patient Safety Day is to promote safety by increasing public awareness and engagement, enhancing global understanding and working towards global solidarity and action.

- People are protected from committing mistakes when positioned in an error-proof environment where systems, tasks and processes they work in are well-designed. Thus, focusing on a system that prevents occurrence of harm is the foundation for improvement. This can only occur in an open and transparent environment where safety culture prevails.
- In this culture prominence is given to safety beliefs, values and attitudes and shared mostly by all in the workplace.

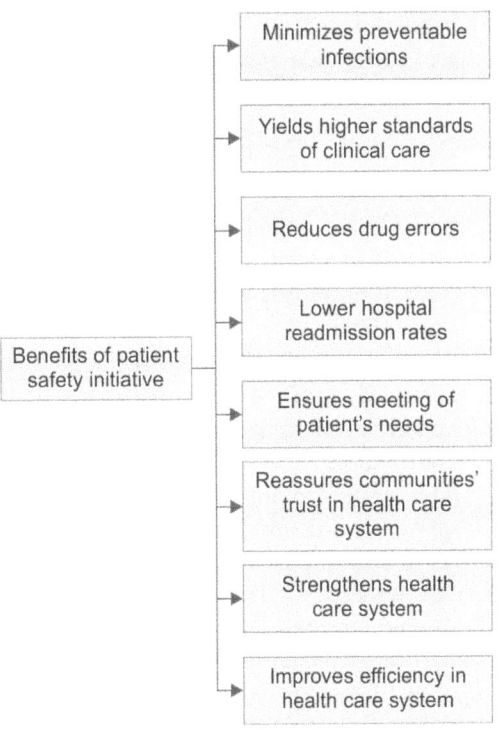

Fig. 5.2: Benefits of patient safety initiative

Benefits of patient safety program/initiative are presented in **Figure 5.2**.

- Patient safety while providing quality health services is a prerequisite for strengthening health care systems and making progress towards effective universal health coverage under sustainable development goal.
- Patient safety program helps minimize preventable infections or injuries.
- Primary benefits of patient safety efforts are that they yield higher standards of clinical care.
- Patient safety efforts can help reduce drug errors at prescription and dispensing stages thereby avoiding further interventions or serious patient harm.
- Patient safety can improve care for patients suffering from chronic diseases and help lower hospital readmission rates.
- A patient safety program can also help ensure that a patient's physical and emotional needs are taken care of during a prolonged stay in healthcare facility.

- Provision for safe services will restore and strengthen communities' trust in the existing health care system.
- Incorporating safety of patients while providing for safe and high quality health services is a prerequisite for strengthening health care systems and making progress towards effective universal health coverage (UHC) under Sustainable Development Goal (SDG).
- Patient safety initiatives involve minimizing physical, mental or emotional harm and safeguarding confidential patient information.
- It is essential to note the impact of patient safety in reducing costs related to patient harm and improving efficiency in health care systems.

To guarantee the successful implementation of patient safety; clear policies, leadership capacity, data to drive safety improvement, skilled healthcare professionals and effective involvement of patients is necessary.

RELATIONSHIP BETWEEN PATIENT SAFETY AND HEALTH INFORMATION TECHNOLOGY (HIT)

Technology innovations have led to significant changes in healthcare system. These innovations best support medical staff and patient safety. Using information technology is a first important step in transforming and changing the healthcare environment to achieve better and safer care.

- Patient safety is a subset of healthcare and is defined as the avoidance, prevention and amelioration of adverse outcomes or injuries stemming from the processes of health care.
- Health information technology (HIT) is the application of information processing involving both computer hardware and software that deals with the storage, retrieval, sharing and use of health care information, data and knowledge for communication and decision-making.
- Health information technology is the area of information technology involving design, development, creation, use and maintenance of information system for the healthcare industry.

Health information technology presents numerous opportunities for improving and transforming healthcare which includes reducing human errors, improving clinical outcomes, facilitating care coordination, improving practice efficiencies and tracking data over time.

Types of Technology used in Health Care

The exponential growth of technology in healthcare has made healthcare personnel increasingly dependent on technology for their daily practice.

- **Common desktop applications**
  - Email
  - Word processors
  - Spreadsheets
  - Internet-based programs
- **Medical devices and equipment's**
  - Imaging technologies such as CT scanning, MRI, Sonography
  - Digital radiology and remote cameras
  - Robotic surgery
  - Monitoring devices such as continuous glucose monitors and falls monitors
  - Automated devices such as bed lifts and sterilization equipment
  - Implants such as pacemakers and prosthetic joints etc.
- **Medical system software applications**
  - Electronic health records
  - Event notification systems
  - Practice management software
  - Digital image repositories and distribution software
  - Use of Information technology (IT) as in electronic reminders, electronic clinical decision support aids, and electronic medication ordering systems

Types of Technology in Enhancing Patient Safety

Innovative medical devices and advanced IT systems have been developed with an intention to improve patient safety. Newer technologies while through good design can reduce patient safety incidents, can also facilitate incident response and provide post event feedback. They can function at both individual clinician level by delivering care and also at systems level by aggregating patient data, or providing access to incident related information.

Medical devices and software designed to improve patient safety range from simple items such as single-use instruments to complex automated systems and software applications. Technologies that can improve patient safety are as follows (**Fig. 5.3**):

- **Smart pumps:** When an error occurs due to incorrect programming of IV pumps with high-hazard drugs, it results in a severe adverse drug event. The likelihood of rectifying the error before the drug reaches the patient is very low. "Smart pumps" are intravenous infusion pumps equipped with dose calculation software designed to identify and correct pump-programming errors (medication error prevention software). These smart pumps allow clinicians to pre-program standard concentrations with upper and lower dose limits for a variety of drugs. This embedded software alerts the operator when the infusion setting is set beyond pre-configured safety limits.
- **Automated medication dispensing cabinets:** Automated medication dispensing cabinets (ADC) are computerized management systems that track medications and supplies. These are electronic drug cabinets that store medication at the point of care with controlled dispensing and tracking of medication distribution.

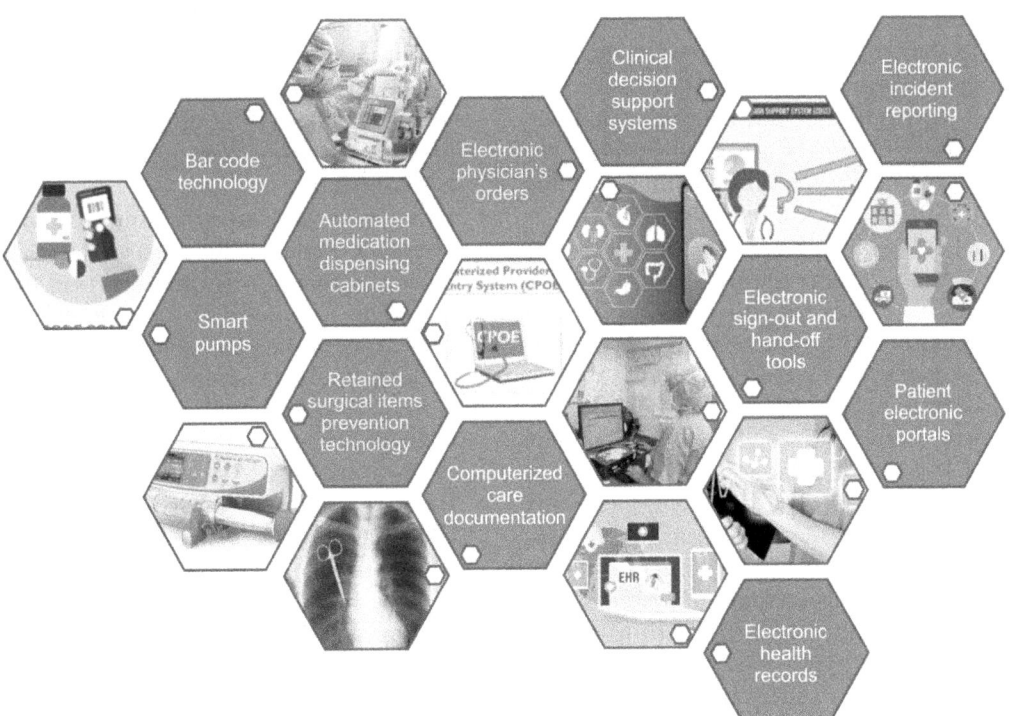

Fig. 5.3: Types of technology in enhancing patient safety

These work as medication inventory management tools that automate medication dispensing process thereby keeping a better track of medication dispensing and patient billing. These reduce medication preparation errors in critical care setting.

- **Bar code technology:** Bar code technology is designed to avert medication errors by ensuring that each patient receives proper medication at the appropriate time. Medication administration systems utilizing this technology integrate electronic medication administration records with bar code technology. Bar codes hold patient related data such as name, drug, dose, route, and time of administration. Bar code scanners placed in patient's room are linked to computerized databases containing patient's drug regimen. This database is in turn linked to patient master file, electronic medication administration record, central pharmacy database etc. The nurse scans the bar code on both the medication package and patient's identification wristband thereby checking for a match. Only on getting a system confirmation for the match is the medication administered. However, if the nurse gets a mismatch alert she terminates the medication process thereby preventing a possible medication error.
- **Electronic physician's orders or E-prescribing or computerized physician order:** Initially introduced to improve the safety of medication orders these are now programmed to allow electronic ordering of tests, procedures and consultations as well. Computerized physician order entry (CPOE) requires the support of a computer to enter medical orders by a physician, nurse practitioner or healthcare provider. Such systems are usually integrated with a clinical decision support system which serves as an error prevention tool by guiding the prescriber on the preferred drug doses, route and frequency of administration. Some CPOE systems go further by prompting the prescriber to any patient allergies, drug-drug or drug-lab interactions. Some sophisticated systems even prompt the prescriber towards interventions based on clinical guideline recommendation. Direct computer entry of orders can reduce errors associated with handwritten orders.
- **Clinical Decision Support Systems (CDSSs):** These are IT applications designed to improve clinical decision-making by providing health care professionals with patient-specific information. These include a range of tools such as notifications, alerts and reminders to care providers and patients, clinical guidelines, condition-specific order sets, patient specific clinical summaries, document templates, investigation and diagnostic support to enhance decision-making and clinical workflow. CDSSs match patient characteristics against a knowledge base, which is then followed up with computer algorithms generating patient management recommendations. This information is rationally filtered and presented to the health care professional at appropriate times with an intention to enhance the decision-making capacity of the healthcare provider. CDSS improves quality of care and patient safety.
- **Electronic sign-out and hand-off tools:** These tools relate to the process of passing patient-specific information from one caregiver to another, from one team of caregivers to the next or from caregivers to the patient and family to ensure patient care continuity and safety. These are used as standalone or integrated with electronic medical records to ensure a structured transfer of patient information during healthcare provider handoffs.
- **Retained surgical items prevention technology:** Retained items such as sponges, sharps, etc., after surgical procedure are reportable errors that can result in patient harm or death and also increase patient and health care costs. Commonly used technology to prevent

retained surgical items is data matrix code (DMC) and radiofrequency identification (RFID). A RFID system consists of a tag attached to the surgical items and a reader that receives unique radio wave signals from the tags. DMC works on the same principle wherein a unique data matrix tag on each surgical item is scanned by a barcode reader as it enters and leaves the sterile field. Both systems are designed to count sponges by scanning matrix labels attached to each sponge as they go in and out of the patient's body. Each sponge has a unique identifier that enables the machine to know which type of sponge is missing and relay that information to the surgical team. A radiofrequency detection system is one that includes a small passive radiofrequency tag attached to every sponge in addition to a handheld wand or mat that contains a detection system. This allows the surgical team to pass a wand over a patient to determine if there are any sponges left inside the patient.

- **Patient electronic portals:** It is a secure online application that provides patients access to their personal health information and a 2-way electronic communication with their care provider using a computer or a mobile device. Patients can log into their personal accounts to access secure information about their own medical history. It allows the patient to participate in his own treatment and know the status of payments or insurance benefits. Often patient portals enable doctors and nurses to send confidential messages to patients, share lab reports or simply recap what was discussed at a recent visit. Patient portals also offer patients a way to securely and confidentially message their provider to ask follow-up questions. Patient portals improve outcomes of preventive care, disease awareness and self-management.
- **Electronic incident reporting:** Patient safety incidents occur regardless of the commitment, training and professionalism of healthcare providers. Gaining information on the number of incidents, their location and the mode of occurrence if they are to be prevented in future. Electronic incident reporting systems are web-based systems that allow healthcare providers involved in safety events to voluntarily report such incidents. It involves notifying a user or administrator of an abnormal event, process or action identified on a computing device, system or environment. It is a part of the security incident and event management process that alerts and logs all security incidents discovered within an information technology environment. Electronic incident reporting has a standardized reporting format, incident action workflow, rapid identification of serious incidents and trigger events while automating data entry and analysis. Incident reporting system may possibly improve clinical processes as the number of incident notification systems across the world has gone up along with identification and reporting of patient safety incidents.
- **Computerized care documentation:** Computerized documentation of care allows the healthcare team to directly capture data related to service delivery using a computer. To automate and streamline documentation, these systems provide document templates, copy-and-paste functions, and a facility to insert clinical data automatically. The key feature with this form of documentation is that the care information can be entered directly from anywhere within the healthcare system. Also, the information is available real time at all locations having access to the computer-based health record. For example, if a nurse completes an electronic form for the risk of asthma attack during an assessment, a protocol of care can be immediately triggered and delivered to the multidisciplinary care team located elsewhere in the health clinic. Through its design, computerized care documentation can increase the efficiency by eliminating redundant charting, make communication

and care coordination seamless, and data available anywhere within the site of care. In addition, while quality of care can be improved by programming prompts into the computerized system, advanced systems can also incorporate decision aids.
- **Electronic health records (EHR):** Storing health records electronically can improve patient safety by improving communication across the patient journey, reducing loss of patient information and removing errors associated with translation factors such as poor handwriting.

Importance/Advantages of HIT for Patient Safety

The widespread adoption of information technology brings many potential benefits to health care. Some of the advantages of health information technology in patient safety are as follows (**Fig. 5.4**):
- **Improves outcomes of care:** Health IT by transforming patient engagement as consumers of health care allows patients to access their medical records thereby making them feel more informed about their condition. It encourages them to actively participate in shared decision-making. This improves outcomes of preventive care, disease awareness and self-management. Patient engagement tools while improving patient involvement also introduce reliability concerns regarding data.
- **Improves patient care:** Improved access to patient data and greater work efficiency speeds up clinical decisions. Faster the clinician gets the diagnostic reports and quicker his orders are implemented, faster is the patient recovery. With automation all departments in the hospital are interconnected. This coupled with faster information access further improves the quality of patient care. Technological innovations can enhance patient safety by automating tasks, introducing medication alerts, clinical reminders, improved diagnostics and consultations.

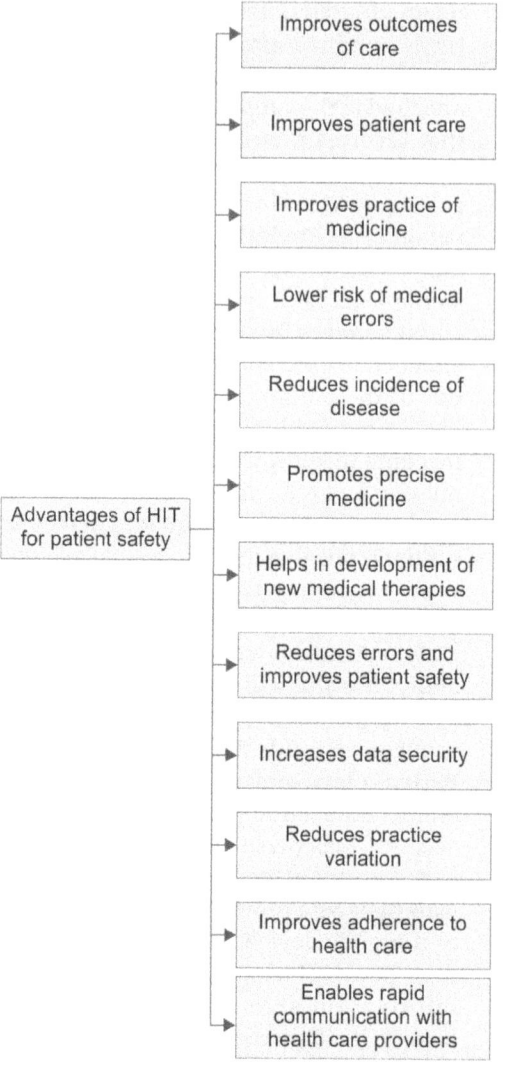

Fig. 5.4: Advantages of HIT for patient safety

- **Improves practice of medicine:** Data gathered through the use of health IT can be used to evaluate the efficacy of therapeutic interventions. It has also led to improvements in the practice of medicine.
- **Lowers risk of medical errors:** Processes on hospital information system are automated with most tasks being assigned to the software to perform. As the tasks are performed with utmost accuracy and minimum human intervention, the scope of error is reduced dramatically.

Computerized physician order entry has helped in overcoming legibility issues, improving order processing times, and lessening the risk of medical errors.
- **Reduces the incidence of diseases:** The ability to use data analytics and big data helps to manage population health management programs and reduce the incidence of expensive chronic health conditions effectively.
- **Promotes precise medicine:** The use of cognitive computing and analytics helps to perform precision medicine (PM) tailored to individual patients. Software performs every task assigned to it with the same accuracy day in and day out without issues like fatigue, miscommunication or lack of focus that are typical of human beings.
- **Helps in the development of new medical therapies:** The ability to share health data among academic researchers helps to develop new medical therapies and drugs.
- **Reduces errors and improves patient safety:** A strong interoperability would allow exchange of patient information and make available the whole picture of patient care. Exchange of data across all health care settings and health care providers would minimize errors and improve patient safety.
- **Increases data security:** All the data is stored on the server or cloud, keeping it safe. Since hospital information system works on login security, not only is the data access restricted to unauthorized personnel but also limited based on the role of the person.
- **Reduces practice variation:** Record uniformity can be designed to reduce practice variations, conduct systematic audits for quality assurance, and optimize evidenced-based care for common conditions.
- **Improves adherence to health care:** A health care provider can search for specific cohorts of patients within a practice to monitor and improve adherence to indicated health care. Telemedicine can improve follow-up for missed appointments, consultations, and diagnostic testing.
- **Enables rapid communication with health care providers:** Electronic medical records facilitate ease of storage and quick retrieval of data enabling rapid communication with the patient in a legible format. HIS facilitates information sharing, improving clinical decision-making, intercepting potential errors, reducing variation in practice, managing workforce shortages and making complete patient data available. A well implemented hospital information system provides instant access to patient's reports and helps in taking timely treatment decisions.

Limitations of Informatics in Patient Safety

Problems with information technology can disrupt the delivery of care and increase the likelihood of new, unforeseen errors that may affect the safety and quality of clinical care leading to patient harm. Technology related adverse events can be linked to any part of the technology system and may involve errors of either commission or omission. These involuntary adverse events are a result of human-machine interfaces or system design. Some of the limitations of informatics in patient safety are depicted in **Figure 5.5**.
- **Consumes more time:** Computerized physician order entry consumes more time to place an order. EHRs have led to clinicians spending more time entering data than conversing with patients.

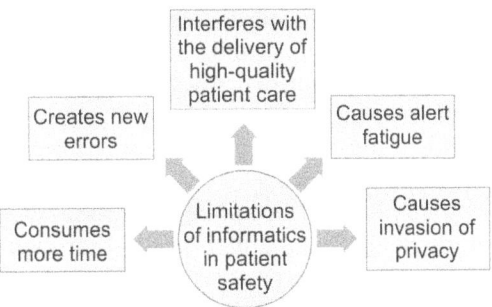

Fig. 5.5: Limitations of informatics in patient safety

- **Creates new errors:** With more time required to complete the ordering process, it may upset the routine of the health care provider. While formatting issues may give rise to serious errors; fragmented display, inflexible ordering formats, incompatible orders, and separations in functions may prevent from projecting a complete picture of patient health care needs as they can be a source for errors in orders. Patient data mismatch or punching data into an alternate patient's chart or documenting patient information under the wrong visit may introduce potentially fatal consequences for electronic charting. Automated and self-populating templates designed to save time can unintentionally introduce an error in the medical record. Use of "copy and paste" technique for preparing patient notes from prior visits may also compromise a patient's record if not properly review and edited.
- **Interfere with the delivery of high-quality patient care:** Poorly designed information technology may contribute to miscommunication, delay or distraction. Decision support tools that are not usable may interfere with the delivery of high-quality patient care. Furthermore, adverse events with the potential to cause significant harm such as delayed diagnosis, medication errors and incorrect treatment decisions have been associated with the use of health IT.
- **Causes alert fatigue:** Employing health alerts to warn health care providers of potential problems may cause alert fatigue due to continuous and excessive volume.
- **Causes invasion of privacy:** Use of portable devices that are not password protected make the patient record vulnerable to invasion of privacy.

With health IT becoming an integral part of the field of medicine it has also brought to fore the many concerns along with its potential benefits. With an increase in the implementation and benefits of health IT systems, it is essential to focus on patient safety and quality.

Obstacles in Introducing Technology to Improve Patient Safety

While the introduction of new technologies is strongly advocating the improvement in patient safety, there are also huge challenges in introducing them particularly in new IT applications and systems.

Following are the obstacles in introducing technology to improve patient safety (**Fig. 5.6**).

- **Access to capital and resources for introducing major initiatives:** Introduction of commercial IT patient safety systems can be very expensive. With numerous vendors offering similar products, opting for the right system can be challenging. With no single vendor yet dominant in the

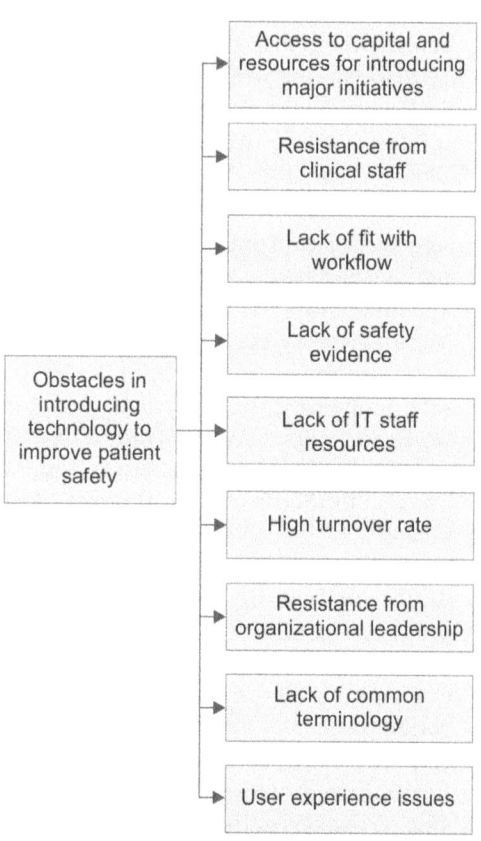

Fig. 5.6: Obstacles in introducing technology to improve patient safety

marketplace, issues around compatibility between systems and long-term support may also arise.
- **Resistance from clinical staff:** Lack of safety prioritization in an organization and/or an environment of uncertainty can bring up resistance from clinicians and administrators, especially towards IT-based innovations. This is further endorsed by recent incidents of high-profile IT system failures.
- **Lack of fit with workflow:** Inadequate integration of newly implemented technology into the workflow can cause disruptions and delays, inefficient use of resources, unnecessary task duplication leading to pointless confrontations resulting from the complexity of human-computer system interaction.
- **Lack of safety evidence:** Only a few studies have demonstrated significant improvement in patient outcomes on introducing IT-based applications.
- **Lack of IT staff resources:** Implementing and managing new IT systems requires considerable investment of time and resources. This can be challenging for many organizations especially those with inadequate resources.
- **High turnover rate:** Complex technologies necessitate deep learning and practice to gain the required level of expertise. High turnover rates among clinical and administrative staff results in only a limited personnel understanding the nuances of the adopted technology which is undesirable. As usefulness of information technology is limited to the data contained in the system, proper staff training and low turnover rate are essential for its successful implementation. Establishments with high staff turnover will find it difficult to harness the dividends fetched by adopting newer technologies.
- **Resistance from organizational leadership:** Exorbitant costs and uncertainty surrounding the effectiveness of new technology can result in resistance being offered by the senior management in introducing new technologies.
- **Lack of common terminology:** Even if the technology is good at recoding and transmitting data effectively, the human element can still make it uncertain and challenging. Clinicians across the country may employ different terminologies for referring to patient problems which may not be in sync with the adopted technologies.
- **User experience issues:** Usability testing allows for the detection and mitigation of issues arising out of faulty design. However, the results can be inconsistent, limiting their scope and usefulness.

There are many barriers to addressing patient safety concerns within a health IT system. An inherent system for mandatory reporting for medical errors related to health IT systems should be in place.

Technological Flaws Compromise Patient Safety

Risks of harm and injury to patients are associated with implementation of health information technology. The primary goal of introducing HIT is to reduce flaws and errors. New risks give rise to unintended consequences which negatively impact patient safety and quality care. Below are the technological flaws which compromise patient safety (**Fig. 5.7**).

- **Poor design:** Poor technological design can result in accidental misuse of equipment resulting in patient safety being compromised.
- **Poor implementation:** Even innovative technologies can fail due to poor implementation. This includes:
  - Implementing systems without consulting the clinical staff
  - Not tailoring the new technology as per requirement
  - Inadequate training to health care providers
  - Improper phasing-in of new initiatives.

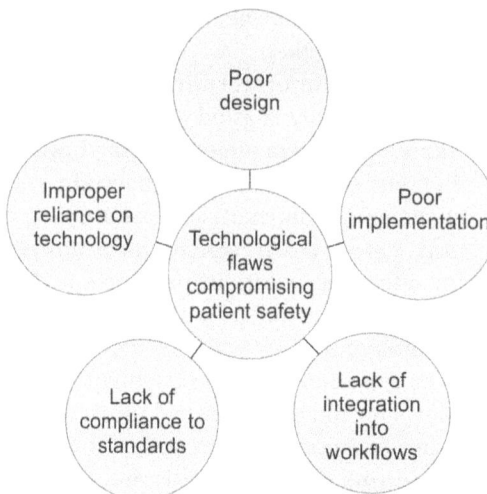

Fig. 5.7: Technological flaws compromising patient safety

- **Lack of integration into workflows:** Any technology must be designed and customized to integrate into the clinical workflows of the organization and end-users. Failure to do so will result in its improper use or it being discarded.
- **Lack of compliance to standards:** Technologies developed in isolation from emerging standards restrain sharing the aggregated data and their interoperability between organizations. This is predominantly the case with electronic medical records and event notification systems.
- **Improper reliance on technology:** Reduced clinical judgment and over reliance on any IT-based system can result in patient safety incidents. For example, faulty default values for doses or routes in a Computerized Physician Order Entry system will produce erroneous orders which the clinicians will trust though contradictory to their clinical judgment. Also, IT compromises on provider/patient interactions and teamwork. Both the above concerns are accepted as being vital in preventing patient safety incidents. Electronic health records also encourage the "cut and paste" culture resulting in large amounts of irrelevant material finding its place into patient records thereby reducing face-to-face contact with patients.
- **Other technology flaws:** Lack of standardized equipment is a cause for unintended incidents.

Recommendations for Organizations Intending to Improve Patient Safety Through IT

In recent years rapid growth of health information technology has improved health care quality and safety. However, healthcare organizations need to be selective in choosing technology which suits their organization structure and process. Some of the recommendations for organizations to improve healthcare quality and safety are given below (**Fig. 5.8**):

- **Health information governance:** Organizations should ensure that their health information system is well coordinated with the patient safety and risk management plan. They must set up a health information oversight mechanism

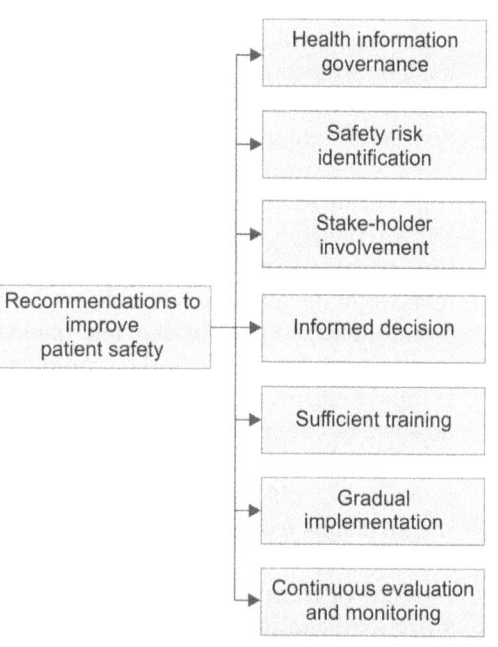

Fig. 5.8: Recommendations to improve patient safety

that includes consumers, investors and sponsors.
- **Safety risk identification:** Organizations need to identify areas where health information technology has a scope to improve patient safety.
- **Stake-Holder involvement:** Stakeholders need to be involved in all phases of health information projects beginning from planning, implementation and evaluation to continuous improvement.
- **Informed decision:** Organizations should review the cost-effectiveness of suggested technologies by evaluating current information technology infrastructure including software and hardware. Utmost care should be exercised while finalizing the design, development and implementation of new systems so as to ensure uptake of systems by clinical staff.
- **Sufficient training:** Organizations need to ensure all relevant line staff receive sufficient training on the use of proposed health information technology.
- **Gradual Implementation:** Rolling out the technology in a gradual stepped approach is crucial to avoid disruption of current processes and systems.
- **Continuous evaluation and monitoring of patient safety outcomes:** Organizations need to measure patient safety outcomes on a continuous basis especially during the initial implementation of technology to ensure that the new technology achieves its intended outcome. Extensive research is required to study the effectiveness of large commercial applications. Health care providers must review and edit automated and self-populating templates designed to save time so as to ensure that they reflect the encounter accurately.
- **Technology optimization:** Organizations need to modify and fine tune the implemented technology based on user feedback and patient safety outcomes. Technologies need to be redesigned to accommodate workflow demands of care processes and the larger context of work setting without imposing unnecessary complexity of clinician intervention for device interaction in clinical decision-making and care delivery. Designing complex technologies requires an understanding of human actions and their contribution to incidents in order to support user tasks in complex healthcare systems.
- **Regular technology updates:** Organizations must ensure that health information technologies are continuously updated so as to comply with recent best clinical practices, regulatory standards, and technical stability.
- World Health Organization patient safety established information technology for patient safety expert working group to examine the role of information technology in improving patient safety in health care. The working group included representatives from high, middle and low-income countries with expertise from clinical medicine, academia, government, health services management and industry. This report by the working group provides an overview of the interplay between IT and issues of patient safety in healthcare. It maps out the boundaries of knowledge in this area and makes recommendations for future research and development.

Developing systems to manage alerts, establish levels of importance and make them unambiguous is a critical patient safety priority.

Role of Various Personnel in Improving Patient Safety

The role of healthcare workers, administrators and technologists is important in developing, implementing and using IT systems effectively.

Role of Healthcare Professionals

Health care professionals should:
- Utilize online resources such as health related databases and practice guidelines to improve practice

- Make proper use of available technology at work
- Lobby for installation of a well proven system at work
- Involve in the development and implementation of technology at work
- Insist on well-designed technologies based on their performance and the context in which they will be used
- Involve in the development of standards for new systems
- Involve in the customization of new technologies as without proper practitioner input and degree of customization the system will lose it future usability
- Ensure the staff are well trained in the use of adopted technologies and
- Provide feedback to staff regarding the introduction and performance of new technologies at workplace and seek suggestions as to how they can be improved

Role of Administrators

The administrator should:
- Insist on well-designed technologies depending the context they will be used in and their performance
- Ensure the involvement of clinical staff in the development and customization of new technologies
- Develop suitable strategies for the implementation of new technologies
- Make adequate budgetary allocations and provide suitable human resources for the implementation of new technologies
- Ensure that the staff are trained in the use of new technologies
- Attempt to standardize the equipment
- Ensure availability of a channel for clinicians and consumers to provide feedback on the implementation of new technologies

Role of Technologists

Technologists should:
- Develop well-designed technologies depending upon the need of the organization
- Ensure participation of clinical staff in the development and customization of new technologies
- Actively seek feedback on the utility and impact of technology on patient care and safety
- Ensure proper maintenance and timely upgrades

FUNCTIONS AND APPLICATIONS OF RISK MANAGEMENT PROCESS

Risks are not only an integral part of any organization but also inherent in the delivery of healthcare. In any healthcare organization, risk management is crucial as it involves human lives. There is a push to implement information technology in healthcare. There are substantial risks associated with this initiative which need to be identified and managed.

Meaning

- Risk means danger or harm. It includes both threats and opportunities.
- Risk is an event happening with potentially harmful outcomes for self and others. E.g., infection, medication errors, IV therapy injuries, patient identification errors etc.
- Risk management is a systematic approach to identifying, analyzing and responding to risks, maximizing the probability and consequences of positive events, minimizing the probability and consequences of adverse events.
- Risk management is the systematic, organized effort to eliminate or reduce the likelihood of harm, damage or loss and maximizing the benefits.
- Risk management is defined as an act or practice of dealing with risk which includes planning for risk, assessing, identifying and analyzing risk areas, developing risk-handling options, monitoring risks to determine how risks have changed and documenting the overall risk management program.

- The American Society of Healthcare Risk Management (ASHRM) defines risk management as the identification, analysis, and evaluation of risk and the selection of the most advantageous method of treating it. This process involves-risk identification, risk analysis, risk treatment, risk control, risk financing, evaluation of risk treatment and strategies.

High-risk Areas in Health Care
- Medication errors
- Complications from diagnostic or treatment procedures
- Falls
- Patient or family dissatisfaction with care
- Refusal of treatment or refusal to sign consent for treatment

Objectives of Risk Management in Healthcare
- To ensure the service user receives good quality care and treatment which is safe and effective
- To protect the assets of the organization
- To ensure staff are able to work in a safe environment
- To reduce the frequency and severity of untoward incidents
- To lead to better communication and co-operation throughout the organization
- To avoid litigation and financial losses
- To introduce cost stabilization

Advantages of Risk Management in Health Care

Increased risks lead to financial losses as non-compliance with regulation and standardization attract litigation. Such instances lead to a drop in hospital reputation and compromised quality of healthcare services in patient care ultimately resulting in dissatisfaction. Risk management provides a protocol for preventing these risks and deal with them as they occur. Some of the top benefits of health care risk management are presented in **Figure 5.9**.

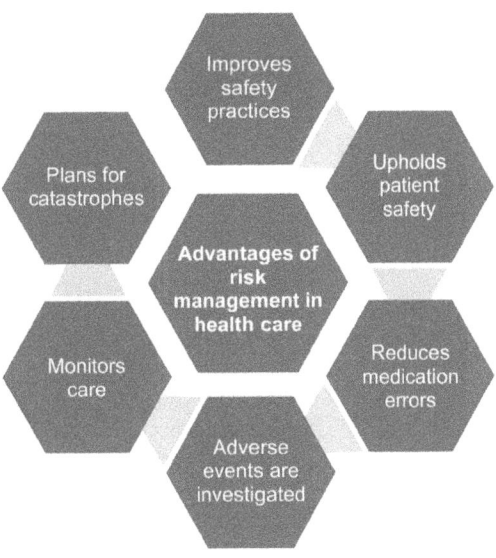

Fig. 5.9: Advantages of risk management in health care

- **Improves safety practices:** Having a ready plan in place promotes calm and measured response besides transparency in staff action. This allows proper implementation and evaluation of corrective actions. Risk management strategies attempt to reduce the number of complaints and claims, raise clinical standards and improve health and safety practices.
- **Upholds patient safety:** By employing risk management, healthcare organizations are able to uphold patient safety, safeguard organization's assets, carry out accreditation, avail reimbursements, maintain, brand value and community standing proactively and systematically. The most important aspect of risk management in health care is that it protects patient records. Some types of risk management in healthcare prevent data breaches, focus on privacy policies and make sure patient information is kept safe from others.
- **Reduces medical errors:** When hospitals adopt a strong risk management process they experience fewer errors, fewer inappropriate services, fewer re-admissions and fewer patient complaints. This improvement in care and patient

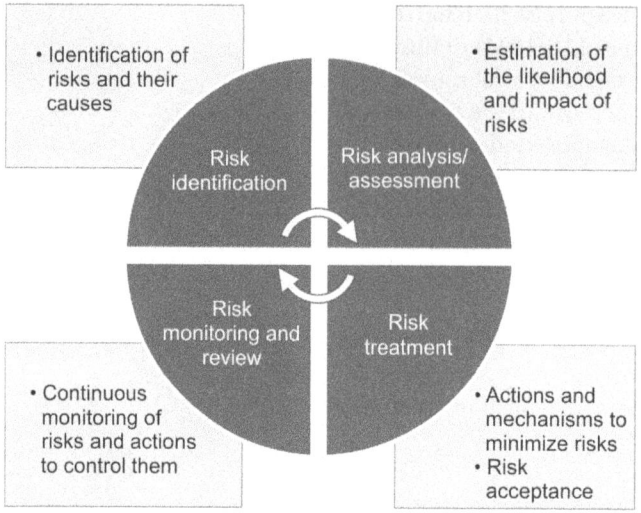

Fig. 5.10: Stages of risk management cycle

experience contributes to profit growth of the organization.
- **Adverse events are investigated:** By employing risk management adverse events are easily detected and openly investigated.
- **Monitors care:** Risk management allows collection of high-quality data to monitor clinical care and early identification of poor clinical performance. It also allows for learning of lessons from complaints.
- **Plans for catastrophes:** Another major advantage of risk management is that it helps to plan for catastrophes. We never know when organizations might experience an emergency which may range from natural disasters to data leaks and more. Common emergency in healthcare are usually related to disease outbreaks. It is vital to have a plan in place for these outbreaks. Risk management plans help with damage control and reduction in patient health risks.

Stages of Risk Management Cycle

Risk management in healthcare consists of clinical and administrative systems, processes and reports employed to detect, monitor, assess, mitigate and prevent risks. The risk management task involves identifying high-risk areas in healthcare operations management that could cause harm to all the stakeholders-patients, visitors and employees implementing risk mitigation programs and creating a robust reporting framework for probable adverse events. The goal of risk management is to lower the probability of risk and alleviate risk impacts. Four stages of risk management cycle are presented in **Figure 5.10**.

Risk Identification

It is the first stage in the entire risk management process. There is a need to first identify if there is potential for harm to self or others. Various steps include:
- Identifying the extent and nature of risks
- Identifying the circumstances under which risks arise
- Identifying the causes and potential contributing factors
- What is the likelihood of harm being occurred to others?
- How often is it likely to occur?
- What are the possible outcomes should the harm occur?
- Who is at risk?
- How immediate is the risk?

- Under what circumstances is the risk likely to increase/decrease?

Comprehensive framework for risk assessment covers eight risk domains:
1. Operational
2. Clinical and patient safety
3. Strategic
4. Financial
5. Human capital
6. Legal and regulatory
7. Technological
8. Environmental and infrastructure-based hazards

As risk management involves managing uncertainty amidst constant emergence of new risks it is challenging to identify all the threats in a healthcare organization. Through use of data, institutional support and engaging all the stakeholders viz. patients, staff and administrators, the healthcare risk managers can unravel the potential threats that would otherwise be hard to anticipate.

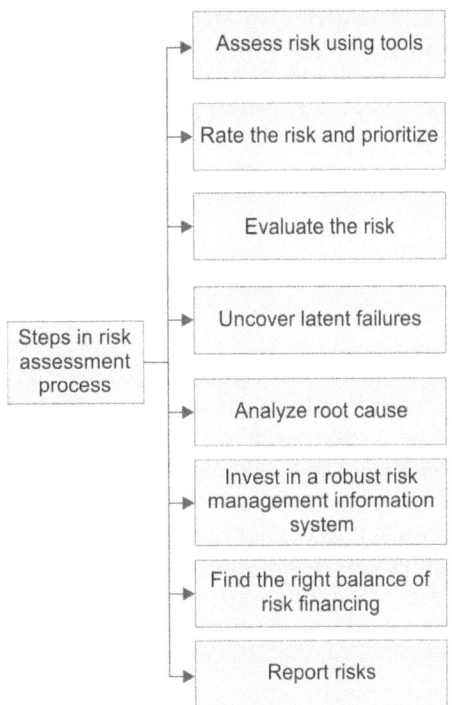

Fig. 5.11: Steps in risk assessment process

Risk Assessment

Risk assessment process aids decision-making by prioritizing the management of risks. It involves analysis and evaluation of the identified risk and a decision to accept the risk or treat the risk, avoid the risk, transfer the risk or control the risk. Various steps involved in risk assessment are presented in **Figure 5.11**.

- **Assess risk using tools:** Risk assessment includes assessment of the extent of actual or potential impact of risk (using risk assessment tools), the likelihood of occurrence and the existing control measures.
  Examples of risk assessment tools:
  - *Multiple risks:* Provide a framework for examining all risks
  - *CRMT:* Clinical Risk Management Tool/ Working with Risk
  - *FACE:* Functional Analysis of Care Environments
  - *GRiST:* Galatean Risk Screening Tool
  - *RAMAS:* Risk Assessment Management and Audit Systems
  - *GIRAFFE:* Generic Integrated Risk Assessment for Forensic Environments
  - *START:* Short-term Assessment of Risk and Treatability
  - Risk of suicide or self-harm
- **Rate the risk and prioritize:** Once the risk is identified, it is vital to score rank and prioritize the risk based on its likelihood and impact of occurrence followed by allocation of resources and assigning of tasks based on these measures. Risk rating should determine the risk management measures required and indicate what intervention should be implemented. Risk can be rated categorically (High/Medium/Low), level of risk may be rated numerically, risk rating = Likelihood × Severity.
- **Evaluate the risk:** Make decisions based on the outcome of risk analysis by listing out the risks requiring treatment and the priorities for that treatment.
- **Uncover latent failures:** Active failures are noticeable and easily evident. For example,

a nurse giving an erroneous medication dose. Latent failures on the other hand are concealed. For example, poor lighting making it hard for the nurse to read the patient chart, the nurse hurrying due to presence of too many high-acuity patients etc.
- **Analyze root cause:** Occurrence of an event should be met with quick response and a thorough investigation carried out to address the immediate patient safety issues so as to mitigate future risk.
- **Invest in robust risk management information system (RMIS):** Risk management platforms provide tools for documenting incidents, tracking risk, reporting trends, benchmarking data points etc. RMIS can thus significantly improve risk management by improving performance through available and reliable systems while simultaneously catering to overall cost reduction by automating routine tasks.
- **Find the right balance of risk financing/transfer/retention:** Risk financing involves organization's methods for efficiently and effectively funding loss that results from risk.
- **Report risks:** Events such as medication errors, malfunction of medical devices, wrong-site injection, wrong part surgery, workplace injuries, medication errors, etc., need to be documented, coded and reported. Procedure for reporting risk are as follows:
  - *Discovery:* Nurses, physicians, patients, families, or any employee or volunteer may report actual or potential risk.
  - *Notification:* Risk manager receives the completed incident form within 24 hours of occurrence of the incident.
  - *Investigation:* Risk manager or representative investigates the incident immediately.
  - *Consultation:* Risk manager consults with the referring physician, risk management committee member, or both to obtain additional information and guidance.
  - *Action:* Risk manager should clarify any misinformation to the patient or family, explaining what exactly happened.
  - *Recording:* Risk manager should ensure that everything is recorded including incident reports, follow-up, and actions taken.

Risk Treatment

Roberts & Holly 1996 suggested **four levels** of management response necessary for minimizing risk.
1. *Primary measures* are proactive and aim to prevent occurrence of harm
2. *Secondary measures* are taken during and immediately after an adverse incident and may include development of a crisis contingency plan, stand by arrangements to ensure an urgent response, more intensive care and possible admission to the hospital.
3. *Tertiary measures* are taken to reduce the risks which arise as a consequence of any adverse incident.
4. *External legislations and guidelines* may be imposed to improve risk management practices.

Healthcare Risk Management Plan

Healthcare organizations are required to have a well set up and accepted on-going risk management plan in place. It is the guiding document for the organization to strategically identify, manage and mitigate risk. Health care risk management plans communicate the purpose, scope and objectives of the organization's risk management protocol. The fundamental components in healthcare risk management plan are given in **Figure 5.12**.
- **Educate and train employees:** Risk management plans are required to specify employee training requirements including orientation of new recruits, ongoing and in-service training, annual review, competency validation and event specific training.
- **Address patient and family grievances:** To promote patient satisfaction and reduce

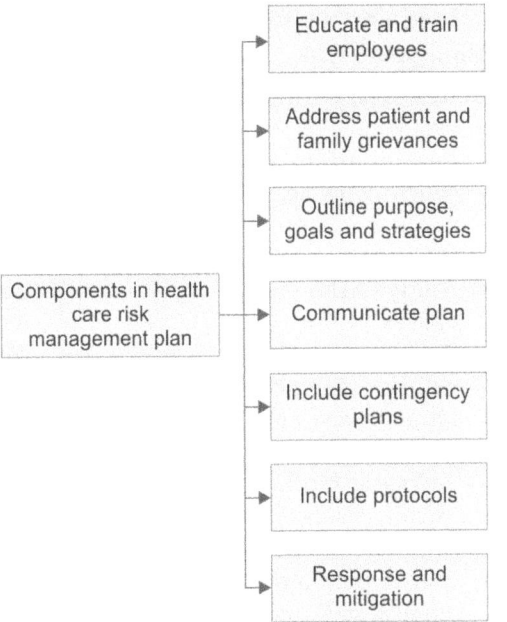

Fig. 5.12: Components in health care risk management plan

likelihood of litigation, the risk management plan should include procedures for documenting and responding to patient and family complaints. Response times, staff responsibilities and prescribed actions need to be expressly mentioned and communicated.

- **Outline purpose, goals and strategies:** Risk management plans should clearly define the purpose and benefits of the healthcare risk management plan. Specific goals to reduce liability claims, sentinel events, near misses and the overall cost of the organizations' risk should also be expressly communicated. Reporting on quantifiable and actionable data should also be covered comprehensively and permitted by the plan.
- **Communicate plan:** A healthcare risk management plan should include how and with whom to communicate the risk. Further the plan should endorse a secure and no-blame culture with anonymous reporting capabilities.
- **Include contingency plans:** Risk management plans should have a provision for contingencies which may include wide failures and catastrophic situations such as malfunctioning of electronic health record systems, security breaches and cyber-attacks. The plan needs to include emergency preparedness for issues such as disease outbreaks, long-term power loss or cyber-attacks.
- **Include protocols:** Every healthcare organization must have a quick and easy-to-use system for documenting, classifying and tracking possible risks and adverse events along with mandatory reporting.
- **Response and mitigation:** Planning for healthcare risk must also include collaborative systems for responding to reported risks, follow-up, reporting and repeat failure prevention.

Healthcare risk management plan needs to be an ongoing one with frequent updates and improvements based on emerging risks, lessons learned, latest information, modifications in healthcare system and practice of medicine. The plan should have a provision for communication and training every time the updates are made.

Risk Monitoring and Review

Risk is not static but dynamic and evolutionary. It is therefore essential to continuously monitor and review the risk management control system. Risk management measures need to be monitored to ensure that they are being implemented as planned. Risk monitoring includes areas of assessment and maintaining a risk register.

Areas of Assessment

- Number of incidents reported
- Grades of incidents and risks identified
- Categories of risks
- Level of root cause analysis activity across the service
- Status reports in relation to the update of safety statements and other quality improvement documents

Risk information can be collected from safety statements, results and recommendations of clinical audits, findings and recommendations from internal audit reports, findings and trends from incident analysis reports.

Risk Register

Risk register is an essential tool for the ongoing monitoring and management of identified risk issues. Risk register must contain the following details:
- Type of risk
- Context
- Risk rating
- Agreed corrective measures/action plan
- Persons responsible and
- Review dates

Risk Review

It should be concerned with evaluating whether the measures implemented have reduced or eliminated the risk. This will involve a reassessment of risk and the cycle should continue through the rating implementation and monitoring stages thereby continuing the risk management cycle.

Role of Healthcare Risk Manager

Risk managers in the healthcare organizations are trained to identify, evaluate and mitigate risks to patients, staff and others. Following are the roles of a risk manager:
- Communicating with stakeholders
- Documenting and reporting on risk and adverse circumstances
- Creating processes, policies and procedures for responding to and managing risk and uncertainty
- Continuous monitoring of the healthcare risk continuum
- Other roles such as insurance claims management, event or incident management, patient safety, provider quality management etc.
- The risk manager should interact with quality assurance committee, safety committee, clinical committee, administrative committee and board of directors

Role of a Nurse Administrator in Minimizing Risk

- Identify potential risk for injury or accident
- Review current organization monitoring system as incident report, audits, committee minutes, policies and procedures related to risk management
- Analyze the frequency, severity and causes
- Review and appraise safety aspects of patient care procedure
- Monitor laws and code related to patient safety and care
- Reduce as much risk as possible
- Identify needs of the patient and family
- Evaluate the result of risk management
- Provide periodic reports to administrators, medical staff, and board of directors
- Establish a formal and standardized incident reporting process

Role of a Nurse in Minimizing Risk

- Use a risk management framework in routine activities
- Perform clinical supervision
- Involve in professional development
- Follow clinical guidelines and protocols
- Practice good communication and documentation
- Involve service users in their care and treatment
- Report and record incidents and concerns

Risk Management Program Elements

Risk management program can be implemented along with following programs:
- Safety/security programs
- Occupational Safety and Health Administration (OSHA) requirements/employee health program
- Infection control
- Informed consent procedures
- Clinical standard of care/negligence
- Medical waste and needle disposal
- Medical record documentation
- Accreditation standards

- Complaint/grievance management
- Employment practices guidelines

Though risk can no way be eliminated completely, it definitely can be minimized by ensuring good communication, providing training and support to staff and ensuring patient safety.

Hospital Risk Management Process

Risk management is a critical function at healthcare organizations. With the right people, processes and systems, healthcare organizations can become more proactive in managing risk which will help build resilience for future disruptions. Steps involved in hospital risk management process are (Fig. 5.13):

- **Implementing robust strategies for patient care and safety:** It involves equipping hospital staff by training, encouraging strong communication and healthy interactions, providing counseling services and conducting competency assessments adequately. Additionally, patient specific strategies include preventing medication errors, doing follow-ups on missing diagnostic results, tracking appointments and ensuring physical safety.
- **Making effective utilization of patient data:** Utilization of patient data aids in providing value added patient care services by using:
  - Reliable clinical decision-making tools supported by robust quality standards and meaningful healthcare criteria.
  - Seamless information exchange across all departments of the hospital including radiology, laboratory, preoperative, inpatient and outpatient units to make accurate patient information available in a timely and secure mode.
  - Capabilities of medical reconciliation of electronic health records of hospitals to prevent adverse health effects of patients.
  - Consolidated patient registries which clearly depict treatment roadmap and identify gaps for analyzing and implementing care management techniques thereby enhancing quality of patient care and impacting cost.
- **Promoting patient participation and engagement proactively:** It involves demonstrating the value of patient-centric services and value-based care for patients clearly.
- **Identifying adverse events accurately:** The hospital organization should have adequate reporting tools to review this associated data in a single integrated repository and have a streamlined process to collaborate all concerned stakeholders in real time, enable feedback mechanisms and monitor the entire process through automation.

A comprehensive and streamlined approach to hospital risk management process not only facilitates patient safety initiatives but also reduces the risk of readmissions. This has a profound impact on attaining overall patient satisfaction.

HEALTHCARE RISK MANAGEMENT AND TECHNOLOGY

American society for Healthcare Risk Management stresses the use of technology

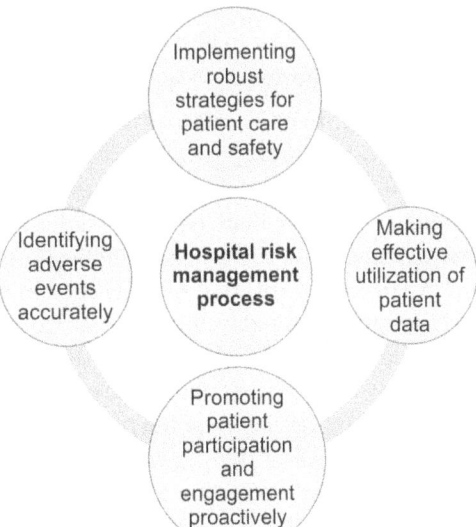

Fig. 5.13: Hospital risk management process

to synchronize risk mitigation efforts across the organization. Implementing integrated healthcare risk management software allows organizations to adapt to uncertainties, collect data and automate processes thereby turning data into insight, all within a secure IT environment efficiently and securely. This contributes to a direct reduction in fatalities on account of human error. Healthcare risk management software can accomplish this in five specific ways:

1. **Flexible design and support:** With healthcare risk management becoming more and more complex, the supporting technology must be all that more flexible and adaptable. Healthcare risk management software allows complex laws and standards to be funneled into a logical workflow enabling employees across various departments to understand their individual roles. As processes start functioning, tasks and data remain accounted for thereby reducing superfluous errors.
2. **Streamlined data collection:** Technology can integrate data tools such as data surveillance, patient safety event reporting, missing reporting etc. This adds clarity to what constitutes an incidence and simplifies the incident collection process. With clear instructions employees are more likely to recognize incidents, near misses and unsafe conditions for what they are and follow through with reporting them. A flexible risk management solution allows for reporting in any location and on any device via a web browser, a secure portal on an organization's intranet or a mobile phone.
3. **Automated processes and communication:** Healthcare risk management software connects people directly to data leading to clear, straightforward plans of action. Automation also provides efficiency thereby increasing accuracy by providing predefined rules. These predefined rules help to reduce human error and built-in automatic reminders or notifications for sign-offs and other tasks keeping each team member accountable. A risk management system not only helps reduce human error but also allows employees from across the organization to return their focus to the most important priority.
4. **Data aggregation and healthcare analytics:** With the help of big data and smart analytics, predictions about possible complications can be made. For example, an incident report may indicate that a patient received the wrong dose of medication. Analysis can reveal the how and why it happened and unearth its root cause. This helps in development of more well-rounded preventive actions and save lives.
5. **Security patient information:** Cloud based risk management software can help in secure filling of patient information and its exchange.

With threats and challenges evolving constantly, organizations can benefit from flexible technology with manageable role-based security.

Role of Technology in Health Care Risk Management

Healthcare organizations require an integrated, real-time view of all risks across the organization to make fast, accurate and strategic decisions. Benefits of technology in risk management program are as follows:

- **Improve the quality of patient care:** Through integrated technology data can be shared, discussed and analyzed easily. This allows small warning signs to be picked up before they can become big problems for the patients and the organization. With simplified data collection and automation in place, staff are freed up to look deeper and focus on trends so as to make better strategic decisions for improved patient quality.

- **Facilitates compliance:** Integrated technology software consolidates all the risks and information into one location, tracks each step of the action plan and automatically follows-up with appropriate parties.
- **Establishes consistency:** Integrated technology breaks down information silos (information management system that is unable to freely communicate with other information management systems) and creates a common approach to addressing all types of risk. This helps to visualize risks and the interrelationships, analyze data and gain actionable insights to those who can make a difference.
- **Elevates resilience:** Integrated technology can help to better mitigate hazards and take advantage of opportunities.
- **Streamlines processes:** Integrated technology breaks down silos (a part of a company, organization, or system that does not communicate with, understand, or work well with other parts), eliminates duplicate efforts and facilitates communication and collaboration across the organization. This helps in preservation of resources, better protection to patients and building of a safety culture.

The right technology is essential for effective healthcare risk management. An integrated risk management solution allows to seamlessly manage all safety and risk management initiatives from one place. It improves the accuracy, speed and actionability of data while reducing risks.

REVIEW QUESTIONS

Long Essays (10 Marks)

1. Describe various types of technology used in health care to enhance patient safety.
2. What is the meaning of patient safety? Describe the role of various personnel in improving patient safety.
3. Explain the stages of risk management cycle and describe advantages of risk management in health care.
4. Explain the role of technology in health care risk management.

Short Essays (5 Marks)

1. Explain nature of patient safety.
2. Describe adverse events in health care safety.
3. Narrate patient safety issues.
4. Explain benefits of patient safety initiative.
5. Enumerate advantages of HIT for patient safety.
6. Explain limitations of informatics in patient safety.
7. What are the obstacles in introducing technology to improve patient safety?
8. Explain technological flaws that compromise patient safety.
9. Describe recommendations to improve patient safety through information technology.
10. What are the steps in risk assessment process?
11. Describe components in health care risk management plan.
12. List out the steps involved in hospital risk management process.

Short Answers (2 Marks)

1. What is patient safety?
2. Medication errors.
3. Meaning of healthcare associated infections.
4. What is the meaning of risk management?

MULTIPLE CHOICE QUESTIONS

1. Which of the following denotes a failure in the treatment process that may lead to potential harm to the patient?
   a. Health care associated infections
   b. Medication errors
   c. Radiation errors
   d. Resistance to antibiotics

2. Which of the following denotes a health care associated infection?
   a. Infections people get while they are receiving health care for another condition
   b. Unsafe transfusion practice
   c. Missed opportunity to make a correct diagnosis
   d. Infection not diagnosed early to save a patient life

3. Which of the following technology enhances patient safety?
   a. Internet based programs
   b. Software
   c. Automated medication dispensing
   d. Desktops

4. Which of the following is a computerized management system for controlled dispensing of medication?
   a. Smart pumps
   b. Automated medication dispensing
   c. Bar code technology
   d. E-prescription

5. Which of the following is equipped with dose calculation software designed to identify and correct infusion errors?
   a. Smart pumps
   b. Automated medication dispensing
   c. Bar code technology
   d. E-prescription

6. In which of the following are scanners placed in patient's room linked to computerized databases containing patient's drug regimen.
   a. Smart pumps
   b. Automated medication dispensing
   c. Bar code technology
   d. E-prescription

7. Which of the following includes notification, alerts, reminders, clinical guidelines and condition specific order sets to care providers?
   a. Smart pumps
   b. Automated medication dispensing
   c. Bar code technology
   d. Clinical decision support systems

8. Which of the following technology passes patient specific information from one care provider to the next to ensure care continuity?
   a. Smart pumps
   b. Automated medication dispensing
   c. E-prescription
   d. Electronic sign-out and hand-off tools

9. Which of the following technology helps in the identification of retained surgical items?
   a. Smart pumps
   b. Radio frequency identification
   c. Bar code technology
   d. E-prescription

10. Which of the following technology helps a patient to log into his personal account to access secure information about his own medical history?
    a. Patient electronic portal
    b. E-prescription
    c. Bar code technology
    d. Smart pumps

11. Which of the following is a web-based system that allows healthcare providers involved in safety events to report such incidents voluntarily?
    a. Patient electronic portal
    b. Electronic incident reporting
    c. Bar coding
    d. Computerized care documentation

12. Which of the following device streamlines documentation and provides document templates?
    a. Electronic health records
    b. Electronic physician orders
    c. Electronic sign out tools
    d. Electronic incident reports

13. Following is not a limitation of information technology
    a. Consumes more time
    b. Streamlines documentation
    c. Creates new error
    d. Interferes with care delivery

14. Following are the obstacles in introducing technology to improve patient safety except
    a. Resistance from clinical staff
    b. Lack of safety
    c. Lack of resources
    d. Reduces practice variation

15. Which of the following is a systematic approach to identifying, analyzing and responding to risks, maximizing positive events and minimizing consequences?
    a. Risk management
    b. Risk identification
    c. Risk diagnosis
    d. Risk analysis

16. Which of the following is the first step in risk management cycle
    a. Risk identification   b. Risk assessment
    c. Risk evaluation   d. Risk analysis

ANSWER KEY

| 1. a | 2. a | 3. c | 4. b | 5. a | 6. c | 7. d | 8. d | 9. b | 10. a |
| 11. b | 12. a | 13. b | 14. d | 15. a | 16. a | | | | |

Clinical Knowledge and Decision-making

UNIT 6

INTRODUCTION

Quality health care relies on co-operation of health care providers as they need to exchange their knowledge for providing quality care to patients. Health care delivery relies heavily on knowledge and evidence-based medicine.

Knowledge management (KM) is viewed as a way to provide the right information, to the right person, at the right time with the potential of attaining a greater competitive advantage. As an interdisciplinary concept, KM regroups concepts from Information Technology Management, Philosophy, Cognitive Sciences, and Organization Studies. The current concept of KM however emerged in the early 1990s within various fields like business administration, public policy, information systems management, library, and information sciences.

Meaning and Definitions of Knowledge Management

Knowledge management refers to all management activities necessary for effective creation, capturing, sharing, and managing knowledge.

Knowledge management is "a set of principles, tools and practices that enable people to create knowledge, and to share, translate and apply what they know to create value and improve effectiveness". *(WHO, 2005)*

Knowledge management is the systematic process and strategy for finding, capturing, organizing, distilling and presenting data, information and knowledge for a specific purpose and to serve a specific organization or community.
—*Dennis J King, US Department of State*

Knowledge management is a professional practices term encompassing the many unique but related facets of creating, organizing, sharing, and using information and experiences.
—*The knowledge for Health Project USAID*

Key Concepts of Knowledge Management

Knowledge management has always been the central question in human societies. KM is described as the systemic, modeling, exchanging, operationalizing, and integration of information to enhance quality. The key concepts of knowledge management are presented in **Figure 6.1**.

- **Systematic process:** KM consists of standardized procedures to collect, store, distribute and use knowledge. The essence of KM is to get the right knowledge to the right people at the right time.
- **Explicit and implicit:** KM is of two types viz., explicit and implicit. Explicit knowledge refers to the visible information available in literature, reports, patents, technical specifications, communication with customers, suppliers, competitors, etc. It can be embedded in rules, systems,

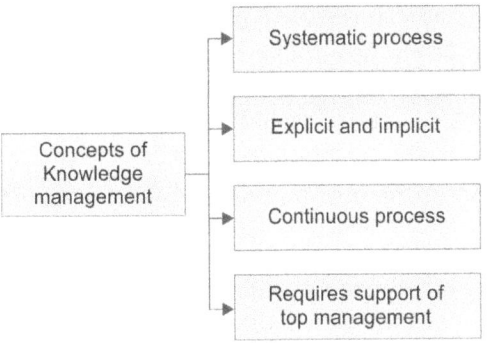

Fig. 6.1: Concepts of knowledge management

policies and procedures, etc., of the organization. Implicit knowledge on the other hand refers to personal knowledge residing in the minds of people as a result of their personal beliefs, values, perspectives, and experience.

- **Continuous process:** KM is a continuous process as the world economy is dynamic and full of challenges. It requires constant creation of new skills and capabilities and improvement of existing ones.
- **Requires support of top management:** KM requires whole-hearted support of top management to provide cultural and technical foundation for the origination and implementation of KM practices.

Components of Knowledge Management

Components for KM can be broadly categorized into three classes: people, processes, and technology (**Fig. 6.2**).

1. **People:** Those who create, share and use knowledge, and collectively comprise the organizational culture that nurtures and stimulates knowledge sharing. The biggest challenge in KM is to ensure participation by the people or employees in the knowledge sharing, collaboration and re-use to achieve organizational results. The key to success in knowledge management is to provide people visibility, recognition and credit.

2. **Processes:** It includes methods to acquire, create, organize, share and transfer knowledge. It is important for processes to be as clear and simple as possible and well-understood by employees across the organization.

3. **Technology:** These are mechanisms that store and provide access to data, information, and knowledge created by people in various locations. KM technology solutions provide functionality to support knowledge-sharing, collaboration, workflow and document management across the enterprise and beyond into the extended enterprise. These tools typically provide a secure central space where employees, customers, partners, and suppliers can exchange information, share knowledge and guide each other and the organization toward better decisions. Knowledge should be available from wherever it is needed to all those authorized

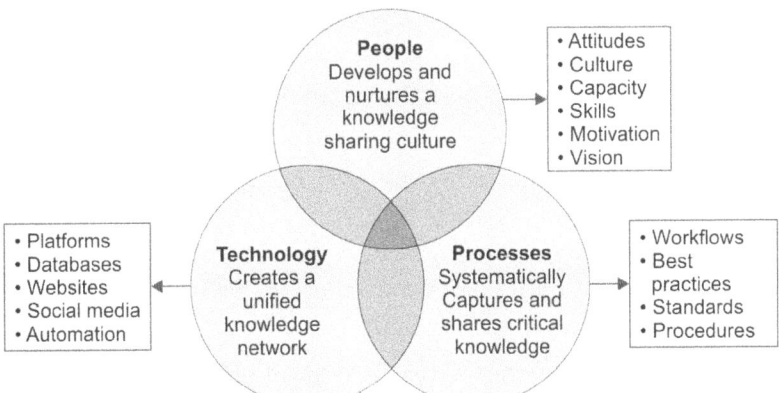

Fig. 6.2: Components of KM

to receive it. Language should be simple and appropriate making both input and output easy.

Stages of Knowledge Management

Knowledge management process comprises of six basic steps that are assisted by different tools and techniques. These steps when followed sequentially transform data into knowledge (**Fig. 6.3**).

Data: Data is a raw form of information that is acquired from many sources. It needs to be cleaned and processed.

Information: Raw data is analyzed and summarized. When data is presented in an understandable way using graphs, tables or figures it is referred to as information.

Knowledge: Information is interpreted and reviewed to generate knowledge. It is presented in combination with intelligence, evidence and qualitative data to enable decision-making.

- **Collecting:** Data collection is the most important step in knowledge management process for which many methods and tools are used. The data collection procedure should be properly documented by data collectors during the collection process. This step also includes data extraction mechanisms and data storage methods. Many organizations use software database applications for this purpose. Relevant and accurate data collection is more important as clinical decisions are made based on this knowledge.
- **Organizing:** The data collected needs to be organized. It is based on certain rules which are laid out by the organization. If there is much data in the database, techniques such as "normalization" can be used for organizing and reducing duplication.
- **Summarizing:** In this step, the collected data is summarized for easy interpretation. Many software packages, charts and tables are used to summarize the data. Data can be presented in tabular or graphical format and stored appropriately.
- **Analyzing:** In this stage, information is analyzed so as to explore relationships, redundancies and patterns. An expert or an expert team should be assigned for this purpose as the experience of the person/team plays a vital role. Usually, reports are created after analysis of information.
- **Synthesizing:** At this point, information transforms into knowledge. The results of analysis (usually the reports) are combined

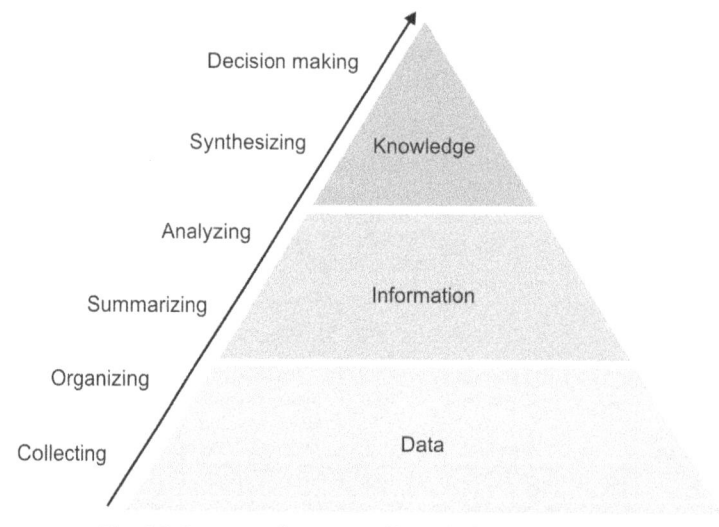

Fig. 6.3: Stages and process of knowledge management

together to derive various concepts and artifacts. A pattern or behavior of one entity can be applied to explain another, and collectively the organization will have a set of knowledge elements that can be used across the organization. This knowledge is then stored in the organizational *knowledge base* for further use. This knowledge base can be accessed from anywhere through the internet.
- **Decision-making:** At this stage, the knowledge is used for decision-making. As an example, when estimating a specific type of project or task, the knowledge related to previous estimates can be used. This accelerates the estimation process while adding high accuracy to it.

Process of Knowledge Management

The process of knowledge management is universal for any organization though the resources used (tools and techniques) can be unique to the organizational environment. Knowledge management process is about acquisition, creation, packaging, and application or reuse of knowledge (**Fig. 6.4**). The process of knowledge includes:
- **Knowledge acquisition:** It includes finding existing knowledge, understanding requirements of organization and searching from multiple sources to acquire knowledge.
- **Knowledge creation:** Knowledge is created by research activities, writing books or articles, etc.
- **Packaging:** Created knowledge is edited and published for others to know.
- **Applying and or using existing knowledge:** Created knowledge is used for medical diagnosis and providing care, etc.
- **Reuse of knowledge for a new purpose:** Created knowledge can be used for product development process, software development, etc.

Knowledge Management Tools

Also called knowledge management solutions or knowledge based software these tools streamline the process of capturing, organizing and sharing/spreading knowledge throughout the organization.

Information technology tools facilitate the capture and distribution of knowledge. Different IT artifacts support the creation, storage, retrieval, transfer and application of knowledge. These are knowledge repositories, databases, electronic bulletin boards and e-mail services. These technologies are important components of knowledge management systems that have become central to health care.

HEALTH CARE KNOWLEDGE MANAGEMENT

Knowledge is an intangible asset for the health care sector which helps to improve health care in various areas such as rehabilitation facility, specialized clinic, hospital, etc. In health care organizations managing knowledge is very crucial.

Healthcare Knowledge Management (HKM) can be characterized as the systematic creation, modeling, sharing, operationalization and translation of healthcare knowledge to improve the quality of patient care.

Dimensions of Knowledge Management

Knowledge management can be understood under two dimensions: internal and

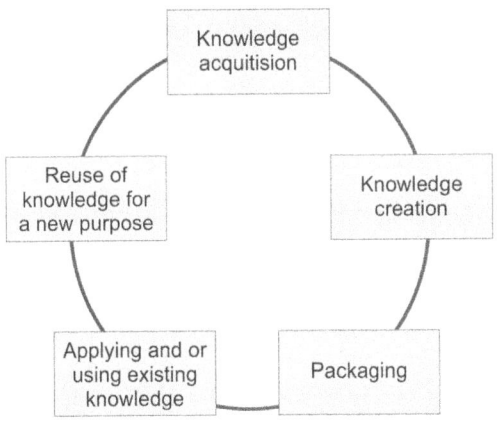

Fig. 6.4: Process of knowledge management

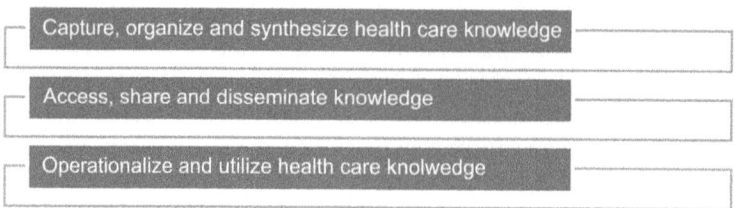

Fig. 6.5: Activities of health care knowledge management

external KM. Internal KM is for health care workers to understand protocols, new studies and research, and procedures. External KM is to help serve patients better.

Goals of Healthcare KM
- To promote and provide optimal, timely and effective healthcare knowledge to health care professionals so as to ensure high-quality, well-informed and cost-effective care to patients.
- To help healthcare professionals take effective patient care decisions.
- To advance innovative knowledge for the improvement of quality and efficiency of healthcare delivery system.
- To address knowledge gaps experienced by health care stakeholders.
- To deploy knowledge-centric solutions/incorporate knowledge management solutions in the clinical area.

Activities of Health Care Knowledge Management
Activities of health care knowledge management are presented in **Figure 6.5**.
- Capture, organize and synthesize different modalities of health care knowledge to comprehend and validate accessible healthcare knowledge resources.
- Access, share and disseminate current and care-specific knowledge to healthcare stakeholders in a usable format.
- Operationalize and utilize health care knowledge within clinical workflows to provide practical patient care services such as decision support, care planning, care decision, etc.

Types of Healthcare Knowledge
Healthcare knowledge is complex, both in form and function. Knowledge type refers to the domains of knowledge. The following knowledge types directly contribute to clinical decision-making and care planning (Fig. 6.6).
- **Patient knowledge:** It involves description of the health status of the patient. Patient observations and physician inferences are coded in the medical records to provide complete picture of the patient.
- **Practitioner knowledge:** It is practice related implicit knowledge held by a practitioner and exercised whilst discharging patient care. Practitioner acquires knowledge through learning, observation and experience.
- **Medical knowledge:** It is the core domain of knowledge which includes theories about

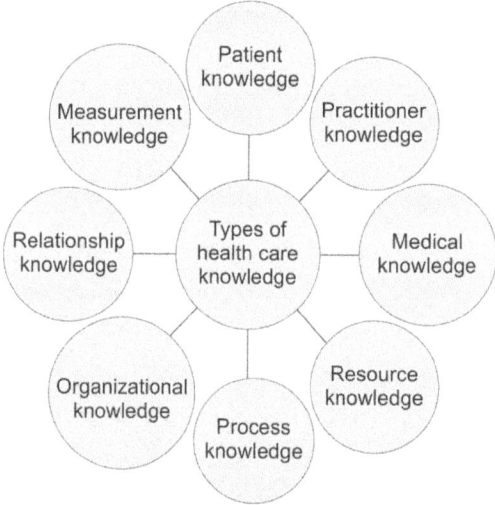

Fig. 6.6: Types of health care knowledge

health and healthcare, healthcare delivery models and processes.
- **Resource knowledge:** It is the quantification of care delivery resources and infrastructure available within a healthcare setting. These include medical diagnostic devices and tools, drugs, nurses, support staff, hospital beds, surgical facilities, and so on. It is important for practitioners to have up-to-date resource knowledge to make decisions about diagnostic and treatment interventions.
- **Process knowledge:** It includes institution specific care pathways (workflows). Process knowledge specifies the standardized way to treat a patient whilst addressing practical considerations such as resources needed to treat the patient as per care pathways.
- **Organizational knowledge:** It includes organizational structure and policies exercised in a health care institution. It entails knowledge flows within the organization, i.e., how the information flows from one source to another, who is required to report to whom, what the decision-making hierarchy is, what the composition of care team is, what the roles and responsibilities of various health care members are and how to make and respond to information requests. Organizational knowledge is particularly important while deploying HKM solutions as their successful deployment needs to be congruent with the organizational and process knowledge.
- **Relationship knowledge:** It includes communication mechanisms and contacts between multiple departments and institutions for the purpose of patient information sharing.
- **Measurement knowledge:** It details the criterion and standards to measure quality of health care delivery process and associated health outcomes. This knowledge helps to set meaningful performance, efficiency and safety benchmarks.

Modalities of Healthcare Knowledge Management

Knowledge modalities refer to representation or medium in which the knowledge exists. The various healthcare knowledge modalities are as follows:
- **Tacit knowledge** of practitioners manifested in terms of their problem-solving skills, judgment and intuition.
- **Explicit knowledge** which includes evidence-based medical literature, reviews, case studies, clinical practice guideline and so on.
- **Practitioner's clinical experiences** (both recorded and observed) and lessons learned through practice.
- **Collaborative problem-solving** discussions or consultations between practitioners.
- **Operational knowledge** in terms of clinical pathways and protocols.
- **Educational resources** in terms of medical education content for practitioners and health education content for patients.
- **Formal decision support** (symbolic) knowledge is encapsulated as symbolic decision rules obtained from domain experts and/or decision models induced from data and stored in knowledge bases.
- **Social knowledge** in terms of community of practice and its communication patterns, interests and expertise of individual community members.
- **Data-induced observations** derived from clinical observations, diagnostic tests and therapeutic treatment records.

Benefits of Knowledge Management in Healthcare

Knowledge management in health care presents lots of opportunities to share knowledge internally and foster an environment of continuous learning for medical staff. When knowledge management system is in place it is easy to collaborate with other health care providers. Knowledge can be easily updated and optimized

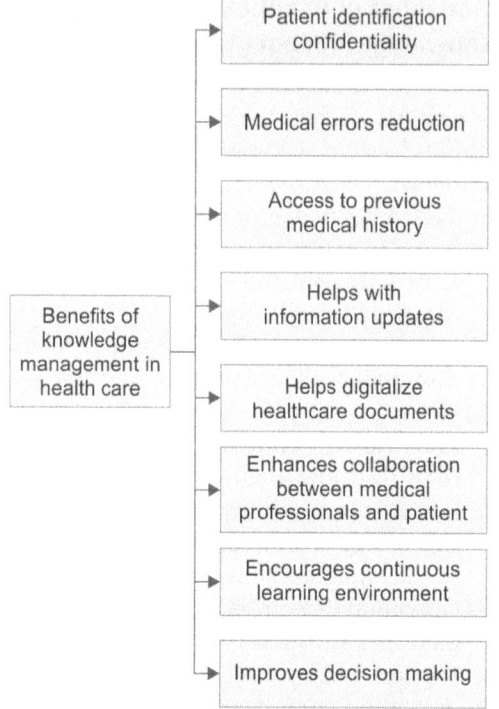

Fig. 6.7: Benefits of knowledge management in health care

for search. Sharing of knowledge not only allows maintenance of highest standards but also reduces the likelihood of mistakes at work. Knowledge management can assist healthcare needs in following areas (Fig. 6.7):

- **Patient identification confidentiality:** Patients are required to share their personal information such as age, address and ailments they are suffering from. Lack of proper security such as properly encrypted knowledge management software to protect doctor-patient confidentiality amounts to a breach of privacy for all the parties involved. Even if a patient does sign up to provide the necessary information, it is vital to protect their privacy at every step.
- **Medical errors reduction:** Medical care is a field where even a trivial mistake could result in a life-or-death situation. Knowledge management can facilitate medical error reduction and consequently their cost by providing a decision support for practitioners. This can be achieved by case-based and/or rule-based reasoning. Knowledge base software helps correct information across the organization and ensure that a single change is reflected across the informational database. Knowledge management software with cloud storage can be very helpful in this case. In addition, restrictive access can be put in place so as to allow only authorized personnel to enter details.
- **Access to previous medical history:** Previous medical history of ailments that a patient has decides upon his future medical treatment. With knowledge base health care centers one can attach the previous medical history information to the present patient data. This makes the next course of action easier for the practitioners and the patient.
- **Helps with information updates:** Both practitioners and patients should be aware of new developments in health care. Knowledge management system helps with information updates within and outside the organization through websites and self-service portals. It not only notifies professional and healthcare call center executives but also allows patients or those who have a member of the family who can benefit from it to see through their self-service portals.
- **Helps digitalize healthcare documents:** With knowledge-based platforms that have cloud storage there is no need to enter records and data over and over again thus allowing digitizing of data with ease. It also allows storing and accessing of patient information across various branches of the healthcare center with minimal effort.
- **Enhances collaboration between medical professionals and patient:** In a complex field such as health care, co-operation between different health care providers is vital for the delivery of quality care. Knowledge management solution allows care providers to document and share symptoms, treatment and other

information that may be helpful while keeping the patient's identity anonymous. Besides collaboration and learning from each other's past and present cases, co-operation provides a chance for innovation.
- **Encourages continuous-learning environment:** Health care providers must learn continuously to figure out a way to provide up-to-date and effective patient care. Through a knowledge management platform health care providers can participate in continuous education courses and new research activities.
- **Improves decision-making:** Knowledge management is a way to capture, distribute and use an organization's information. Knowledge management solutions can help the decision-making process by providing accurate and comprehensive information in a matter of minutes.

Role of Knowledge Management in Improving Decision-making in Clinical Context

- Health care is experiencing exponential growth in the scientific understanding of diseases, pathology, treatment and care pathways. New healthcare knowledge is being generated at a rapid pace as a result of which it is changing constantly.
- This growth of knowledge is not congruent with effective dissemination and application in current clinical practice.
- This large volume of health care knowledge dispersed across different mediums is making it extremely difficult for healthcare professionals to be aware of and apply relevant knowledge for making the best patient care decisions. This disorganized information leads to confusion among health care providers.
- Health care professionals are constantly overwhelmed with new knowledge as they struggle to find actionable information in the time of need.
- In the health care industry right information can save lives only if professionals have the ability to access it quickly irrespective of time and location. Utilization of this knowledge has a profound impact on patient care and health outcomes.
- Most of the doctors base their decisions on personal knowledge and experiences as they rarely have time to track down and consult other professionals.
- Patient care decisions should be based on best available knowledge applied in line with point-of-care patient data and compliance with patient's therapeutic preferences.
- Key to successful clinical decision-making depends on the timely availability of correct and relevant knowledge with respect to the clinical context.
- Appropriate decision-making requires a lot of information. With knowledge management process clinicians can access a great amount of knowledge within a short period of time.
- Use of knowledge management solutions enables a system to create single source of truth for an organization. This information can be used as a knowledge base and ensure that the most accurate information is available. It improves clinician confidence.
- An advanced and meticulous organized healthcare knowledge management solution enables doctors to search for and identify symptoms, procedures and other valuable information immediately that could forever change the lives of patients for the better.
- Health care knowledge is central to clinical decision-making throughout the diagnostic therapeutic cycle. This healthcare knowledge empowers professionals with decision-making.
- Healthcare knowledge management solutions allow hospitals to standardize their procedures completely and provide easily accessible training on these procedures. This reduces the potential mistakes due

to lack of education or training. In some organizations knowledge management solution has a powerful search engine and a mobile application that allows doctors, nurses and medical technicians to access procedures at a moment's notice while performing the procedure or just before the procedure.

- Knowledge management provides data that is both additional and advanced for making informed decisions. It provides comprehensive and curated knowledge that enables individuals to make decisions quickly and with greater confidence. When all relevant data is displayed in one place it allows the decision-makers to evaluate the content and focus on the pertinent information quickly.
- If an organization wants to make better decisions having access to information is crucial.
- Health care knowledge is employed to primarily support clinical decision-making. Knowledge management is applied to arrive at correct diagnostic decision and derive the most therapeutic regimen in the clinical area.
- Decision-making process can be enhanced by incorporating advanced technology such as artificial intelligence (AI) and natural language processing (NLP) to better understand the intent of the request.

Relationship between Knowledge Management and Nursing Care Performance

- Nurses are the largest group of health care professionals who not only play a key role in all health care settings, but also make major contributions to improve health care.
- Nurses' knowledge provides the basis for daily decision-making in patient care.
- If nurses are unable to access and apply current and relevant knowledge needed for patient care it can result in extending substandard care.
- For improved quality care there is a strong need to support and enable the activities of nurses that improve knowledge flow in hospitals.
- Knowledge management can improve quality care by helping nurses deal with fragmented knowledge existing in medical environment.

Barriers to Knowledge Management

With healthcare professionals continuously learning about new diseases, treatments and care pathways, the field of healthcare generates a lot of knowledge. To capture this growing knowledge the healthcare industry is trying to adopt knowledge management. It is also the best strategy to improve the quality of patient care significantly. KM helps the healthcare industry to create, identify, acquire, develop, disseminate and utilize health care knowledge. Implementation of KM in healthcare is not an easy process as there are numerous barriers to it. Barriers to successful KM can be categorized into three categories viz. technology factors, organizational factors and human factors.

1. **Technological factors:** Technical factors include infrastructure constraints, user-hostile system and dissatisfying training. Also the use of system implies extra effort. All this may lead to poor acceptance by employees.
2. **Organizational factors:** The exchange of implicit knowledge often fails due to linguistic hurdles. Other factors include expensive initial investment, lack of senior management support, lack of incentives for documentation and dissemination of knowledge, unfavorable knowledge management culture in the organization, etc.
3. **Human factors:** One of the most important barriers in this area is lack of awareness, uncertainty, distrust, reluctance of clinicians to use information and communication technology tools on daily basis mainly due to lack of time and lack of motivation of employees to share knowledge.

STANDARDIZED SOFTWARE LANGUAGES/TERMINOLOGIES USED IN HEALTH INFORMATICS

A standardized clinical terminology or software language is a compilation of terms used in clinical assessment, management and care of patients. Standardized terminology includes agreed definitions that adequately represent the knowledge behind these terms and link with a standardized coding and classification system.

Benefits of Terminology Standards

Most of the communication between health information systems relies on structured vocabularies, terminologies, code sets and classification systems to represent health concepts. Benefits of use of terminology standards are:

- Structured and standardized data is essential for the effective utilization of Electronic Health Records as it makes health information meaningful and possible to share electronically or exchange across various health care provider settings. The use of standardized terminology facilitates standardized data sets that help in linkage of information in one data set to other data sets for analysis.
- Terminology standards are a fundamental requirement for effective communication. They denote concepts in an unambiguous manner between the sender and receiver of information.
- Standard terminology provides a foundation for interoperability by improving the effectiveness of information exchange.
- The use of standard terminology is a logical step in health IT.
- It facilitates communication among nurses and other health care workers.
- Structured terms provide a means for organizing information and serve to define the semantics of information using consistent and computable mechanisms.
- Structured coded data entry is helpful for documentation of clinical details, billing and retrieval of medical records.
- It provides decision support and shared understanding across continuum of care.
- It improves patient safety, quality care and evidence-based practice.
- It helps in evaluation of health care provided.
- It enables research reporting and synthesis.

Classification of Health Care Terminology Standards

Health care terminology standards are grouped based on purpose such as billing, clinical, laboratory, and pharmacy terminology standards.

- Healthcare billing terminology. Examples are ICD, DRGs, and CPT Code.
- Clinical terminology. Examples are SNOMED CT, NLM, HL7, FHIR, etc.
- Laboratory Terminology. Examples are LOINC®.
- Pharmacy Terminology. Examples are First Databank, Multum, Micromedex, Medi-Span, RxNorm.

Common Terminology Standards used in Health Information and Technology

Terminology standards used in health informatics are:

LOINC

- Logical Observation Identifiers Names and Codes (LOINC) is a universal code system for identifying health measurements, observations, and documents.
- These codes represent the "question" for a test or measurement.
- LOINC codes can be grouped into Laboratory and Clinical tests, measurements and observations.
- LOINC includes terms for laboratory test orders and results, clinical measures such as vital signs, standardized survey instruments and other patient observations.
- It comprises of more than 71,000 observational terms that primarily represent laboratory and clinical observations. It is available free of cost and used extensively

within the U.S. health IT systems for the exchange of clinical information.

UCUM

The Unified Code for Units of Measure (UCUM) is a code system intended to include all units of measures used in international science, engineering and business to facilitate unambiguous electronic communication of quantities together with their units.

SNOMED CT

- Systematized Nomenclature of Medicine-Clinical Terms (SNOMED CT) is a comprehensive clinical health terminology product, owned and distributed by SNOMED International.
- It enables the consistent, processable representation of clinical content in electronic health records.
- These codes often represent the "answer" for a test or measurement to the LOINC "question" code.
- When implemented into health IT, SNOMED CT provides a multidisciplinary approach to consistently and reliably represent clinical content in EHRs and other health IT solutions. SNOMED CT is important in the development and implementation of health IT, as it supports the development of high-quality clinical content. It also provides a standardized way to record clinical data that enables meaning-based retrieval and exchange.

RxNorm

- RxNorm provides normalized names for clinical drugs and links its names to many of the drug vocabularies commonly used in pharmacy management and drug interaction software. By providing links between these vocabularies, RxNorm can mediate messages between systems not using the same software and vocabulary.
- RxNorm now includes the National Drug File-Reference Terminology (NDF-RT) from the Veterans Health Administration.

NDF-RT is a terminology used to code clinical drug properties including mechanism of action, physiologic effect and therapeutic category.

RadLex

RadLex is a unified language of radiology terms for standardized indexing and retrieval of radiology information resources. It unifies and supplements other lexicons and standards such as SNOMED-CT and DICOM. It is managed by the Radiological society of North America.

MEDCIN

MEDICIN is a medical terminology maintained by Medicomp Systems that encompasses symptoms, history, physical examination, tests, diagnoses and therapies.

ICD-10

ICD-10 is the 10th revision of the International Statistical Classification of Diseases and Related Health Problems (ICD), a medical classification list by the World health Organization (WHO). It contains codes for diseases, signs and symptoms, abnormal findings, complaints, social circumstances, and external causes of injury or diseases.

CPT®

Current procedural terminology (CPT®) is a code set maintained by the American Medical Association (AMA). It is used to bill outpatient and office procedures.

HCPCS

The health care common procedure coding system (HCPCS) is a set of healthcare procedure codes based on CPT that is leveraged for Medicare reimbursement.

CDC CVX and MVX

The Centers for disease control and prevention (CDC) provide a number of code sets for vaccines [Vaccines Administered (CVX)] and manufacturers [Manufacturers of

Vaccines (MVX)]. These codes can be used in immunization messages.

NDC

The National Drug Code (NDC) is maintained by the Food and Drug Administration (FDA) which provides a list of all drugs manufactured, prepared, propagated, compounded or processed for commercial distribution.

SNOMED CT to ICD-10-CM Map

Implementation of electronic health records resulted in generation of huge volumes of clinical data. Historically, clinical terminology is used to represent clinical data. These elements are varied among different systems. Not having standard terminology creates difficulty in sharing data and performing computer-based decision support. Overtime multiple standards of terminology have been developed and adopted in health care at different times for different purposes. Due to this a need for mapping between controlled terminologies arose. One such cross-terminology mapping is SNOMED CT to ICD-10-CM cross-map. The purpose of SNOMED CT to ICD-10-CM cross-mapping is to support semi-automated generation of ICD-10-CM codes from clinical data encoded in SNOMED CT for reimbursement and statistical purposes. The map can be used in real-time by healthcare providers and coding professionals for retrospective coding purposes.

Alternative Billing Concepts (ABC) Codes

- ABC codes are produced and maintained by ABC coding solutions.
- ABC codes include descriptions of integrative health care services, remedie and supplies.
- An ABC code is a five-letter string followed by a two-character code modifier.
- The string identifies service, remedy or supply item while the code modifier identifies the practitioner type.
- ABC codes may be used by health care practitioners and insurers for updating medical records, billing, processing claims and managing benefits.

Standard Nursing Terminologies

- Realizing that the standardization of nursing care documentation was a critical component to support interoperable health information, the ANA in 1989 created a process to recognize languages, vocabularies and terminologies that support nursing practice.
- Currently, the ANA recognizes two minimum data sets, two reference terminologies and eight interface terminologies for facilitating documentation of nursing care and interoperability of nursing data between multiple concepts and nomenclatures within IT systems (**Table 6.1**).
- Minimum data sets are sets of data elements with standardized definitions and codes collected for a specific purpose such as describing clinical nursing practice or nursing management contextual data that influence care.
- Interface terminologies (point-of-care) are actual terms/concepts used by nurses for describing and documenting care

Table 6.1: ANA Recognized Standard Nursing Terminologies

Interface terminologies
• Clinical Care Classification (CCC) System
• International Classification for Nursing Practice (ICNP)
• North American Nursing Diagnosis Association International (NANDA-I)
• Nursing Interventions Classification System (NIC)
• Nursing Outcomes Classification (NOC)
• Omaha System
• Perioperative Nursing Data Set (PNDS)
• ABC Codes

Minimum data sets
• Nursing Minimum Data Set (NMDS)
• Nursing Management Minimum Data Set (NMMDS)

Reference terminologies
• Logical Observation Identifiers Names and Codes (LOINC)
• SNOMED Clinical Terms (SNOMED CT)

of patients (individuals, families and communities).
- Reference terminologies are designed to provide common semantics for diverse implementations which ideally enable clinicians to use terms appropriate for their discipline-specific practices, then map those terms through a reference terminology to communicate similar meaning across systems.

Clinical Care Classification (CCC) System

- The CCC, previously known as Home Health Care Classification (HHCC) was originally created by Virginia Saba and colleagues in 1991 to document nursing care in home health and ambulatory care settings.
- CCC system facilitates the electronic documentation of nursing plans of care in a new way. It is specifically designed for clinical nursing documentation at the point of care.
- CCC provides a standardized framework and a unique coding structure for assessing, documenting and classifying patient care by nurses and other clinical practitioners.
- **CCC includes two sets of terminology:** 1. Nursing diagnoses and 2. Nursing interventions. These terminologies are classified using a coded framework consisting of 21 care components that are displayed around the six steps of the nursing process. The six steps are assessment, diagnosis, outcome identification, planning, implementation, and evaluation.
- Nursing diagnoses are enhanced using the three modifiers: improved, stabilized or deteriorated to document expected and actual outcomes.
- Nursing interventions are expanded using the four modifiers: assess/monitor, care/perform, teach/instruct, and manage/refer to document the type of action for each nursing intervention creating 792 nursing interventions.
- Each nursing intervention consists of a core concept and a type action modifier making the coding of terminology flexible and adaptable.

International Classification for Nursing Practice (ICNP)

ICNP is an international terminology that provides description and comparison for nursing practice and allows for cross-mapping between other terminologies. The ICPN is defined as a classification of nursing phenomena, nursing actions and nursing outcomes that describes nursing practice.

Vision
To have nursing data readily available and used in health care information systems worldwide.

Aim
To improve health care delivery.

Elements of ICPN
- Nursing phenomena-nursing diagnoses
- Nursing interventions
- Nursing outcomes

Objectives
- To establish a common language for describing nursing practice in order to improve communication among nurses and with others.
- To describe the nursing care of people in a variety of settings.
- To enable comparison of nursing data across clinical populations, settings and geographic areas.
- To stimulate nursing research.
- To provide data on nursing practice to influence policy.

Advantages
- ICPN classifies patient data and clinical activity in the domain of nursing thereby making it helpful in decision-making and policy development.
- Improves communication and statistical reporting practices across health services thus increasing nursing visibility.

- Provides a structured and defined vocabulary as well as a classification for nurses.
- Provides agreed set of terms for recording observations and interventions of nurses across the world.
- Provides a framework for sharing nursing data and comparing it with nursing practice across settings.
- Describes nursing care of people in a variety of settings thereby enabling comparison of nursing data across clinical populations, settings and geographical areas and time.
- Supports evidence-based practice.
- Brings different nursing terminology together.
- Ensures that nurses have the information tools they need to meet the changing health care needs of individuals.
- As ICNP is owned and copyrighted by the International Council of Nurses (ICN), those wanting to use ICNP need to obtain permission from the ICN.

North American Nursing Diagnosis Association International (NANDA-I) Terminology

An international language for nurses:
- NANDA became NANDA-I in 2002 to provide a shared language for nurses to address health problems, risk states and readiness for health promotion.
- Nurses to communicate with each other and professionals from other health disciplines about "what" nurses are focused on and phenomenon that nurses are directing interventions toward.
- Presently NANDA includes more than 216 nursing diagnoses.
- This facilitates the development, refinement, dissemination and use of standardized nursing diagnostic terminology.
- Provides evidence-based terminology into clinical practice.
- NANDA-I has a global reach to nurses through its website, published materials, conferences and network groups.

Nursing Interventions Classification System (NIC)/Nursing Outcome Classification (NOC)

- It is one of the standardized languages recognized by the American Nurses Association (ANA), a comprehensive research-based standardized classification of interventions that nurses perform.
- It is included in the Unified Medical Language System (UMLS) in the National Library of Medicine (NLM) and in the Cumulative Index of Nursing and Allied Health Literature (CINAHL).
- The classification includes interventions that nurses carry out on behalf of patients, both independent and collaborative, and direct and indirect care.
- NIC interventions include both physiological and psychological interventions for illness treatment and prevention, for individuals, families, and communities.
- Each intervention as it appears in the classification is listed with a label name, a defined set of activities to carry out the intervention and background readings.
- It includes 565 interventions grouped under thirty classes and seven domains. The seven domains are: physiological : basic, physiological : complex, behavioral, safety, family, health system, and community.
- Each intervention has a unique number (code).
- It is used for clinical documentation, communication of care across settings, evaluating outcomes, conducting effective research, measuring nursing productivity, evaluating nursing competencies, facilitating reimbursement, and designing curriculum.
- It integrates data across systems and settings.

Omaha System

- The Omaha System is a research-based, comprehensive practice, and documentation of standardized taxonomy designed to describe patient care with rational

components such as an assessment component, care plan and an evaluation component.
- It is designed to enhance practice, documentation, and information management.
- It is intended for use across the continuum of care for individuals, families, and communities.
- It provides a structure to document patient needs and strengths, describes multidisciplinary practitioner interventions and measures patient outcomes in a simple and user-friendly yet comprehensive manner.
- It enables collection, aggregation and analysis of clinical data.
- It supports quality improvement, critical thinking and communication.
- It speeds up evidence-based research practices.
- It links clinical data to demographic, financial, administrative and staffing data.

Perioperative Nursing Data Set (PNDS)

- PNDS is a "standardized language that addresses the perioperative patient experience from pre-admission until discharge. It is the only perioperative nursing language recognized by ANA.
- It provides a consistent method for classifying and documenting perioperative patient care across the surgical continuum, allowing for the monitoring and benchmarking of patient outcomes and operating room efficiency.
- It describes the nursing diagnoses, interventions and patient outcomes.
- The PNDS provides a framework to standardize clinical documentation within an EHR.

Nursing Minimum Data Set (NMDS)

- The NMDS is a set of elements developed consistent with the general concept of a Uniform Minimum Health Data Set (UMHDS) and specifically intended for the collection of essential nursing care data.
- It is important to have data to describe what nurses do, to whom they deliver care, and what the effectiveness and cost of that care are. Harriet Werly and Norma Lang in 1985 developed NMDS with this view which was later recognized by ANA in 1999.
- The NMDS is defined as a minimum set of data elements with uniform definitions and categories about specific dimensions of nursing designed to meet the information needs of multiple data users in the health care system.
- It includes 16 items organized into categories of nursing care (diagnoses, interventions and outcomes), patient demographics and service elements (e.g., facility identifier, nurse identifier, admission, and discharge dates).
- The main purposes are to establish comparable nursing data across clinical populations, settings, geographic areas, and time; describe nursing care of patients/clients and their families in a variety of settings; demonstrate or project trends regarding nursing care provided and the allocation of resources to patients/clients based on their health problems or nursing diagnoses; stimulate nursing research through links to data existing in nursing and other health care information systems; and provide data about nursing care to influence clinical, administrative, and health policy decision-making.

Nursing Management Minimum Data Set (NMMDS)

- NMMDS is a research-based management data set that specifically identifies variables essential to nursing administrators for decision-making about nursing care effectiveness.
- It provides standard administrative data elements, definitions and codes to measure the context of nursing care required by nurse administrators to make management decisions.
- NMMDS has structured around 18 elements associated with nursing environment, nursing care resources, and financial

resources. Elements in the current health system provide evidence for nursing leaders to measure and manage decisions leading to better patient care, staffing and financial outcomes.
- It also enables the reuse of data for clinical scholarship and research.

Benefits of Standardized Languages in Nursing Practice

- Better communication among nurses and other health care providers
- Increased visibility of nursing interventions
- Improved patient care
- Enhanced data collection to evaluate nursing care outcomes
- Greater adherence to standards of care
- Assistance in assessment of nursing competency

Implications of Standardized Language for Nursing Education, Research, and Administration

In addition to enhancing the care provided by direct care nurses, standardized language has implications for nursing education, research, and administration.

- Nurse educators can use the knowledge inherent in standardized nursing languages to educate future nurses. Such a system can be used to describe the unique roles of the nurse.
- Nurse educators can teach students the use of systems such as the CCC and Omaha when in community health fields, or the NANDA, NIC, NOC terminology when in acute care settings.
- References to the primary resources upon which each intervention is based are listed at the end of each individual intervention to provide information supporting each intervention.
- By referring to the references associated with these nursing standards, nurse educators can role model the use of standardized language to help students recognize the body of knowledge upon which the standards are built.
- Tying the standardized language to education and practice will enhance its implementation and expand practicing nurses' knowledge of interventions, outcomes, and languages.
- Armed with an appreciation for the value of standardized language, students can champion further development and the use of standardized nursing languages upon their entry into professional practice.
- The use of standardized languages can provide a launching point for conducting research on standardized languages.
- Research conducted by two teams of educators at the University of Iowa on the NIC and NOC are excellent examples of the research that can be done on the standardized nursing languages using computerized databases designed for research.

Issues Related to use of Standardized Languages in Nursing

- Licensing fees, copyrights and associated pricing challenges
- Not having sufficient resource-intensive mapping requirements and maintenance
- Lack of alignment on terminology standards for nursing content definition
- Lack of customized development and implementation of EHR system
- Incomplete Electronic Documentation of Nursing Care

REVIEW QUESTIONS

Long Essays (10 Marks)
1. Write the meaning of knowledge management. Describe components and stages of knowledge management.
2. What is health care knowledge management? Describe benefits of knowledge management in health care.
3. Explain the role of knowledge management in improving decision-making in clinical context.
4. What is standardized clinical terminology? Describe the benefits of terminology standards.
5. Narrate common terminology standards used in health information and technology.
6. Describe ANA recognized standard nursing terminology.
7. Explain the implications of standardized language for nursing education, research and administration.

Short Essays (5 Marks)
1. What are the key concepts in knowledge management?
2. Describe the process of knowledge management.
3. Explain the process of knowledge management.
4. Describe the modalities of healthcare knowledge management.
5. Explain the relationship between knowledge management and nursing care performance.
6. Narrate barriers of knowledge management in health care.
7. Classification of healthcare terminology standards.
8. Explain international classification for nursing practice.
9. Describe NANDA-I.

Short Answers (2 Marks)
1. What is knowledge management?
2. What is health care knowledge management?
3. Goals of health care knowledge management
4. List types of healthcare knowledge
5. LOINC
6. RxNorm
7. ICD10
8. CCC
9. List the issues related to using standardized language in nursing

MULTIPLE CHOICE QUESTIONS

1. _____ knowledge management is embedded in rules, systems, policies and procedures of the organization.
    a. Explicit knowledge management
    b. Implicit knowledge management
    c. Systematic knowledge management
    d. Continuous knowledge management

2. Following are all components of knowledge management, except:
    a. Technology
    b. Process
    c. People
    d. Organization

3. Which of the following is a raw form of information?
    a. Information
    b. Knowledge
    c. Data
    d. Knowledge management

4. When raw data is analyzed and summarized it is called as
    a. Data
    b. Knowledge
    c. Information
    d. Decision

5. Information is interpreted and reviewed to generate _____
   a. Data
   b. Information
   c. Knowledge
   d. Wisdom

6. In which of the following stages of knowledge management does information transform to knowledge?
   a. Collection stage
   b. Organization stage
   c. Summarizing stage
   d. Synthesizing stage

7. Patient knowledge includes _____
   a. Health status of the patient
   b. Theories about health care
   c. Care delivery resources
   d. Care pathways

8. Which of the following includes medical knowledge?
   a. Health status of the patient
   b. Theories about health care
   c. Care delivery resources
   d. Care pathways

9. Which of the following includes resource knowledge?
   a. Health status of the patient
   b. Theories about health care
   c. Care delivery resources
   d. Care pathways

10. Which of the following includes process knowledge?
    a. Health status of the patient
    b. Theories about health care
    c. Care delivery resources
    d. Care pathways

11. Which of the following terminology facilitates the electronic documentation of nursing care plans?
    a. Clinical care classification system
    b. Health care common procedure coding system
    c. RxNorm
    d. Logical observation identifiers names and codes

ANSWER KEY

| 1. a | 2. d | 3. c | 4. c | 5. c | 6. d | 7. a | 8. b | 9. c | 10. d |
| 11. a | | | | | | | | | |

E-Health: Patients and the Internet

UNIT 7

INTRODUCTION

India's rapidly growing population has increased nearly four times since it gained independence in 1947. Being a developing country with most of the population falling under the lower-middle income group, it currently faces a shortage of doctors, nurses, midwives, and healthcare infrastructure. The existing health care facilities and health care personnel are inadequate to cater to the health care needs of the entire population. Hence, a demand-supply gap is prevailing in the country. Around 70% of the Indian population lives in remote and rural areas lacking access to basic healthcare facilities. This includes less number of primary care doctors practicing in rural and semi-urban areas.

A study of the Indian Pharma Industry has estimated that the penetration of modern medicine in the country is limited to only 30% of the entire population. Many conditions remain untreated or are managed with prescription medicines purchased over the counter or by faith healers. In such situations there is significant potential for e-health to deliver cost-effective and quality health care. In a bid to provide affordable healthcare to the poorest people and bridge the rural-urban health gap successive governments in India are spending on e-health systems.

Meaning and Definitions

- e-Health is an emerging concept in the field of medical informatics and public health. It refers to health services and health-related information delivered or enhanced through the internet and related technologies.
- e-Health refers to using information and communication technology (ICT) such as computers, mobile phones, and satellite communications for health services and information (United Nations Foundation).
- e-Health is the transfer of health resources and health care by electronic means. Healthcare is supported by electronics, informatics, and telecommunications.
- e-Health can be defined as the delivery of health care using modern electronic information and communication technology when health care providers and patients are not directly in contact and their interaction is mediated by electronic means.
- e-Health is the cost-effective and secure use of information and communication technologies in support of health and health-related fields, including healthcare services, health surveillance, health literature and health education (WHO).

Concepts

- e-Health is described as the use of electronic information and communication technology in healthcare sector.

- e-Health illustrates the technical progress to expand health care locally, country wide and universally by using information and communication technology.
- e-Health encompasses all sorts of electronic health data exchange such as tele-medicine, tele-health, etc.
- e-Health includes communication with health care professionals via email, accessing medical records and research health information, etc.
- e-Health is the delivery of health care using modern electronic information and communication technologies. This approach is used when health care providers and patients are not directly in contact and their interaction is mediated by electronic means.
- This approach to health care is increasingly being employed in geographically extended areas where the availability of health care is severely reduced or non-existent and when appropriate qualified medical personnel are not available.
- Services included in this form of approach include physical and psychological diagnosis and treatment, telepathology, vital signs monitoring, electronic prescribing, teleconsultation, etc.
- It includes forms of prevention and education, diagnostic, therapy, and care delivery through digital technology independent of time and place.
- It includes telemedicine, mHealth, telecare, ePublic health, eMental health or telehealth.
- It is a kind of blended care where conventional care is combined with online interventions.
- e-Health mainly focuses on self-care, self-management, and patient participation.
- It focuses on prevention, health education, health care innovations, and curbing rising expenditure.
- e-Health has a goal of providing quality life by uplifting the healthcare system.
- Digital health is an umbrella term for e-Health, telehealth, etc. It has a goal of reaching highest possible people who need help via the digital channel. Digital health uses tools such as telemedicine and smartphone applications.
- Though both mHealth and e-Health perform similar functions and play a role in supporting healthcare with electronics, the primary difference between them is the means by which information is provided.
- mHealth is an abbreviation for mobile health, which utilizes mobile devices such as cell phone or a tablet to support health care practices. With mHealth services, patients are able to log, store and monitor their health records on their personal mobile devices. These applications are helpful in improving the efficiency of health care information delivery. mHealth applications can be helpful for researchers, practitioners, and patients use.
- e-Health consists of a much broader understanding of healthcare practices supported by electronic processes. It includes electronic health records, patient administration system, lab systems, and other records that cannot be stored within mobile health applications. e-Health carries a much broader definition than mHealth.
- Telehealth refers to both clinical and remote non-clinical services including providing of training and continued medical education for practitioners.
- Telemedicine solely refers to remote clinical services.

Core Areas of e-Health According to WHO

- Delivery of health information for health professionals and health consumers through internet and telecommunications.
- Using the power of information technology and e-commerce to improve public health services such as educating and training of health workers.
- Use of e-commerce and e-business in health systems management.

Goals of e-Health

Goals of e-Health are:
- To improve quality and efficiency in health care services
- To improve accessibility and capability of the health sector
- To reduce costs

Purposes of e-Health in India

e-Health can improve delivery of healthcare services and management of public health system. Ministry of Health and Family Welfare (MoHFW) is promoting e-Health, i.e., use of information and communication technology in the direction of making available services to citizens and citizens empowerment through information dissemination to bring about significant improvement in public healthcare delivery.

The main purpose of e-Health is to improve efficiency in health care delivery, extend healthcare to rural areas and provide better quality at low cost. The other purposes are:
- To ensure availability of services on a wider scale
- To provide healthcare services in remote and inaccessible areas through telemedicine
- To address the health human resource gap by efficient and optimum utilization of existing human resources
- To improve patient safety by accessing medical records and reducing healthcare costs
- To monitor geographically dispersed tasks
- To provide help in evidence-based planning and decision-making
- To improve efficiency in imparting training and capacity building

Characteristics of e-Health

The 'e' in the e-Health not only means 'electronic' but represents a number of e's that characterizes what e-Health is all about. The characteristics of e-Health are as follows (Box 7.1):

> **Box 7.1: Characteristics of e-Health**
> - Efficiency
> - Enhances quality
> - Evidence based
> - Empowerment of consumers and patients
> - Encouragement
> - Education
> - Enables information exchange and communication
> - Extends scope
> - Ethics
> - Equity

- **Efficiency:** One of the main benefits of e-Health is to improve efficiency in health care thereby reducing costs. This can be achieved by avoiding unnecessary duplication or unnecessary diagnostic or therapeutic interventions through enhanced communication possibilities between health care establishments and patient involvement.
- **Enhances quality:** Increasing efficiency includes improving quality. e-Health may enhance the quality of health care by allowing comparisons between different providers, involving consumers as additional power for quality assurance and directing streams to the best quality providers.
- **Evidence based:** e-Health interventions are evidence-based in the sense that their effectiveness and efficiency should not be assumed but proven by rigorous scientific assessment and evaluation.
- **Empowerment of consumers and patients:** By making the knowledge bases of medicine and personal electronic records accessible to consumers over the internet, eHospitals not only open new avenues for patient-centered medicine, but also enable evidence-based patient choice.
- **Encouragement:** Patient participation is encouraged through more proactive care. e-Health provides encouragement for a new link between the patient and the health expert, and towards a true co-operation where choices are made mutually.

- **Education:** Physicians are educated and consumers provided with health education and preventive information online. This provides a platform to expand knowledge through information.
- **Enables information exchange and communication:** e-Health enables information exchange in a standardized way between health care establishments. It also creates an environment for easier exchange of information and easy communication between the consumer and the service provider.
- **Extends scope:** Through e-Health the scope of health care is extended beyond its conventional boundaries in both geographical and conceptual sense. e-Health enables consumers to easily obtain health services online from global providers. These services can range from simple advice to more complex interventions or pharmaceutical products.
- **Ethics:** e-Health involves new forms of patient-physician interaction thereby posing new challenges and threats to ethical issues such as online professional practice, informed consent, privacy and equity issues.
- **Equity:** Making health care more equitable is one of the promises of e-health. However, at the same time there is a considerable threat that e-health may deepen the gap between the 'haves' and 'have-nots'. Underprivileged people who lack money, skills, and access to computers and networks cannot use computers effectively. Such patient populations are least likely to benefit from advances in information technology unless political measures ensure equitable access for all. The digital divide currently runs between rural vs urban populations, rich vs poor, young vs old, male vs female people, and between neglected/rare vs common diseases.

Benefits of e-Health

Improper functioning of the three-tier health care delivery, and inaccessibility of secondary and tertiary government health services are the major hurdles in effective health care utilization. The use of technology offers tremendous opportunity for developing countries like India to advance in health care delivery by utilizing the scarce resources effectively. The vastly underserved health care market combined with high mobile phone penetration and rapidly growing smartphone adoption creates an enabling environment condition for e-Health adoption in India. As developing countries are confronted with health-related problems, e-Health is an opportunity for marked improvement in the field of public sector health care. Various benefits offered by e-Health are presented in **Box 7.2**.

> **Box 7.2: Benefits of e-Health**
> - Improves patient monitoring
> - More informed patients
> - Provides insight
> - Encourages healthy habits
> - Easier decision-making for healthcare professionals
> - More accessible and equal health care
> - Reduces medical errors
> - Helps to create more efficient hospitals and health clinics
> - Ensures cost effective care
> - Saves time
> - Accomplishes health priorities
> - Lowers administrative burden

- **Improves patient monitoring:** Technology enables easy monitoring of patient conditions with an option to record their progress in real-time. Patient information can be communicated easily, thereby bridging the gap between health care providers and patients.
- **More informed patients:** Through ICT, patients can access guide books and self-practice manuals from reliable sources. This allows the patients to make better decisions as they have the power to manage their own health.
- **Provides insight:** Digital healthcare environment provides patients a greater insight into their health. This gives them

an opportunity to gain greater control over their own health.

- **Encourages healthy habits:** People can download health-related apps and keep a track of their walking, eating, and sleeping habits. This encourages a healthier lifestyle among the entire population which may include increasing physical activity, better nutrition, avoiding risks, and wider use of preventive care.
- **Easier decision-making for healthcare professionals:** ICT aids in detection of illness at an early stage. It also aids in identifying optimal treatment more easily.
- **More accessible and equal health care:** Access to health is no longer limited by time and space. More equal opportunities are being provided to everyone.
- **Reduces medical errors:** e-Health allows healthcare providers to work more effectively, determine the right treatment more quickly and avoid mistakes.
- **Helps to create more efficient hospitals and health clinics:** e-Health streamlines the health system, minimizes human errors, and cuts administrative costs. It provides better care by improving all aspects of patient care including safety, effectiveness, patient-centeredness, communication, education, timeliness, efficiency, and equality. Communication is much easier as it bridges the gap between the patient and the health service provider.
- **Ensures cost effective care:** e-Health ensures cost-effective care by reducing paperwork, duplication of cost, unnecessary travel, etc.
- **Saves time:** e-Health provides quick access to patient records and information for efficient health care. Patients can have online consultations or even schedule their personal visits. This reduces wastage of time.
- **Accomplishes health priorities:** e-Health is crucial in accomplishing health priorities which include universal health coverage and sustainable developmental goals.
- **Lowers administrative burden:** Reduces paperwork, permits sharing of information securely and easily with colleagues.

Limitations/Barriers and Challenges

- Due to poor digital literacy and trouble in learning and using software, available information can be difficult to access and understand
- Shortage of IT and clinical resources, and skilled personnel for the use of technology
- Financial constraints, additional cost for getting internet connectivity
- Ethical issues such as lack of privacy, security and confidentiality
- Unsuited services, unavailability or lack of basic electronic services and infrastructure in remote areas
- Additional workload
- Time-consuming to bring electronic health records up-to-date

Facilitators for Using e-Health Services

- Improved communication
- Improved motivation
- Need to be integrated into routine care
- Involvement of all the stakeholders in implementation
- Having user-friendly software
- Easy-to-use services
- Utilization of available services

USE OF INFORMATION AND COMMUNICATION TECHNOLOGY (ICT) TO IMPROVE PERSONAL AND PUBLIC HEALTH

The use of ICT in health is defined as e-Health. It encompasses broader concepts like mHealth, telemedicine, health information system, electronic health records, etc. ICT has a great potential to improve the quality of health services in the country as it provides a pathway for accessing health information and efficient health services.

Use of ICT in Health Care

The emerging role of ICT has created a huge impact on health care. It enhances quality of care, improves patient security and data protection, and reduces operating and

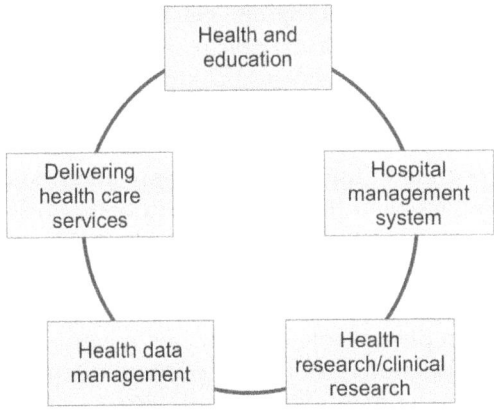

Fig. 7.1: Use of ICT in health

administrative costs. With telecommunication devices becoming more user-friendly and being used by a large section of the population, communication gap has been bridged to an appreciable extent. Accessibility to information has become simpler by use of ICT making the end user feel more relaxed while availing the healthcare services. The use of ICT in health can be categorized into five main streams which include (Fig. 7.1):

1. **Health and education:** ICT makes education accessible and available meaning people can seek, learn and communicate with others easily in a short span of time. Health education creates awareness among the public about communicable and non-communicable diseases, preventive measures, and available diagnostic and therapeutic interventions. This provides them the liberty to choose among the best hospitals and doctors for treatment and live their life in a healthy way.

2. **Hospital management system:** Hospital management system is a computer system that enables hospitals to manage information and data related to all aspects of healthcare-processes, providers, patients thereby ensuring completion of processes swiftly and effectively. The hospital database management has greatly evolved since its introduction in 1960, with an ability to integrate the existing facilities, technologies, software and systems in a hospital. ICT helps the hospital management in the following areas:
   - Improve patient safety and satisfaction
   - Get updated with latest technology
   - Gain knowledge of population health and statistics
   - Strengthen the work force

3. **Health research/clinical research:** It refers to research related to learning more about human health. It aims to find better ways to prevent and treat diseases. ICT in health care research helps in finding possible preventive measures to eradicate and reduce spread of diseases. Research enables invention of new technology which can limit the spread of diseases. This saves lives of many individuals by providing treatment in advance.

4. **Health data management:** Health care data management is the compilation of patient data from multiple sources across providers and organizations. The fundamental use of ICT in hospitals is the electronic storage of medical data. It allows health care providers to enter patient information into a singular database where it can be securely stored, analyzed and shared. Through ICT data can be transferred to both patients and doctors. While patients can have immediate access to medical records for use anywhere and anytime, doctors can use them for consultation purposes. Electronic health records have made it possible to digitize paper health records thus making health care delivery quick, coordinated, transparent and secure.

ICT offers various ways to improvise the healthcare system. Intelligent use of ICT can bring about greater changes in the health care system and elevate it to the next level thereby playing an important role in country's development.

5. **Delivering health care services:** With the advancement of telemedicine and tele-counselling it is now possible to deliver health care services in rural and remote areas of the country. Health information

systems have made it possible to monitor health data in real time.

Activities covered under e-Health in India

Government of India has been increasingly focusing on e-Health to bring about improvement in Indian Public health care delivery by progressively using information and communication technology under the overall objective of digital India. Core activities covered under e-Health are:
- Supporting the use of information and communication technology in health development.
- Providing supervision and technical provision to member states for incorporating e-Health solutions through a synchronized, multi-stakeholder and multi-sector approach.
- Monitoring the developments to notify policy and practice and report frequently on the use of e-Health in the region.
- Support multi-sectoral partnership and management between diverse organizations.

e-Health activities are carried out through national health portal, online services, hospital information system, e-office, telemedicine, etc. (**Fig. 7.2**).

e-Health Government-led Initiatives in India

The Indian Ministry of Health and Family Welfare, Ministry of Communication and Information Technology as well as certain state governments and the Indian Space Research Organization (ISRO) are playing a significant role in the development of e-Health in India.

The National Informatics Center is a premier information Technology Organization of the Indian Union Government in Informatic Services and Information and Communication technology application. NIC is a part of Ministry of Electronics and Information Technology, Government of India. It is playing a pivotal role in steering e-governance applications in the governmental departments at national, state and district levels across the country, enabling the improvement in government services. Almost all Indian-government websites are developed and managed by NIC.

To steer 'digital India' ahead, MoHFW has taken up various e-Gov initiatives in Health care sectors in India. The division is named as e-Health division.

e-Health initiatives have a vision to deliver better health outcome in terms of:
- Access
- Quality
- Affordability
- Lowering of disease burden
- Efficient monitoring of health entitlements to citizens
- The scope of these initiatives is to make all medical facilities available at all times from any part of the world through Web service, mobile services, SMS or call center services. Main intention is to cover online medical consultation, online medical records, online medicine supply management and pan-India exchange of patient information.

Some of the initiatives led by ministry and State Government are as follows:
- **The India health Information Network Development (I-HIND):** I-HIND is a web-based network connecting all health care establishments in both public and private sectors.
- **National Health Portal:** In order to create awareness about health care among the Indian population, the Ministry of Health

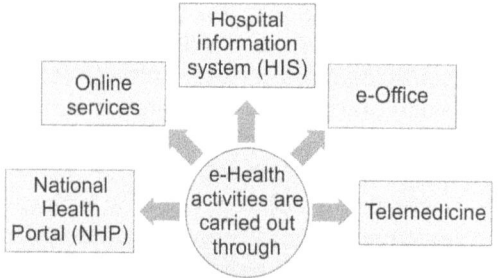

Fig. 7.2: Activities carried out through e-Health in India

and Family Welfare is creating the first national portal on health which will be a reference source for information on health issues, treatment centers and other vital information.
- **Health literacy program:** The Ministry is working on a health care literacy or education program for health care service providers in rural areas. It includes skill development programs for health care workers such as ASHA workers, community workers and support staff at Primary Health Center (PHCs).
- **Electronic health cards:** Government is taking the initiative of providing health card to every child in the country as a birth certificate to capture the individual's health records from the time of birth itself.
- **Electronic health records:** MoHFW has envisaged the establishment of a system where electronic health records of all citizens will be created, made available and accessible online to facilitate continuity of care.
- **Hospital Information System (HIS):** HIS is being implemented for computerized registration and capturing EHRs of patients in public health facilities up to PHC level. HIS implementation will be done as follows:
    - *e-Hospital:* National Informatics center (NIC) has developed the eHospital project with a vision to improve the delivery of hospital health care services to citizens across the country. It is implemented in many hospitals. The modules of eHospital includes; patient registration, billing and accounts, radiology/imaging, blood bank management, OT management, pharmacy management, electronic medical records, birth and death registrations, store and inventory, dietary services, laundry services and personal management.
    - *E-Sushrut:* A hospital information system (HIS) has been developed with the objective of streaming the treatment flow of a patient in the hospital.
- **Integrated disease surveillance program:** This network connects all district hospitals and medical college hospitals within a state to facilitate teleconsultation, tele-education, training of health professionals, and monitoring of disease trends.
- **National cancer network:** It has been implemented by connecting 25 regional cancer centers with peripheral hospitals for facilitating the National Cancer Control Program.
- **My health record:** It provides a single online personal medical record storage platform to citizens of India enabling them to manage their own medical records in a centralized way. My health record can be accessed from anywhere and anytime by both patients and physicians alike.
- Other initiatives include a teleophthalmology project, a national telemedicine grid, a national OncoNET project, a National medical College Network and National Digital Medical Library Consortium. The Ministry of Communication and Information Technology in collaboration with the state governments has established more than 75 nodes all over India. One of these nodes is the telemedicine network in West Bengal for diagnosis and monitoring of tropical diseases.
- The state government of Rajasthan in collaboration with ISRO has established a telemedicine network which not only connects medical colleges and district hospitals but also six mobile vans outfitted with e-Health equipment.
- The state government of Karnataka has formed an autonomous trust to run 'The Karnataka State Telemedicine Network Project'. It has set up about 30 nodes till date.
- The Government of India, in a joint initiative with the African Union launched the Pan-African e-network project to support tele-education, telemedicine, e-governance, infotainment, resource-mapping and meteorological services. The project connects the nodal centers in India

with 53 nations in Africa through the use of electronic ICT to provide telemedicine to its African counterparts.

Online Services

- **Online Registration System (ORS):** It is a framework to link various hospitals for online registration, payment of fee and appointment, online diagnostic reports, etc. As on date many hospitals are on board ORS.
- **MeraAspatal (patient feedback system):** It is an IT based feedback system to collect information on patients' level of satisfaction.

Online Consultation-Telemedicine

- **National Medical College Network (NMCN):** It is established with the purpose of providing e-Education and e-Healthcare delivery, wherein 50 Government Medical Colleges are being interconnected. Facilities included at these centers are:
    - State-of-the-art digital lecture theater with integrated 3D projection
    - Telemedical video collaborative environment
    - Centralized multipoint control unit
    - Centralized web casting/streaming solution
- **National Telemedicine Network:** It provides telemedicine services to remote areas by upgrading existing Government healthcare facilities such as medical colleges, district hospitals, primary health care centers and community health centers.
- **Teleradiology (NIC-Delhi):** CORS (CollabDDS Online Radiology Services) is a web interface among different health communities for resolution of radiological and dental issues. The main objective of this project is to provide online radiology interpretation of reports and continue medical education for medical officers in an effort to lessen the lack of radiologists at primary health care institutions. CORS is accessible to local as well as remotely situated doctors for seeking guidance from expert radiologists. Using CORS, doctors can either upload patient information to experts or even conduct real-time collaboration with them.
- **SATCOM based Telemedicine nodes at pilgrim places:** Telemedicine nodes at pilgrimage places has been envisaged using Space Technology Tools for telemedicine facility. Through this program specialty consultation is provided to the devotees visiting the following places:
    - Kashi Vishwanath Temple, Varanasi (UP)
    - Maa Vindhyavasini Mandir, Vindhyachal Dham, Mirzapur (UP)
    - Sheshnag, Amarnath Pilgrimage (J&K)
    - Pampa Hospital, Ayyappa Temple at Sabarimala, Kerala

    Tele-consultation can be obtained from any of the superspecialty nodes setup across the country such as PGIMER (Chandigarh), SGPGI (Lucknow), AIIMS (Delhi), JIPMER (Puducherry), etc.
- **JIPMER BIMSTEC-Strengthening regional health care:** The aim of JIPMER Bay of Bengal Initiative for Multi-sectoral Technical and Economic Cooperation (BIMSTEC) telemedicine network is to improve regional cooperation in the field of healthcare by strengthening Telemedicine based patient care services and sharing medical knowledge among BIMSTEC countries.
- **Tele-evidence:** Tele-evidence is a modality that allows doctors to testify in the judicial process by utilizing the video conferencing facility without actually visiting the courts. The tele-evidence facility streamlines the process of doctors appearing in courts in response to summons thereby saving time.

Office Automation

- **E-Office:** In response to the long-felt need for efficiency in Government processes and service delivery mechanisms, MoHFW has initiated the implementation of e-office. It is done with the purpose of significantly improving the operational efficiency of the

Government by transitioning to a 'Paper Less Office'. This will not only reduce the processing delays but also establish transparency and accountability.
- **Video conferencing facility:** This has been implemented to:
  - Increase the efficiency of officers
  - Speeding up office procedures
  - Make work more collaborative
  - Discuss important matters irrespective of geographical locations

Center for Health Informatics

The Center for Health Informatics (CHI) has undertaken various activities relating to e-Governance/e-Health for improving the efficiency and effectiveness of healthcare system. Center for Health Informatics has developed portal/dashboards for the following projects.

- **Health and wellness centers (HWC):** The center for Health Informatics, MoHFW has implemented the project for monitoring Health and Wellness Centers (HWCs) under Ayushman Bharat Scheme.
- **CPHC-NCD (Comprehensive Primary Health care—Non-Communicable Disease) program:** For this project all the necessary infrastructure, software, sitting space, call center setup and other assistance will be provided by the MoHFW through CHI.
- **LaQshya:** It is an initiative intended to improve the quality of care in Labour Room and maternity operation theaters. CHI has developed a portal/dashboard for this program.
- **National program for health care for elderly (NPHCE):** CHI has developed a portal/dashboard for monitoring this program
- CHI is assisting Rashtriya Bal Swasthya Karyakram (RBSK) by making out-bound calls to beneficiaries.
- National Health Portal (NHP) (www.nhp.gov.in) was set up to improve health literacy and provide access to health services.
- **Pradhan Mantri Surakshit Matritva Abhiyan (PMSMA) (https://pmsma.nhp.gov.in):** CHI has developed PMSMA portal/dashboard and created a helpdesk for supporting the program.
- CHI has developed budget dashboards of MoHFW for tracking the budget provisions, allocations and expenditure.
- CHI has developed an online reporting mechanism for monitoring total number of digital and physical transactions for hospitals across the country.
- CHI tracks the progress and action taken to achieve the National Health Policy.
- CHI tracks the physical and financial progress of all AIIMS across the country.
- CHI has taken the following mHealth initiatives:
  - mCessation (Quit Tobacco) to reach out to tobacco users to quit tobacco use.
  - mDiabetes for creating awareness on healthy lifestyle, exercise and drugs.
  - CHI has developed and installed health information kiosks at various central and state government hospital premises for providing quality health-related information to all the citizens.
  - CHI has also involved in providing effective Cyber security in health, incidence response resolution and cyber crisis management.
  - Other initiatives include media campaigns and enabling digital payments.

e-Health infrastructure

For health care to reach the masses and support growing demand for healthcare services in India, e-Health's infrastructure needs to undergo drastic changes. The following infrastructure is required for e-Health:
- **Physical infrastructure:** It includes hospitals, clinics, doctors' offices, and community service centers.
- **Transport infrastructure:** The wired and wireless transport layer and its components such as transmission and networking equipment and handsets.

- **Digital infrastructure:** Enabling platforms and software solutions which enable standardized, media-rich data capability that can be accessed from remote locations. There is a wide range of available software applications, diagnostic devices, and content.
- **Human infrastructure:** Trained medical practitioners at all levels.
- **Policy infrastructure:** Ensuring a policy environment which provides rules for the exchange of information.

DIGITAL HEALTH SERVICES IN INDIA

Digital health refers to the use of information technology and communications to manage health and wellness. The key applications of digital health are presented in **Figure 7.3**.

Telemedicine

It is the use of telecommunications technology to provide health care. It provides health care services remotely. *'Tele'* is a Greek word meaning 'distance' and *'mederi'* a Latin word meaning 'to heal and become a whole'.

Definitions

- **Telemedicine:** Telemedicine is 'the delivery of healthcare services where distance is a critical factor, by all healthcare professionals using information and communication technologies for the exchange of valid information for diagnosis, treatment and prevention of disease and injuries, research and evaluation and for the continuing education of healthcare providers, all in the interest of advancing the health of individuals and their communities (WHO)'.
- **Telehealth:** Telehealth is the use of electronic information and telecommunication technologies to support long-distance clinical healthcare, patient and professional health-related education and training, public health and health administration.
- **Telemedicine consultation center (TCC):** Telemedicine consultation center refers

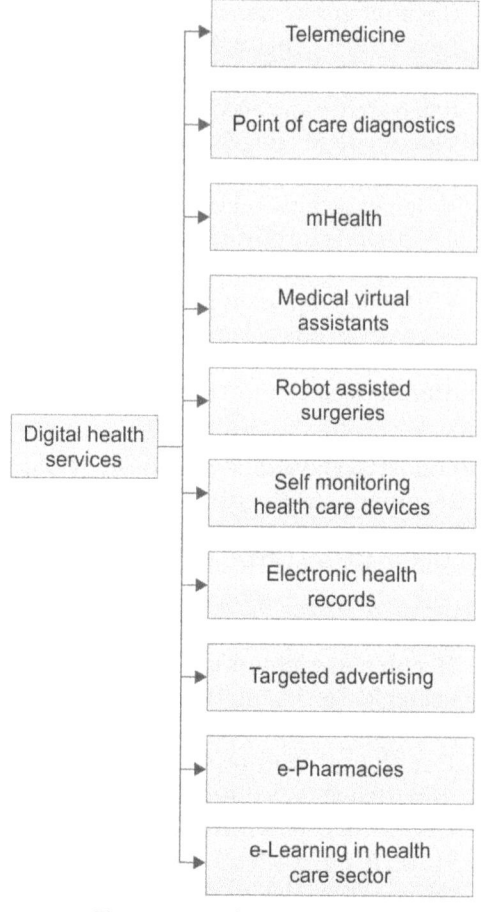

Fig. 7.3: Digital health services

to the site where the patient is present. In a telemedicine consultation center, equipment for scanning/converting, transformation and communicating the patient's medical information is available.
- **Telemedicine specialty center (TSC):** Telemedicine specialty center refers to the site where the specialist is present. He can interact with a patient present in a remote location, view his reports and monitor his progress.
- **Telemedicine system:** It consists of an interface between hardware, software and a communication channel to eventually bridge two geographical locations for exchange of information and enabling tele-consultancy between the two locations.

Current Scenario of Telemedicine in India

- Telemedicine services in our country come under the combined jurisdiction of Ministry of Health and Family Welfare and the Department of Information Technology.
- The Telemedicine division of MoHFW, GOI has set up a National Telemedicine Portal for implementing telemedicine.
- To ensure safe data transmission during telemedicine practices, MoHFW developed a set of Electronic Health Record standards in 2013 which was later revised in 2016. Telemedicine practices in India have been extended to the fields of traditional medicine.
- The National Rural AYUSH Telemedicine Network aims to promote the benefits of traditional methods of healing to a larger population through telemedicine.
- **Village Resource Center (VRC):** The VRC concept has been developed by ISRO to provide a variety of services such as tele-education, telemedicine, interactive farmers' advisory services, tele-fishery, e-governance services, weather services, and water management. VRC provides connectivity to specialty hospitals and brings the services of expert doctors to the villages.
- **AROGYASREE:** This project is the initiative of Indian Council of Medical Research. It is an internet-based mobile telemedicine service that integrates multiple hospitals, mobile medical specialists and rural mobile units or clinics to provide telemedicine services.

Types of Telemedicine Applications

Three basic types of telemedicine are presented in **Figure 7.4**:

1. **Store and forward or asynchronous telemedicine:** Here the sender takes information or digital image, stores the information and sends it to the receiver through a computer. The receiver can review the data according to his convenience. It is used in non-emergency situations where

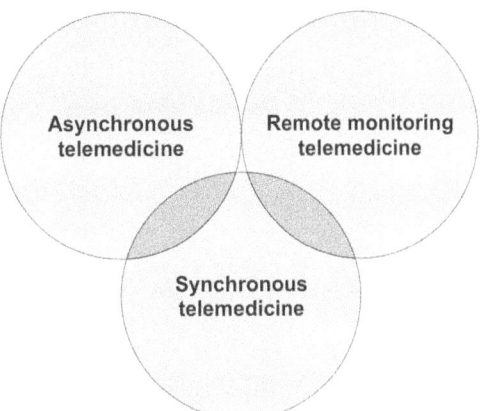

Fig. 7.4: Types of telemedicine applications

consultation is made in the next 24 to 48 hours and sent back. Teleradiology, telepathology and teledermatology are a few examples.

2. **Real time or synchronous telemedicine:** Here both the sender and the receiver are online at the same point of time enabling live transfer of information. It is used when face-to-face consultation is required. The patient or nurse practitioner or telemedicine coordinator is present at the original site while the specialist is present at the referral site which is mostly an urban medical center. Videoconferencing equipment at both locations allows a real-time consultation to take place. All specialties of medicine are conducive to this kind of consultation.

3. **Remote monitoring telemedicine:** Here technological devices are used to monitor health and clinical signs of a patient remotely.

Telemedicine centers are placed in primary health care centers, secondary health care centers and tertiary health care centers.

Application of Telemedicine in Public Health

Over the past several decades the use of wireless broadband technology has become more advanced and cell phone and internet use universal. Patient education with images and videos, transfer of medical images like

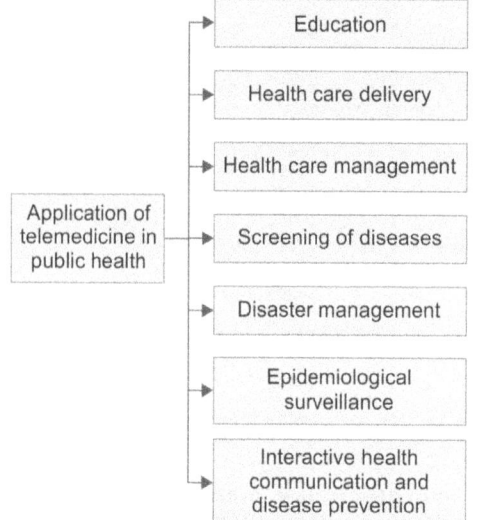

Fig. 7.5: Application of telemedicine in public health

X-rays and scans, real-time audio and video consultations became a reality. Improvement in internet infrastructure made telemedicine stress free and cost-effective. The use of existing computing devices, smartphone cameras, and wearable biosensors has made adoption and practice of modern-day telemedicine manageable and convenient. It does not require any form of training too. The core application of telemedicine is presented in **Figure 7.5**.

- **Education:** It includes tele-education, teleconferencing and tele-proctoring. Through tele-education and distance learning, training can be provided to rural health care professionals. Tele-proctoring uses telemedicine technology to provide surgical oversight from a remote expert surgeon to an on-site surgeon. In a teleconference, meeting among health care professionals occurs through telecommunication where they discuss and interact among themselves.
- **Health care delivery:** Telemedicine allows remote health services to reach needy people through mobile health clinics.
- **Health care management:** Telemedicine is used in preventive and promotive health care services. It includes tele-consultation and tele-follow up services.
- **Screening of diseases:** Telemedicine is used in screening diseases. For, e.g., diabetic screening project, ophthalmology screening, etc.
- **Disaster management:** Portable telemedicine system with satellite connectivity and customized telemedicine software is useful during a disaster period as all other modes of connectivity are disrupted.
- **Epidemiological surveillance:** Geographic Information System (GIS) provides the basic architecture and analytical tools to perform spatial-temporal modeling of climate, environment and disease transmission. It
  - Helps in understanding the spread of vector-borne diseases
  - Provides new insights into geographical distribution and gradients in disease prevalence and incidence
  - Provides valuable insight into population health assessment
  - Provides valuable information of different populations at risk based on risk factor profiles
  - Helps in differentiating and delineating risk factors in the population
  - Plays a pivotal role in anticipating epidemics
  - Is an essential tool in real-time monitoring of diseases
- **Interactive health communication and disease prevention:** Information technology and telemedicine can be used to inform, influence and motivate individuals on health, health-related issues and adoption of healthy lifestyles. The various approaches are:
  - It can relay information to individuals as well as to the population as a whole.
  - It provides easy access to health for those living in remote areas.
  - It simplifies the health decision-making process between health care providers and individuals regarding prevention, diagnosis or management of

health conditions. This exposes the user to a broader choice base.
- It promotes and maintains healthy behavior in the community.
- It helps in information exchange and emotional support. Online internet applications enable individuals with specific health conditions, needs or issues to communicate with each other, share information and provide or receive emotional support.
- It promotes self-management of health problems.
- It is an important tool for evaluation and monitoring of health care services.

With the advent of telemedicine, distance is no longer a hurdle in providing healthcare to remote areas. Telemedicine services can now be made available to all irrespective of time, place, social status or gender.

Telemedicine programs are actively supported by the following organizations or agencies:
- Department of information technology
- Indian Space Research Organization
- NEC Telemedicine program for North-Eastern States
- Apollo Hospitals
- Asia heart Foundation
- State Governments

Challenges
- Financial unavailability
- Lack of basic amenities
- Patients' fear and unfamiliarity
- Lack of awareness among health professionals
- Technical constraints

Point-of-care diagnostics (POCD)
It is the emerging trend in medical device industry. Also known as remote testing, it includes a broad range of products such as biosensors, portable x-rays, handheld ultrasounds and smartphone based POCDs. These devices are generally automated technologies which run on artificial intelligence and machine learning algorithms that enable simplification of complex diagnostic procedures to provide immediate diagnostic results.

Advantages
- Enables accurate diagnostics in resource limited setting.
- Facilitates disease management, monitoring and real time diagnosis of diseases.
- Implantable such as sensors help with continuous monitoring of a particular health condition, which directly aids the medical decision-making of the patient.
- Enables physicians to provide telehealth services after diagnosis through POCD devices without requiring patients to physically travel and undergo diagnostic tests at medical facility.

mHealth
mHealth (Mobile health) is the provision of digital health services on a mobile platform. It is the use of mobile phones and other wireless technology in medical care.

Definitions
Use of mobile and wireless technologies to support the achievement of health objectives (WHO).

Use of mobile and wireless devices such as cell phones, tablets to improve health outcomes, health care services and health research (National Institute of Health).

Types of Apps
Apps are divided into three categories:
1. **Disease and treatment-related apps:** These apps support diagnosis and treatment, help in disease and epidemic outbreak tracking, remote monitoring of disease conditions, etc.
2. **Wellness management apps:** These apps help in fitness, lifestyle, diet, nutritions, and stress management.
3. **Other apps:** Apps related to communication and training of health care professionals, providing education and awareness, helpline, etc.

Application of mHealth in Public Health

mHealth is a set of apps, devices, connections that allow the user to be mobile. Various applications of mHealth are presented in **Figure 7.6**.

- **Remote monitoring:** Remote monitoring provides physicians with an early detection system thereby reducing the incidence of higher and more costly health care interventions, cost of transportation and time.
- **Remote consultation:** Healthcare apps assist in remote consultation and remote monitoring. Individuals with limited ability to travel to see a care provider and those living in rural areas are more benefited.
- **Interactive applications:** Use of interactive web applications tailored to specific conditions, applications related to tacking tools, automated alerts based on clinical conditions, medications, and treatment plans provide personalized health care.
- **E-mail exchange of information:** Physicians can send e-mail requests regarding follow-up care, prescription renewals, referrals, etc. This exchange of e-mails can strengthen the patient-physician relationship and engage the patient more fully in his or her care. This process strengthens the medical decision-making and self-management.
- **Teleconferencing:** Development of virtual care teams by conducting teleconferencing with primary care doctors, educators, caregivers, and family members.

Benefits

Major benefits of using mobile devices to educate consumers about preventive health services, disease surveillance, treatment support, epidemic outbreak tracking, and chronic disease management are:
- Convenience
- Increased access to health care
- Better outcome for patients
- Reduced cost of care
- Improved personalized health care
- Communication with the physician or care team without actual face-to-face meeting
- Secure messaging

Disadvantages

- Privacy policies such as data breach, privacy violation
- Inaccurate device measures resulting in generation of erroneous information

Medical Virtual Assistants

Virtual Medical Assistant (VMA) conducts administrative tasks to assist healthcare providers. A healthcare virtual assistant is an individual who works remotely and can help a healthcare provider with routine tasks such as managing the front office, setting appointments, patient engagements, etc. Virtual assistants work from a remote location without being physically present on the hospital premises. Development in technology with the advancement of high-speed internet has made it easier for many to work remotely.

Activities of Virtual Medical Assistant

The following administrative tasks are carried out by a virtual medical assistant (**Figure 7.7**):
- **Manages the practice calendar:** Creates a schedule that includes appointments in advance, cancellations and sending appointment reminders to patients with

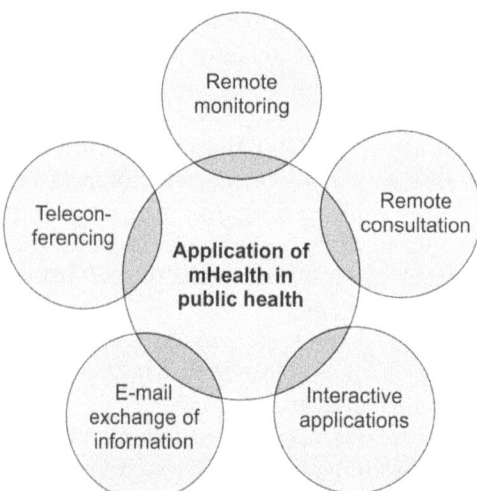

Fig. 7.6: Application of mHealth in public health

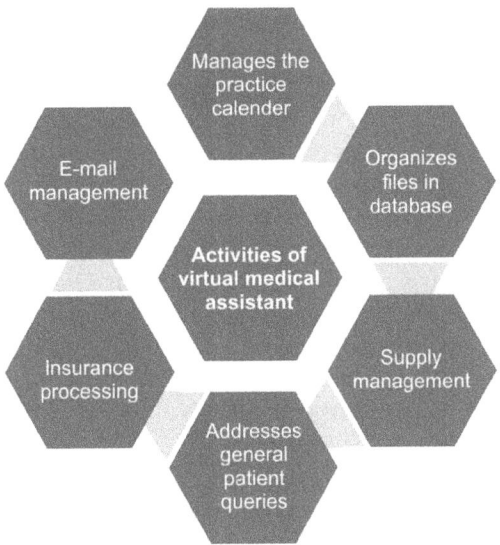

Fig. 7.7: Activities of virtual medical assistant

upcoming visits. It also fixes up meetings and events, manages follow-ups and checks on patients after appointments.
- **Organizes files in database:** VMA while tracking information of each patient also builds an accurate medical history for future diagnosis.
- **Supply management:** VMA keeps track of supplies at practice and orders new items when necessary.
- **Addresses general patient queries:** Responds to general patient queries related to administration such as payments, facilitates referrals or document transcripts.
- **Insurance processing:** VMA carries out pre-authorization of consultations with insurance or medical aid and completes the paperwork for claims.
- **E-mail management:** Manages the email inbox by clearing out emails and responding to messages.
- Other activities include medical billing and coding, prescription refills, transferring physical forms into a digital format.

Advantages
- Health care providers can focus on their jobs and improve skills in practice
- Healthcare providers can give quality care and spend time with patients
- Is cost effective as it saves on the cost of having a full time employee
- Improves patient satisfaction
- Improves workflow and practice is smooth

Virtual Assistant Technologies
- Automated calling systems and interactive voice response systems (IVRS)
- mHealth apps
- Health portals and health kiosks

Robot Assisted Surgery
Robotic surgery involves the use of a robotic surgical system to perform operations on patients. It can either be done solely or performed alongside traditional open surgical procedure. It uses highly advanced computer-controlled instruments to perform complex surgeries in a minimally invasive way that enhances the capabilities of surgeon's hands.

It allows surgeons to perform procedures in hard-to-reach areas through small incisions. Robotic surgical instruments make use of a laparoscopic approach with precision cutting instruments and 3-D visual cameras which enable or assist the surgeon in performing complex surgeries with an unobstructed view and precision. This specialized technology enhances magnification and enables precise movements. Surgeons require formal or special training through minimally invasive and robotic surgery fellowships.

Technology consists of
- **Patient cart:** Patient cart is kept next to the patient's bed where he is being operated upon. It holds the camera and the instruments that are required for the surgery. These include surgical arms with tiny instruments and wrists at the tip.
- **Vision cart:** It enables seamless communication between all the components.
- **Surgical console:** It is a place where the surgeon sits and controls the robot's arm movements throughout the surgery.

The computer console where the doctor is seated provides the surgeon with a high-definition, magnified, 3D view of the surgical site.

These components work together in allowing the surgeon to view what is happening, then mimic the movements to guide the instruments.

Common Surgical Procedures Carried Out with Robotic Assistance

Robot surgery is commonly used by urologists, gynecological surgeons, general surgeons, and colorectal surgeons. Robotic surgery may be used for the following surgical procedures:
- Coronary artery bypass
- Cutting away cancer tissue from sensitive parts of the body such as blood vessels, nerves, etc.
- Gallbladder removal
- Hip replacement
- Hysterectomy
- Total or partial kidney removal
- Kidney transplant

Robotic Surgery Procedure

- Surgeon makes one or more small incisions
- Ports (thin tubes) are placed through these incisions
- A robot is attached to these ports and instruments placed through them
- A long thin camera (endoscope) is placed through one of the ports
- The camera provides high-definition images in 3D during the surgery
- Surgical instruments are placed through other ports which allow the surgeon to perform the operation
- Surgeon controls the robotic arm while sitting at the console
- The assistant stays next to the surgeon to help change the instruments when needed

Advantages

- Enables surgery through small incisions
- Better assistance in performing delicate surgeries
- **Precise and accurate surgeries:** The robotic arms' movements are more exact than a human hand. Range of motion is greater as the robotic arms rotate instruments in tight spaces in ways that otherwise are not possible.
- **Better visualization:** A sophisticated camera provides magnified high-definition views of the surgical area. It also has 3D capabilities for imaging that are superior to the naked eye.
- Faster recovery time
- Reduced loss of blood
- Less pain during recovery
- Lower risk of infection
- Shorter hospital stays
- Smaller scars

Disadvantages

- Only available in centers that can afford the technology and have specially trained surgeons
- Risk of nerve damage and compression

Future applications are capsule endoscopy wherein the patient swallows a tiny camera allowing the health care provider to take pictures of the digestive tract. Other applications are removing plaque from arteries, taking tissue biopsies, attacking cancerous tumors directly, and delivering targeted medicines.

Self-monitoring Health Care Devices

A rise in the prevalence of various chronic diseases coupled with greater awareness amongst the common people regarding self-monitoring health care devices has led to the use of these devices. Self-care monitoring devices are used for measuring and monitoring various vital parameters of a patient. These devices monitor blood sugar levels, heart rate, hypertension, and other conditions. These devices measure, monitor, display, and document physiological information at regular intervals via sensors or other input devices attached to the patient. Monitors and sensors are now being integrated into wearables which allow them to detect various physiological changes in the body such as tracking weight, sleep patterns, diet, and exercises. These devices detect various health problems besides alerting the users.

Advantages
- Assist in better patient compliance and disease management
- Portable and user-friendly devices are more likely to encourage patients to adopt a more active role in keeping track of their health

Commonly used self-monitoring health care devices include:
- Blood pressure monitors
- Body temperature monitors
- Cardiac arrhythmia devices
- Sleep apnea monitors
- Blood glucose monitors
- Pedometers

Electronic Health Record (EHR)
An EHR is a digital version of the patient's health record. EHRs help eliminate the problems associated with physical records such as loss and lack of accessibility. EHR can be stored centrally and accessed at any point of time irrespective of where or when the information is collected. EHRs enable doctors to view their patient's complete medical history even if they are treating the patient for the first time. This helps reduce duplication of tests and facilitates the secure exchange of information. This in turn helps the patient and health care facilities manage costs (Refer to Unit 4 for a detailed discussion on electronic health records).

e-Pharmacies
e-Pharmacy or online pharmacy is a pharmacy that operates over the internet and fulfills orders through mail, courier or delivery persons. Various models that have been adopted include online-only pharmacies and physical pharmacies with an online presence. Online pharmacies allow pharmacists to cater to a large group of patients as the inherent geographical restrictions on physical pharmacies are removed in the online mode.

e-Learning in the Healthcare Sector
Continuous medical education and continuous nursing education is a mandatory requirement under the regulation governing doctors and necessary for doctors and nurses to keep in touch with the current trends and developments in the field of medicine and nursing. e-Learning is a more convenient platform for healthcare professionals to attend such programs. e-Learning saves time and costs and is accessible from anywhere.

Targeted Advertising
Wearables (electronic devices designed to be worn on the user's body) and information provided by users generate information related to the user's medical history and health conditions. This information can be used by companies to provide targeted advertising of products to users who are more likely to purchase or use such products. For example, glucose monitoring products could be advertised to diabetic patients based on their medical history provided by them. Targeted advertising however throws up various legal and ethical issues.

AYUSHMAN BHARAT DIGITAL MISSION

In pursuance of the National Health Policy, 2017 MoHFW introduced the National Digital Health Mission (NDHM) on August 15, 2020 to create a digital health ecosystem. Later it was renamed as Ayushman Bharat Digital Mission (ABDM). It is now applicable nationwide for which participation is voluntary.

Aims
- Establish a federated health information architecture
- Establish a health information exchange
- Establish a national health information network by 2025

ABDM Components

Following are the main components of ABDM (Fig. 7.8):

- **Health ID:** Creation of a Digital Health ID for all citizens through which health data can be stored, accessed, and shared. This Health ID may be linked to Aadhaar and mobile number of the individual. The health ID will enable the individual to store all health-related information and records electronically and access it from anywhere irrespective of time and location. Additionally, sharing credentials of the health ID will allow healthcare professionals to access the health data and past records of the individual with consent.
- **Health facility registry:** Participating entities of the ABDM must first register as a healthcare provider. Both public and private health facilities such as hospitals, clinics, diagnostic laboratories, and imaging centers, pharmacies can register under the ABDM. Upon registration, policies under the ABDM shall be binding and the health facility shall digitize their systems accordingly. The list of registered entities is stored in a repository to help individuals find health services digitally and with ease.
- **Health care professional's registry:** In addition to the registration of facilities, individual healthcare providers may register themselves under the ABDM. Professionals involved in healthcare services, both modern and traditional can get online presence and visibility. Healthcare professionals who sign up to ABDM's registry can view patient's records online and also treat them online.
- **Health records:** Health records have been executed as a mobile application system to let individuals add and maintain their health data. The user can also share the data with doctors, healthcare facilities, and others.
- **Consent manager:** While exchange of health information is enabled by the consent manager, the gateway which supports health data accesses requests and manages the consent preferences of users of the ABDM interfaces.

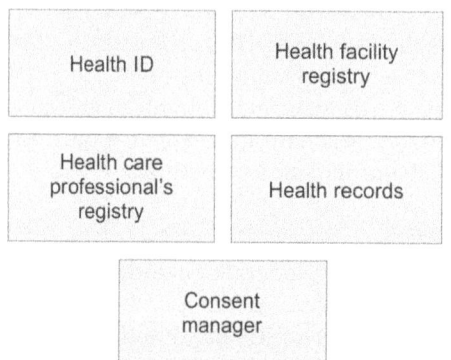

Fig. 7.8: Components of ABDM

PUBLIC HEALTH INFORMATICS

Public health informatics (PHI) uses information science and technology to improve health. The primary focus of public health informatics is the application of information science technology to promote the health of all populations, not just specific individuals.

Meaning and Definitions

- Public health informatics refers to using informatics in public health data collection, analysis, and actions.
- It is the systematic application of information, computer science, and technology in areas of public health including surveillance, prevention, preparedness, and health promotion.
- It is the application of informatics to public health practice intelligently and focused on preventive and promotive health.
- Public health informatics has been defined as the systematic application of information and computer science and technology to public health practice, research, and learning (Yasnoff et al., 2000).

Concepts of PHI

- It utilizes applications that prevent disease and possible injury by changing the environment or weakening the conditions that put large group of people at risk.

- It does not limit itself to particular contexts such as social, behavioral or environmental issues. Instead it considers how to effect prevention at all vulnerable points in the path of disease, disability or injury.
- It focuses on populations than individuals. The focus is on health of the community as opposed to that of the individual patient.
- It is oriented to prevention rather than diagnosis and treatment—prevention of spread of illness or even quarantining some individuals to protect others
- It is governmental in context, i.e., involves governmental agencies
- It requires the application of knowledge from numerous disciplines particularly information science, computer science, management, organizational theory, psychology, communications, political science, and law.
- ICT related tools such as Geographical Information System (GIS), telemedicine, patient's information system, decision support system, electronic health records (EHRs) form the basis of a public healthcare set up.
- The scope of PHI is conceptualization, design, development, deployment, refinement, maintenance and evaluation of communication, surveillance, and information system relevant to public health.

Principles of Public Health Informatics

There are four basic principles in public health informatics (**Fig. 7.9**):

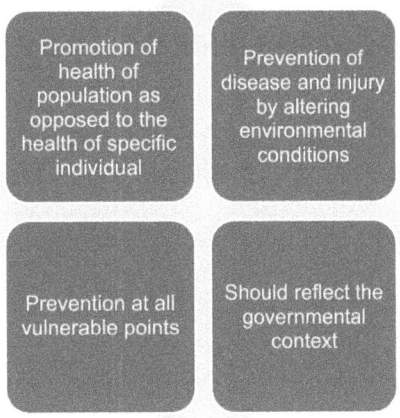

Fig. 7.9: Principles of public health informatics

1. **Promotion of health of population as opposed to the health of specific individual:** As a discipline, public health informatics should focus on the health of the population and the community as opposed to that of the individual patient. In a health care setting the major unit of attention is an individual with a specific disease or condition. In public health, consideration is for the community as the patient may require 'treatment' such as quarantine or disclosure of the disease status of an individual to prevent further spread of illness. It also requires attention to environmental factors such as water quality and automotive safety, etc. that affect the health risk of entire populations rather than specifically identifiable individuals.

2. **Prevention of disease and injury by altering environmental conditions:** Public health informatics should be on applications of information science and technology that prevent disease and injury by altering the conditions or the environment that put populations of individuals at risk. Traditional health care largely treats individuals who present with a disease, while public health seeks to avoid the conditions that led to the disease in the first place.

3. **Prevention at all vulnerable points:** Public health informatics applications should explore the potential for prevention at all vulnerable points in the causal chains leading to disease, injury, or disability. The applications should not be restricted to particular social, behavioral, or environmental contexts. Public health interventions should be cost-effective and acceptable to the people. Examples are vaccinations, solid waste disposal, wastewater treatment, smoke alarms, fluoridation of water, safe housing, etc.

4. **Should reflect the governmental context:** Public health informatics should reflect the governmental context in which public health is practiced. Much of public health operates through government agencies that require direct responsiveness to legislative, regulatory, and policy directives. In addition, some public health actions involve authority for specific measures to protect the community in an emergency. These include closing down a restaurant or contaminated pool or lake, changes to immunization policy, etc.

Scope of PHI

- Epidemiological disease surveillance, epidemic outbreak risk assessment
- Disaster management which includes preparedness, mitigation and response
- Provision of health care in remote areas and screening for diseases. Example, telecardiology, teleophthalmology, etc.
- Electronic medical records/electronic health records
- Updation of health statistics
- Education and training including continuing medical education for health care providers
- Development of decision support systems (DSS) for patients and health care providers
- Improving public health governance by providing greater accessibility of health services to remote areas
- Public health research

ICT Applications in Indian Public Health

The main objectives of PHI are:
- Promotion of health of the whole population which will ultimately promote the health of the individuals
- Prevention of diseases and injuries by changing the conditions that increase the risk for the population

ICT applications prevalent in Indian public health scenario at present are telemedicine, GIS, and EMRs.

Telemedicine

It is defined as the delivery of health care and exchange of health care information across a distance. It is an important domain of public health. The proven public health potentials of telemedicine are:
- Reduced distance and extra strain for rural habitants to travel to a super-specialty hospital in the city
- Cost reduction of treatment and follow-up
- Time saving and timely availability of expert medical services
- Improved prognosis on account of access to standard treatment
- Maintenance of data base with respect to various diseases and locations
- Remote training of medical students by experts in the field
- Updated health information for health care workers and patients
- Decreased response time during the management of epidemic/outbreak or a disaster
- Screening of diseases, e.g., rheumatic heart disease through telecardiology program, etc.

Major telemedicine service providers in India are:
- ISRO, Department of space
- Ministry of communications and information technology, Government of India
- Ministry of health and Family Welfare, GOI and State governments
- All India Institute of Medical Sciences
- Private sector. Example, Apollo Telemedicine Networking Foundation in South Asia; Narayana Hrudayalaya, Bengaluru; Arvind Eye Hospital, Madurai, etc.

Geographical Information System (GIS)

GIS uses map overlay techniques which view data pertaining to demographics, social infrastructure, health care institutions and patient's geo-positioned points. Public health applications of GIS include infectious disease surveillance and control especially the vector borne diseases to meet the demands of outbreak investigation and response, analyzing spatial and temporal trends, mapping populations at risk, stratifying risk factors, assessing resource allocation, planning and targeting interventions and monitoring diseases, and interventions over time.

Electronic Medical Record (EMR) and Electronic Health Record (EHR)

EMR is an electronic record of a specific health-related event of a person. EHR is the electronic record of a person which encompasses all health-related events from birth to till death (womb to tomb health record). Advantages of digitalization of an individual's health or medical record are:
- Helps in reduction of error in medical care
- Easy to maintain for a longer time
- Cost effective
- Easily accessible
- Improves efficiency of health care
- Helps in research

In India the use of EMR is limited to medical college institutions and corporate institutions. Some of the public health experiments in India are Personal Digital Assistants (PDAs) by rural health workers in Rajasthan, Disaster management project of Maharashtra Earthquake Rehabilitation Project, Maharashtra, computerized village offices in Andhra Pradesh and Puducherry.

Challenges

- Lack of technical standards
- Paucity of funds
- Lack of apt public health governance process
- Non-availability of trained manpower in remote rural areas for establishment and maintenance of ICTs required for public health informatics
- Difficulty in developing a coherent and integrated national public health information system
- Reluctance to use newer technology by health care providers
- Unfamiliarity with the use of newer technologies by health care professionals
- Privacy, security, and confidentiality issues

Process of Public Health Informatics

Public health informatics follows the below sequential process:
- Formulation of models for acquiring, representing, processing, displaying or transmitting health informatics
- Developing computer systems to deliver information
- Installing information technology systems
- Evaluating the outcome in terms of effects on overall health care system
- Major functions of public health informatics include electronic disease surveillance, e-registers, electronic lab reporting, early event detection, and program monitoring, and evaluation.

ROLE OF NURSE

Nurses have been working in the field of informatics for the past many decades. It is the application of information technology in nursing including education, management and practice.

Nursing Informatic Definitions

According to American Nurses Association (ANA), nursing informatics is a specialty that integrates nursing science, computer and information science to provide nursing care.

Nursing informatics is the integration of information technology and all aspects of nursing such as clinical nursing, management, research or education (Guenther & Peter, 2006).

Competencies Required for an Informatics Nurse

An informatics nurse should have computer skills, informatics knowledge and informatics skills.

Computer Skills

These include an ability to perform computerized searches and retrieving patient demographics data, use of telecommunication devices, digital documentation of patient care, use of information technologies for providing nursing care, safe use of networks and computer technology for providing nursing care.

Informatics Knowledge

These competencies include recognition of use of nursing data for improving practice, knowing the impact of computerized information management on the role of a nurse, determination of limitations and reliability of computerized patient monitoring systems.

Informatics Skills

- These competencies include interpretation of information flow within the organization, development of standards and database structures to facilitate clinical care, education, administration and research.
- It also includes the development of innovative and analytic techniques for scientific research in nursing informatics.

Responsibilities of a Nurse Informaticist (NI)

Nursing informatics is a combination of technology and patient care that acts as a bridge between a health care organization's system, its providers and clinical staff. With their specialized training both as a registered nurse and information technology specialist, nurse informaticists understand how all the pieces fit together and provide valuable input for system designing from a provider standpoint. Responsibilities however vary depending upon the organizational needs. The main responsibilities of a nurse informaticist are:

- **Educate staff on changes to electronic medical or health records:** The important role of a nurse informaticist is to educate the workforce about the reasons for using electronic health records and help the nursing workforce document and submit accurate data. NI develops the educational material and implements the educational sessions with regard to implementation of EMR.
- **Understand and communicate the need for nursing informatics:** Increased understanding improves nurses' confidence in the system's data. This knowledge helps the health care professionals understand how specific data play an important role throughout the care process and decision-making.
- **Implement new technology and processes:** Implementation of new technology creates a change in the clinical process. Without proper training, the implementation of new technology can fail to gain adoption. This results in compromised patient safety and team members getting frustrated. An effective nurse informaticist guides and educates the new process of implementation, ensures testing completion and provides hands-on training.
- **Provide support:** Nurse informaticist supports nurses, consumers, other health care team and stake-holders in their decision-making to achieve desired outcomes.
- **Improve workflow through communication and information technology:** Nurse informaticist works along with other health care team members and helps improve and develop health care technology. They bridge the gap between patient care and IT teams and provide a voice for clinicians.
- **Develop information systems based on current standards of care:** Nurse informaticists help ensure EHRs are optimally designed to fit the organization's workflow and easy for providers to use.

NI ensures the technology is compatible with practice guidelines. NI also helps in implementation of these systems and train professionals for effective use.
- **Ensure information systems remain updated:** NI retrieves and reviews information frequently to improve patient safety.
- **Develop evidence-based procedures for optimal care delivery:** NI conducts research to create new informatics knowledge for optimal care delivery.

REVIEW QUESTIONS

Long Essays (10 Marks)
1. Define e-Health and describe the characteristics and benefits of e-Health.
2. Describe the use of information and communication technology to improve personal and public health.
3. What is e-Health? Explain the various activities covered under e-Health in India.
4. Describe e-Health government-led initiatives in India.
5. What is digital health? Explain digital health services in India.
6. Write in detail on various telemedicine applications in public health and supported organizations for telemedicine program.
7. Explain in detail on application of mHealth in public health.
8. What are self-monitoring health care devices? Explain their advantages.
9. What are the aims and components of Ayushman Bharat digital mission.
10. Write a note on meaning, concepts, principles, scope and applications of public health informatics.

Short Essays (5 Marks)
1. What are the challenges in implementation of public health informatics in India?
2. Responsibilities of a nurse informaticist
3. Point-of-care diagnostics
4. List various types of apps used in health care
5. Concept of e-Learning in health care sector
6. Explain concepts of e-Health
7. Core areas of e-Health
8. What are the purposes of e-Health in India
9. Describe characteristics of e-Health
10. What are the challenges in implementation of e-Health
11. Use of ICT in health care
12. Write a note on e-Health infrastructure
13. What are the activities of virtual medical assistant
14. List common surgical procedures that are carried out with robotic assistance

Short Answers (2 Marks)
1. e-Health
2. m-Health
3. Telehealth
4. Telemedicine
5. What is EHR
6. Digital health
7. e-Pharmacies
8. Arogyasree
9. Medical virtual assistant

MULTIPLE CHOICE QUESTIONS

1. Which of the following denotes transfer of health resources and health care by electronic means?
   a. mHealth
   b. e-Health
   c. digital health
   d. telecommunication

2. In which of the following services are patients able to log, store and monitor their health records on their personal mobile devices?
   a. mHealth
   b. e-Health
   c. ePharmacy
   d. telecommunication

3. Which of the following includes both clinical and remote non-clinical services?
   a. mHealth
   b. e-Health
   c. telemedicine
   d. telehealth

4. Which of the following includes only clinical services?
   a. mHealth
   b. e-Health
   c. telemedicine
   d. telehealth

5. Which of the following is a major barrier in implementation of e-Health in India?
   a. Poor digital literacy
   b. Ethical issues
   c. More time consuming
   d. Added workload

6. Which of the following denotes tele-evidence?
   a. A modality via which doctors can testify in the judicial process
   b. Digital consultation can be obtained from any of the super specialty nodes
   c. Tele-medicine consultation can be provided to devotees visiting pilgrim places
   d. Tele medicine services to the remote areas

7. Which of the following digital health services uses mobile phones and other wireless technology in medical care?
   a. mHealth
   b. ePharmacy
   c. telemedicine
   d. telehealth

8. Which of the following apps helps in fitness, lifestyle, diet, nutrition and stress management?
   a. Treatment apps
   b. Wellness apps
   c. Diagnosis apps
   d. Communication apps

9. Which of the following is a benefit of medical virtual assistants?
   a. Conducts administrative tasks to assist healthcare providers
   b. Works in hospital with high-speed internet to help health care providers
   c. Assists doctors in providing care
   d. Assists nurses in providing care

10. Which of the following allows surgeons to perform procedures in hard-to-reach areas through small incisions?
    a. Button hole surgeries
    b. Endoscopic surgeries
    c. Robotic surgery
    d. High speed surgeries

11. All of the followings are self-monitoring health care devices except
    a. Blood pressure monitoring
    b. Pedometers
    c. Blood glucose monitors
    d. Optometry

ANSWER KEY

1. b	2. a	3. d	4. c	5. a	6. a	7. a	8. b	9. a	10. c
11. d									

Using Information in Healthcare Management

UNIT 8

INTRODUCTION

Most important premise in the current health environment is the use of information systems and technology to improve quality and safety of patient care. Many healthcare organizations are utilizing information technology to provide quality healthcare services to their patients. Nurses being a significant component of patient care, are recognized as one of the most important users of health information system. In recent years, nursing departments have begun using information technology for executing their daily tasks.

NURSING INFORMATION AND NURSING INFORMATION SYSTEM (NIS)

Meanings and Definitions

Nursing information includes data collected by nurses, data used by nurses, data about nursing activity and data about the nursing resources.

Nursing information system is a part of the healthcare information system that deals with nursing aspects, particularly the maintenance of the nursing record.

Nursing information system refers to the application of computer science and information science to manage operations involved in the nursing profession.

Nursing information systems are computer systems that manage clinical data from a variety of healthcare environments and made available in a timely and orderly fashion to aid nurses in improving patient care.

Purposes of Nursing Information System

Nursing information systems are stand-alone or divisions of hospital information system (HIS) that allow nurses to access clinical information to and from other healthcare providers. This information is used to better support nurses in their daily tasks. Purposes of nursing information system are:

- To make available relevant patient data in a useable form for extending comprehensive nursing care
- To process information for supporting management functions such as receiving and supplying data from departments, make policy and operating decisions, patient care decisions
- To provide a comprehensive automated information processing system for all phases of the nursing process. The introduction and development of this systems affects the overall processing of information in hospitals
- To provide better care to patients while exploring the possibility of assessment and exchange of clinical information with other healthcare providers

- To improve clinical data integrity and satisfy user needs
- To improve access to healthcare information, readability of nursing documents, avoidance of repetition while carrying out documentation, better support of workflow and greater compliance to the legalities
- To develop care plans for patients

Key Principles in Guiding Nursing Information System

The following principles provide basis for future development of computer systems that will support nurses in various activities:
- Information should be person-oriented.
- Information will be derived from operational systems.
- Information will be secure and confidential.
- Various systems should be integrated with each other.
- Information will be shared across the organization.

Components of Nursing Information System

Nursing profession depends on accurate and timely access to appropriate information for performing various professional activities related to patient and community care. Nursing information system integrates technical knowledge, quality control and, clinical and administrative services to patient care. Applications of NIS can be described under two major headings: clinical practice and nursing administration (**Fig. 8.1**).

Clinical Practice

Many new clinical practice devices and IT systems have been developed with an aim to improve patient care, some of which are described below:
- **Computerized care documentation:** This system allows the nurses to enter information about nursing care services delivered to a patient via a computer directly, with the major advantage being that the entry can be done from anywhere within the organization. Also the information is available at any location with access to computer-based health record on a real-time basis. It includes progress notes, nurses' notes, TPR charts, medication charts, laboratory reports, diet sheets and other support staff documentation. For example, no sooner does a nurse complete an electronic form of medication hypersensitivity during an assessment, a care protocol can be immediately triggered and delivered to the multidisciplinary care team located elsewhere in the health organization.
- **Electronic health record:** It is a digital record of health information. It contains past medical history, vital signs, progress notes, diagnoses, medications, immunization dates, allergies, lab data and imaging reports. It also contains other relevant information such as insurance information, demographic data and data from personal wellness devices. A patient's vital signs, admission and nursing assessments, care plans and nursing notes can be entered into the system either as structured or free text. These are stored in central repository and retrieved when needed. Storing health records electronically can improve patient safety through better communication across the patient journey, reduce loss of patient information and eliminate errors.
- **Electronic medication administration record (eMAR):** It is an electronic medication administration record technology that automatically tracks medications from order to administration using assistive technologies in conjunction with an electronic medication administration record. The physician makes an electronic entry detailing a patient's medication order which then appears in the pharmacy software package for editing and verification by a pharmacist. Verified orders are available in the nursing staff's point-of-care. A virtual list of medications due along with administration timeframe for each medication is displayed. Nurses can continue with the administration on

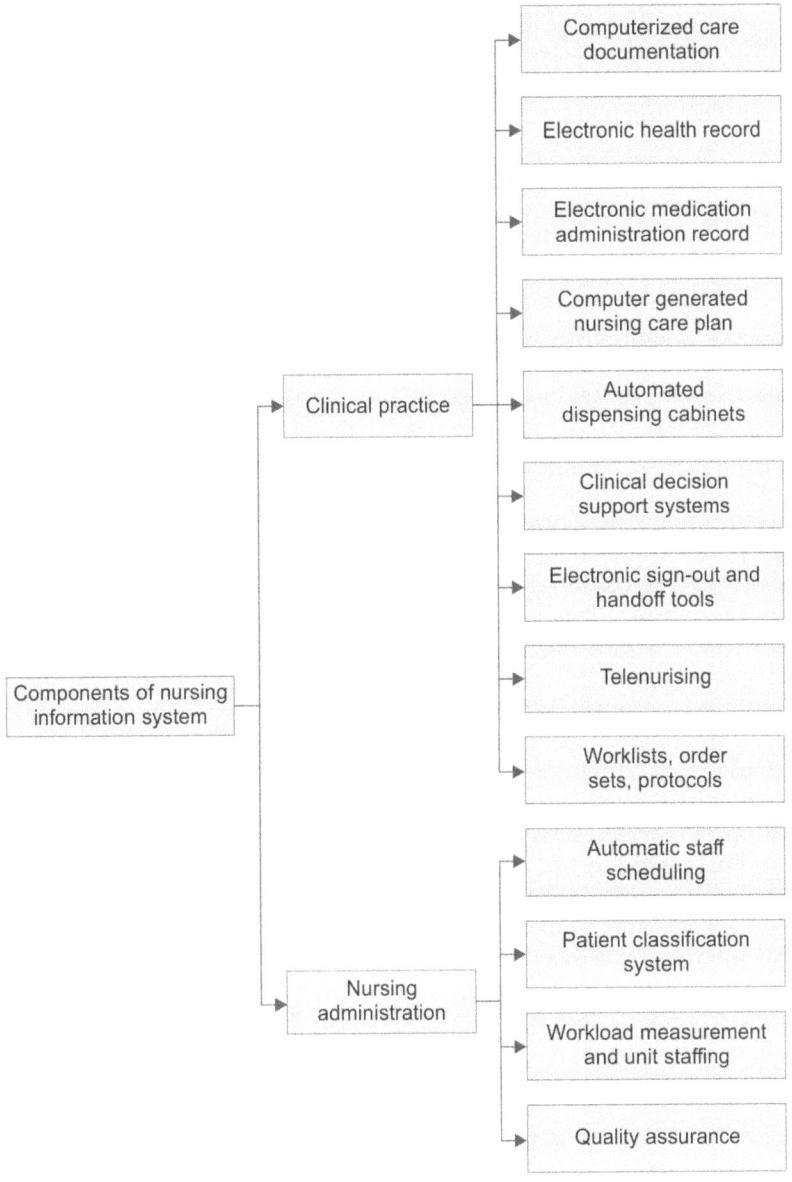

Fig. 8.1: Components of nursing information system

getting order verification by scanning the medication and the patient wrist band. The handheld barcode reader registers each medication. The software while documenting the actual administration of medication verifies for its correctness, time of administration and dosage. eMAR reduces medication errors, increases patient safety and improves the workflow efficiency of nurses and other healthcare personnel. Besides alerting the nurse about the next dose it also cautions about the medications.

- **Computer-generated nursing care plans and critical pathways:** A computer can generate a list of possible nursing diagnosis for a patient with certain signs and symptoms. The newer computer programs

display recommended interventions for selected diagnosis and expected outcomes. This program helps in planning patient care, communicating patient care needs among the nursing and support teams, document changes in patient condition and his response to treatment.
- **Automated dispensing cabinets:** These are computerized drug storage devices that allow medications to be stored and dispensed near the point-of-care, while controlling and tracking drug distribution.
- **Clinical decision support systems (CDSS):** It includes a range of tools to enhance decision-making and the clinical workflow. These include notification alerts and reminders to care providers and patients, clinical guidelines, condition-specific order sets, patient specific clinical summaries, document templates, investigation and diagnostic tools. CDSSs match patient characteristics against a knowledge base based on which computer algorithms then generate patient management recommendations. This information is intended to enhance the decision of the healthcare provider which is rationally filtered and presented to the healthcare professional at an appropriate time. CDSS improves quality of care and patient safety. Decision support module can be added to nursing information systems for providing prompts and reminders. They also provide linkages between signs/symptoms, etiological factors and patient populations. Online access to medical resources can also be made available through this support module.
- **Electronic sign-out and handoff tools:** Sign-out or hand-off communication relates to the process of passing patient-specific information from one nursing official to another, from one team of caregivers to the next or from caregivers to the patient and family for the purpose of ensuring patient care continuity and safety. These applications are used as stand-alone or integrated with electronic medical record to ensure a structured transfer of patient information during healthcare provider handoffs.
- **Telenursing:** It is the use of telecommunications technology in nursing to enhance patient care. These include use of electronic channels such as wire and optical fibers to transmit voice, data and video communication signals.
- **Worklists:** These are list of nursing tasks and interventions for each patient, generated to provide instructions to nursing and supporting staff.
- **Order sets, clinical protocols and templates:** Setting up of templates and order sets for standardized clinical protocols in the inpatient area. For example, protocol for myocardial infarction. This facilitates implementing of standard evidence-based guidelines for best practice across the healthcare organization.

Nursing Administration

There are information systems designed for nursing managers to support them in their decisions and planning for service delivery through improved access to information. These manage the clinical and administrative affairs of nursing units, including their resources. Some of the NISs used in administration activities are given below:
- **Automatic staff scheduling:** Staff scheduling involves the optimal allocation of nurses to shifts. Automated nurse scheduling systems are called as shift modules. The system generates daily, weekly, monthly schedules, duty allocation charts, swapping schedules and training details for nurses. Besides saving a considerable amount of time it also economizes on cost. Shift modules are designed to handle absenteeism, overtime, staffing levels and cost-effective staffing.
- **Patient classification systems (PCSs):** PCS also known as patient acuity system, is a tool that provides exact clinical data for forecasting and allocating nursing staff. It classifies patients based on the need for care and nursing activities that are

necessary to meet their care needs during a specific period. It assists nurse leaders determine workload requirements and staff needs.
- **Workload measurement and unit staffing:** Nursing workload management systems assist nursing managers in staffing, budgeting, planning and quality assurance by providing required information.
- **Quality assurance and outcome analysis:** NIS uses certain criteria to monitor quality care, time spent, nursing activities performed to meet the needs of patients.

Benefits of Nursing Information System

Incorporating information technology into patient care has many benefits (**Fig. 8.2**).
- **Improves nurses' documentation:** Clinical documentation is very important in any healthcare system. NIS provides an easy way to record all the necessary data in a systematic and uniform way affecting the patient care services positively. Nurses' data may include daily recording of temperature, pulse, respirations, blood pressure, medication dosage, time and frequency; time schedule for investigations and their results, etc. NIS not only helps reduce the need for redundant paperwork but also enables maintaining patient history that can be easily accessible when required.
- **Better staff management:** Shift modules can be used for arriving at an appropriate skill mix per shift. This helps in lesser time being spent on designing duty rosters and finding an efficient way to handle administrative activities such as workload management, maintaining staff records, handling absences, overtime, staffing levels, cost-effective staffing as well as scheduling shifts, etc. NIS also helps nurse administrators in assessing staffing requirements as well as financial management through budgeting and monitoring of expenses.
- **Helps in efficient decision-making:** Decision support modules provide linkages between signs and symptoms, etiology or related factors and patient population. Some features of NIS enable information management and decision-making through active and passive systems. Passive systems are able to organize and format the data according to present parameters and provide parameter-specific information as and when required. Active systems on the other hand are a step advanced diagnoses on the basis of predefined criteria applied to the patient information.
- **Enhances synchronization:** In nursing, patient data generated in all units is always essential and significant for the decision-making in any unit of a medical facility. Synchronization of data can thus be achieved by integrating NIS with other clinical systems enabling easy and speedy access of documented information to all the

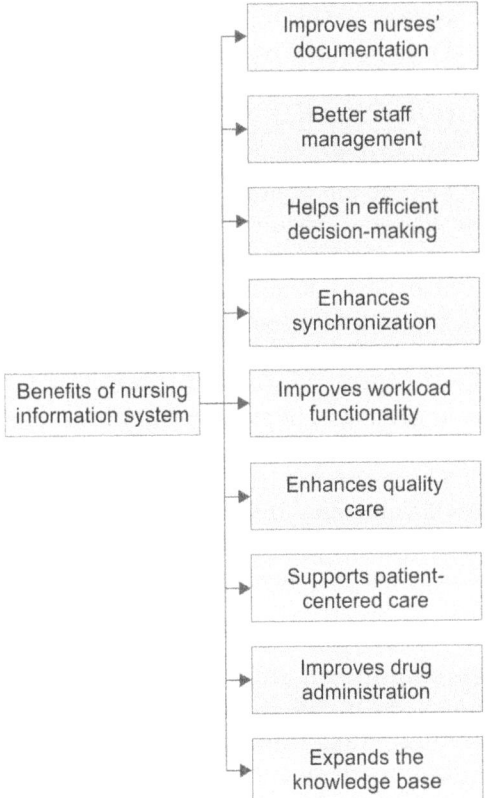

Fig. 8.2: Benefits of nursing information system

appropriate units. Nurses need access to information for program planning, for the operation and supervision of clinical and management interventions and to evaluate the outcomes of care.

- **Improves workload functionality:** Staffing levels and appropriate skill mix per shift can be more easily determined by shift modules. This leads to less time spent in designing and amending rosters.
- **Enhances quality care:** Time spent on care planning is reduced thereby improving the quality of what is being recorded. It improves patient assessment, care planning and evaluation. Greater efficiencies are recorded in patient monitoring and providing personalized care pathways as the time required to wade through paper work is totally eliminated.
- **Supports patient-centered care:** NIS offers greater access to health care, and an increasing capacity to reach patients as per their desire. It impacts overall nursing practice. NIS can also provide options to improve health without having the patient come into the hospital/clinic. A patient can thus gain control over his own health care.
- **Improves drug administration:** Patient charting modules can store admission information, nursing assessments and also nursing notes. These can be retrieved as and when required for drug administration. Electronically prescribed drugs are more legible thereby reducing the likelihood of them being wrongly administered to patients. It reduces medication errors and also streamlines the drug administration process.
- **Expands knowledge base:** Expands the knowledge base of both nurses and patients by making personal health-related information easily accessible.

Implementation of NIS enhances the nurse's ability in organizing nursing care management, documentation and quality nursing care. It can also improve data reporting, communication system and provide clear delegation.

Strategies to Implement Nursing Information System

- Involve nurses, users, other healthcare professionals from all departments in the design, development and testing of information system applications.
- Designate a nurse to co-ordinate the implementation process within the nursing department.
- Establish a user's committee to introduce NIS by involving the key players.
- Identify consultants and other manpower resources available during this process.
- Develop a training program to address the "why" or the rationale for the system, its advantages and disadvantages.
- Employ a nursing informatics expert to educate and train the nurses.
- Provide training prior to and during the implementation phase.
- Provide continuous user support in the operational phase.
- Ensure security, privacy and confidentiality.

NURSING INFORMATICS (NI)

Technology has evolved over the years and so has the job of nursing. With healthcare providers moving to electronic health records, nurses with an interest in technology may also want to move into nursing informatics. Due to the enhanced implementation of technology such as the introduction of electronic medical record (EMR), nursing informatics has been gaining in popularity and the number of informatics nurses growing. With the anticipated emergence of EMRs as the primary tool for documenting and communicating patient information in the near future, the role of an informatics nurse is gaining importance.

Meaning and Definitions

Nursing informatics is a specialty that integrates nursing science with multiple information and analytical sciences to identify, define, manage and communicate data, information, knowledge and wisdom in nursing practice.

Nursing informatics incorporates the field of nursing, computer science and information science so as to develop and maintain medical data systems that are designed to improve patient outcomes as well as boost the overall performance of a healthcare organization.

Use of information technology in relation to any function, within the purview of nursing that are carried out by nurses when performing their duties. —*Hannah et al, 1985*

A combination of computer science, information science and nursing science designed to assist in the management and processing of nursing data, information and knowledge to support the practice of nursing and the delivery of nursing care.
—*Graves and Corcoran, 1989*

Nursing informatics is a specialty that integrates nursing science, computer science and information science to manage and communicate data, information, knowledge and wisdom in nursing practice.
—*ANA, 2008*

Goal of Nursing Informatics

To improve the health of populations, communities, families and individuals by optimizing information management and communication.

Sciences Underpinning Nursing Informatics

- NI is a combination of nursing science, information science and computer science to manage and process nursing data, information and knowledge to facilitate the delivery of health care.
- The combination of sciences creates a unique blend that is greater than the sum of its parts, a unique combination that creates the definitive specialty of NI.
- Computer and information science applied in isolation will have less impact than when they are applied within a disciplinary framework.

Need for Nursing Informatics

- To provide comprehensive and quality care to patients, nurses need to be prepared to use information and telecommunications technology.
- All over the world, health organizations are implementing clinical information systems and electronic health records. Hence nurses are required to acquire adequate knowledge and skills to enable implementation of clinical information systems.
- Around the world, telecommunication infrastructures are being upgraded thereby enabling more people and organizations to use Internet services and video conferencing facilities. Presently video conferencing technology is being widely used in health care. Educating nurses in the rationale and appropriate use of information systems is essential to take advantage of these opportunities.

Nurse Informaticist

Nurse informaticists also known as nurse informatics specialists are specially trained to help manage, interpret and communicate the vital medical data and information that flows in and out of physician's offices, hospitals, clinics and other healthcare facility computer systems.

Informatics Nurse Specialist

A registered nurse with formal, graduate education in the field of informatics or a related field and considered a specialist in the field of nursing informatics.

Informatics Nurse

A registered nurse with an interest or experience working in an informatics field. A generalist in the field of informatics in nursing.

Working Areas

Nurse informaticists work in various settings to aid in managing the use of information

systems, whether or not those healthcare sites or companies directly service patients.
- Nurse informaticists usually work in the information systems department of a health care setting and are skilled in three primary areas viz. computer science, information technology and nursing science.
- They work in hospitals, emergency healthcare centers, technology companies, electronic healthcare records (EHR) companies and many more areas.
- They use computer programs to improve patient outcomes. Many nurse informaticists work as consultants.
- They also work in an administrative capacity and contribute to decision-making on medical information technology.
- Nurse informaticists train nurses on use of technology and on how to enter medical information into a computer system.
- Depending on the setting, nurse informaticists can hold one of several job titles such as informatics nurse, clinical informatics nurse, nurse informatics specialist, chief nursing informatics officer, clinical analyst and health informatics officer.
- Most organizations prefer to hire informatics nurses who possess at least a bachelor's degree in nursing with many seeking a master's degree in health informatics.

Basic Competencies Required for a Nurse Informaticist

A nurse informaticist should have:
- Specific competencies related to use of medical devices in all clinical practice areas and use of telehealth in community.
- The ability to communicate with other interdisciplinary teams as well as the IT team.
- Computer literacy and skills in order to effectively use an EMR and other clinical information systems.
- Capabilities to collect evidence-based research to improve practice.

The World Health Organization has a number of informatics initiatives in place to help meet its e-Health mandate, which includes the eHealth Technology Advisory Group formed solely to support WHO's work in e-Health.

National League for Nursing (2015) also identified the need to prepare students for technological/digital healthcare through nursing education "to teach...about technology to better inform healthcare interventions that improve healthcare outcomes and prepare the nursing workforce".

Skills Required for a Nurse Informaticist

The American Association of Colleges of Nursing 2008 defined specific skills needed for a nurse informaticist as follows:
- Demonstrate skills in using patient care technologies, information systems and communication devices that support safe nursing practice.
- Use telecommunication technologies to assist in effective communication in a variety of healthcare settings.
- Apply safeguards and decision-making support tools embedded in patient care technologies and information systems to support a safe practice environment for both patients and healthcare workers.
- Understand the use of computer information systems to document interventions related to achieving nurse-sensitive outcomes.
- Use standardized terminology in a care environment that reflects nursing's unique contribution to patient outcomes.
- Evaluate data from all relevant sources including technology to inform the delivery of care.
- Recognize the role of IT in improving patient care outcomes and creating a safe care environment.
- Uphold ethical standards related to data security, regulatory requirements, confidentiality and client's right to privacy,
- Advocate for the use of new patient care technologies for safe and quality care.
- Recognize that redesign of workflow and care processes should precede

implementation of care technology to facilitate nursing practice.
- Participate in evaluation of information systems in practice settings through policy and procedure development.

(*Source:* AACN, Baccalaureate Education, 2008)

Standards of Nursing Informatics Practice

The American Nurses Association 2015 identified nursing informatics standards of practice. The identified standards and competencies are provided in **Table 8.1**.

History of Nursing Informatics

Nursing informatics, a new specialty that combines technology and patient care has emerged over the past 20 years to help nurses fully utilize information technology to improve patient care delivery.

- In the 1970s, nursing began to realize the importance of computers in the field of nursing thereby involving in the design, purchase and implementation of information systems.
- In the 1980s medical and nursing informatics specialties emerged.
- 1995 saw the first certification exam for NI being introduced.
- The post-2000 era saw an unprecedented explosion in the number and sophistication of both computer hardware and software.
- Telemedicine became possible and was recognized as a specialty in the late 1990s
- NI has experienced rapid growth in the last 20 years which does not appear to be slowing down
- The American Nurses Credentialing Center (ANCC) recognizes nursing informatics as a specialty with board certification.

Table 8.1: Standards of nursing informatics practice

Standards	Description	Competencies
Standards of practice for nursing informatics		
Standard 1: Assessment	The informatics nurse collects comprehensive data, information and emerging evidence pertinent to the situation	Uses workflow analysis to examine current practice
Standard 2: Diagnosis, problems and issues identification	NI analyzes assessment data to identify diagnoses, problems, issues and opportunities for improvement	Validates the diagnoses, problems, needs, issues and opportunities for improvement with the healthcare consumer
Standard 3: Outcomes identification	NI identifies expected outcomes for a plan individualized to the healthcare consumer	Documents expected outcome as measurable goals
Standard 4: Planning	NI develops a plan that prescribes strategies, alternatives and recommendations to attain expected outcomes	Develops the plan in collaboration with healthcare consumer and key stakeholders
Standard 5: Implementation	NI implements the plan	Uses specific evidence-based actions and processes to resolve diagnoses, problems or issues to achieve outcomes. The informatics nurse co-ordinates planned activities, employs informatics solutions and provides consultation to influence the identified plan
Standard 6: Evaluation	NI evaluates progress towards attainment of outcomes	Conducts a systematic evaluation of outcome

Contd...

Contd...

Standards	Description	Competencies
Standards of professional performance for nursing informatics		
Standard 7: Ethics	NI practices ethically	Applies the code of ethics for nurses with interpretative statements to guide practice
Standard 8: Education	NI addresses the need for education, attain knowledge and competencies reflecting current nursing practice	Demonstrates commitment to lifelong learning
Standard 9: Evidence-based practice and research	NI integrates evidence and research into practice	Demonstrates application and integration of evidence and research into practice
Standard 10: Quality of practice	NI contributes to the quality and effectiveness of nursing and informatics practice	Collects data to analyze and monitor quality of informatics practice.
Standard 11: Communication	NI communicates effectively	Communicates effectively using a variety of methods
Standard 12: Leadership	NI demonstrates leadership in professional practice	Demonstrates leadership skills such as mentoring and problem solving and promotes the organization's mission and vision
Standard 13: Collaboration	NI collaborates with the healthcare consumer and others in the practice of nursing and nursing informatics	Partners with other to effect change
Standard 14: Professional practice evaluation	NI evaluates her own nursing and informatics practice	Promotes self-evaluation, identifies areas of strength as well as areas of professional growth
Standard 15: Resource utilization	NI uses appropriate resources to plan and implement safe practices	Modifies practice as discipline and technology evolves
Standard 16: Environmental health	NI supports nursing practice in a safe and healthy environment	Participates in ways to support healthy communities

- Additionally, nursing informatics provides a career path in leadership as chief nursing informatics officers position across the healthcare system.

Importance of Nursing Informatics

Nurse informatics plays a valuable role in the following areas **(Fig. 8.3)**:
- **Improves quality of care and patient outcomes:** One of the many benefits of incorporating technology into healthcare is that it makes it easier for providers to collect more data and information about their patients. But that data is only useful if it is collected, analyzed and applied and shared effectively which can only happen if providers are able to easily use the EHR system. Nurse informaticists ensure EHRs are optimally designed to fit the organization's workflow and are easy for providers to use. They help healthcare providers to spend as little time as possible to navigate through technology and more time focusing on getting and sharing the right information about their patients.
- **Streamlines clinical processes:** Technology solutions are designed to simplify provider workloads and streamline clinical processes. Nurse informaticists play a pivotal role in the proper setup and implementation of technological solutions.
- **Facilitates organizational change management:** Nurse informaticists are leaders in process and change management.

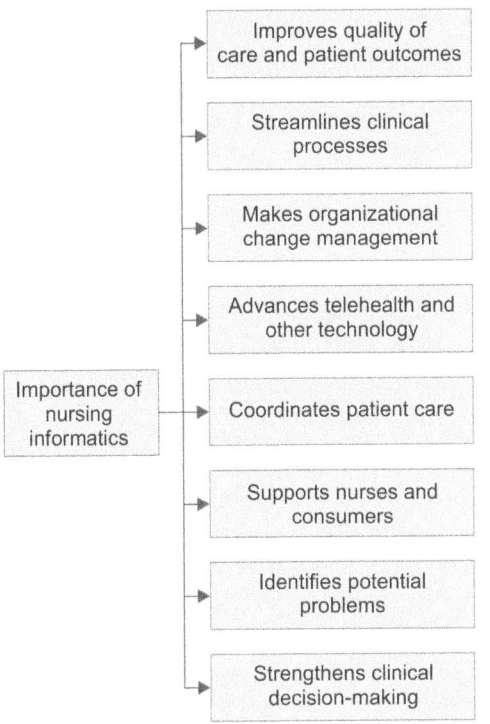

Fig. 8.3: Importance of nursing informatics

They guide others through planned initiatives in unexpected situations. They anticipate situations that are dynamic, facilitate implementation of change, and sustain it by taking charge and advancing progress.

- **Advanced telehealth and other technology:** Nurse informaticists play a major role in evaluating telehealth platforms so as to ensure technology is compatible with practice guidelines, as well as help implement and roll out these systems and train providers on how to effectively use them.
- **Co-ordinates patient care:** Nurse informaticists are trained to take a holistic approach to complex systems. Not only do they have the clinical knowledge necessary to anticipate patient and provider needs but also understand how these systems work. They can more readily anticipate potential failure points in the patient care cycle before they occur. In doing so, nurse informaticists can proactively address these obstacles and ensure a seamless and effective patient experience.
- **Supports nurses and consumers:** American Nurses Association advises that nursing informatics supports nurses, consumers, patients, interprofessional healthcare team and other stakeholders in their decision-making in all roles and settings to achieve desired outcomes. This support is accomplished through the use of information structures, information processes and information technology. Nursing informatics supports the collection, storage, analysis, retrieval, communication and use of information to help nurses to:
  - Care for patients to the highest quality
  - Share data, information and knowledge
  - Compare theory and practice to advance nursing knowledge and practice
  - Support consumers, patients, nurses and other providers in their decision-making in all roles and settings
- **Identifies potential problems:** Nurses holding the job of a nurse informaticist use their clinical background as well as their computer and organizational skills. They act as a bridge between the healthcare organizational system and its providers and clinical staff. Because of their unique training both as registered nurses and information technology specialists, nurse informaticists understand how all the pieces fit together and provide valuable input into how systems should be designed from a provider standpoint.
- **Strengthens clinical decision-making:** As nurses face ever-changing and challenging practice situations; competency in nursing informatics promises to strengthen clinical decision-making skills. Informatics enhances nursing practice, provides quicker access to patient information, improves overall efficiency and reduces potential errors in practice.

As the role of technology in health care continues to expand, the role of nursing informatics is also continuing to expand for effective implementation of these new technologies effectively.

Roles and Responsibilities of Informatics Nurse

Nursing informatics strives to facilitate the unique job responsibilities of nurses through optimized health information technology methods and software tools. Specialists may apply nursing informatics skills to:
- Develop data structures and software tools for nurses to use
- Keep electronic health records aligned with best practice for data management, processing and organization
- Implement analytics to monitor and facilitate nursing processes
- Enable healthcare and IT professionals to communicate with each other more effectively
- Develop and enforce privacy policies in accordance with ethics and regulations
- Educate providers on how to make the best use of electronic health records and clinical decision support systems
- Involve in EHR implementation, documentation optimization, care coordination and population health initiatives.

Essential Responsibilities of a Nurse Informaticist

The day-to-day responsibilities of a nurse informaticist vary depending upon the organizational needs around information management. The American Nursing Informatics Association (ANIA) is the association of professional nurses and associates who use informatics to improve the health of populations. American Medical Informatics Association lists the essential responsibilities of nurse informaticists as follows:
- Improve workflow through communication and information technologies
- Retrieve and review information to improve patient safety
- Contribute to the construction of an interoperable national data infrastructure
- Advance public health by influencing healthcare policy
- Develop information systems based on current standards or care
- Ensure information systems are kept updated
- Educate staff on EHRs and EMRs

EVALUATION, ANALYSIS AND PRESENTATION OF HEALTHCARE DATA TO INFORM DECISIONS IN THE MANAGEMENT OF HEALTHCARE ORGANIZATIONS

Healthcare data is any data pertaining to health of an individual patient or group of people. This health data is gathered from various sources such as electronic health records, personal health records, patient portals, health-related smart phone apps, health surveys, clinical trials, disease registries, etc. This data may also include clinical decision support systems (physician's written notes and prescriptions, medical imaging, laboratory, pharmacy, insurance and other administrative data). It comes from a variety of sources starting from patients, nurses, doctors, support staff, administration, vendors etc. and are recorded in different forms like patient records, patient satisfaction surveys, patient complaint registers, quality care assessments, employee satisfaction surveys, etc. Previously these data were stored in a hard copy format. However, due to digitalization this large amount of data is presently stored in an electronic form.

Healthcare Data Analytics

Health data analytics is the process of performing various analytical operations on current and past data to identify and predict trends or patterns, develop insights, improve outcomes and even better manage the disease.

In health data analytics, healthcare data is acquired, managed, analyzed and interpreted to provide actionable insights.

Need for Data Analysis

- With an increase in use of electronic health records and electronic means of data collection and storage, there is a significant amount of data being collected in real time.
- These datasets also called big data are complex and voluminous. They are a host to diversity of data types spread among multiple healthcare systems, health insurers, researchers, government entities etc.
- This big data cannot be processed using traditional software, hardware, management tools and storage options.
- Cloud storage is a necessity when dealing with big data. It is built to secure sensitive patient information. It is also cost-efficient and has been helpful in lowering the healthcare costs.
- The healthcare industry while generates tremendous amount of data, struggles to convert that data into insights that improve patient outcomes and operational efficiencies.
- Effective analysis of these large amounts of organizational data can lead to better decision-making.
- Through this analysis one may make accurate diagnosis, discover more cost-effective interventions, deliver quicker treatments to patients, improve usage of hospital facilities, help in effective planning and ensure proper allocation of resources for improving patient outcomes.
- Health management methods rely on data analytics to identify populations in need of care, measure the care provided to those populations and deliver care to the correct people.

Types of Healthcare Analytics

Healthcare providers use four essential analytics strategies to get most from their data to reach their goals. Each strategy is valuable depending upon the situation. Different situations call for application of different types of data strategy. The main goal of any strategy is to improve patient care and make an operation more efficient. Following important strategies represent data-driven methods for healthcare organization (**Fig. 8.4**):

- **Descriptive analytics:** It is one of the commonly used approaches to data analytics used by healthcare organizations. It uses historical data wherein collected data is aggregated and categorized. It provides simple summaries about the observations, discovers patterns and provides information on whether the outcome was positive or negative. This type of analysis is used for answering questions about what has already occurred. Looking at data based on past and present decisions, healthcare leaders can make more informed decisions about the future.

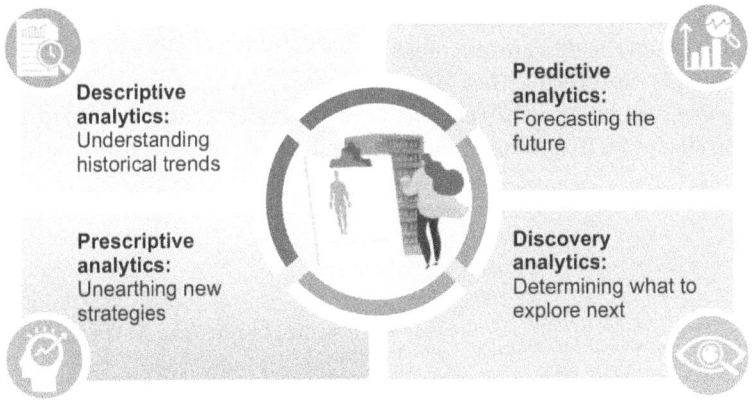

Fig. 8.4: Four types of healthcare data analytics.

- **Predictive analytics:** Predictive analytics uses current and historical data to predict possible future outcomes based on current strategies. It can provide keen insights by using existing data and then using probabilities to forecast outcomes. It uses advanced algorithms designed to uncover trends in data as well as relationships between different datasets such as health outcomes among specific patient demographics. It is a powerful tool for helping healthcare leaders set future strategies. Predictive analytics can be employed to identify those at risk for certain diseases.
- **Prescriptive analytics:** It uses historical data to determine potential solutions for healthcare organizations using advanced algorithms. Prescriptive analytics provide advices or options to medical professionals for successful prevention of patient problems. Information thus provided can help medical professionals determine the best course of action in real-time rather than having them rely on their own instincts and knowledge in stressful situations. Prescriptive analytics not only anticipates what will happen and when it will happen, but also why it will happen. It automatically processes new data to improve prediction accuracy and provide better decision options.
- **Discovery analytics:** It represents cutting edge of health informatics and data analysis. In this method, sophisticated software can develop potential new healthcare outcomes which may include discovering a new drug, identifying new diseases and developing alternative strategies for treatment. It allows medical professionals and healthcare administrators to test a hypothesis.

Benefits of Data Analytics in Health Care

Healthcare data management has the potential to prompt better care if used properly. With the availability of centralized data sets there is immediate access to necessary information wherever and whenever needed. Better data leads to better care. Some of the benefits of data analytics in health care are presented in **Figure 8.5.**

Support Clinical Treatment Decisions

Predictive modeling uses data mining, machine learning and statistics to identify patterns and predict outcomes. The use of predictive analytics can alert healthcare professionals to potential risks. The health data collected can be used for risk scoring, readmission, prediction and prevention and deterioration at the individual patient level. Population health management is impossible without the use of these models. Outbreaks and outcomes can be predicted and in knowing what is to come, preventive measures can be taken. Predictive modeling can even be used in administrative applications to increase efficiency and lower costs for all. It improves accuracy and speed of identifying patients at higher risk of disease. It also promotes preventive measures by giving patients a greater insight into their health and treatment goals.

Reduction in Healthcare Costs

Health care is expensive. Through the use of predictive and prescriptive analytics, healthcare organizations and practitioners

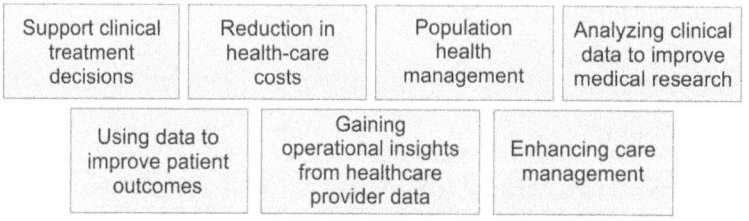

Fig. 8.5: Benefits of data analytics in health care

can get detailed models for lowering costs and patient risk. Healthcare data analytics can manage supply chain costs, prevent equipment breakdowns and decrease fraud. If hospitalization is necessary, data analytics can help practitioners predict risks of infection, deterioration and readmission. This too can help lower costs and improve patient care outcomes.

Population Health Management

Health management methods rely on data analytics to identify populations in need of care, measure the care provided to those populations and deliver care to the correct people. Through data analytics, providers can improve patient outcomes, enhance care management and address social determinants of health. The use of data analytics improves the ability of health organizations to predict the outbreak of disease, improve the prevention of disease, enhance the quality of life and extend the lifespan.

Analyzing Clinical Data to Improve Medical Research

Data analytics techniques gather and analyze clinical data from electronic medical records and public health records. The data analytic results help care providers identify approaches to improve the efficiency of clinical processes and other healthcare operations. This leads to more accurate diagnosis and treatment by personalized healthcare provision. It also provides insight into the cause of disease by linking risk factors with health outcomes. Data analytics techniques are being applied to improve research efforts in many health-related areas by gathering and analyzing clinical data from EHRs, electronic medical records, personal health records and public health records.

Using Data to Improve Patient Outcomes

The main goal of quality improvement in healthcare settings is to provide safe and effective care to patients. To achieve this goal, healthcare providers collect and analyze patient data in real time, develop and apply a systematic approach to improve patient outcomes. Through data analytics, medical professionals can gain insights into patient needs thereby prioritizing on allocation of resources resulting in improved care management. With more types of data becoming available and new tools being developed, results of the analytics become clear and easy for healthcare professionals to access. Data analytics helps healthcare providers to identify the wants and needs of patients. Providing accurate data-driven forecasts in real-time allows healthcare providers to respond more quickly to changing healthcare markets and environments. Big data is often used to address health concerns of large communities of people. By analyzing patient data, healthcare providers can reduce errors and better identify at-risk populations.

Gaining Operational Insights from Healthcare Provider Data

Improved staffing through health analytics: Through healthcare data analytics, management can identify staffing issues, recruit, hire, train and retrain healthcare workers. Data-driven approach to staff management helps managers to develop a greater insight into the productivity of individual workers and teams and the cost effectiveness of staff decisions. This allows the hospital to adjust staffing ratios in a way that reduces its labor costs without affecting the quality of care provided or patient outcomes.

Enhancing Care Management

Through data analytics organizers can consider physical and social determinants of health that may impact individuals and focus on well care rather than waiting for a patient to become ill. For example, through data analytics providers can assess which processes are the most effective methods for wellness and prevention within value-based care models.

Through data analytics and population health management, systems can identify populations in need, stratify risk and track patient progress. This allows analytics to better understand environmental factors that could influence an individual's health. The hospital uses metrics called the social vulnerability index and the community need index to assess and target where the medical care facilities are needed the most.

Data analytics in healthcare can be applied to every aspect of patient care management. The ability of data analytics to convert raw healthcare data into actionable intelligence is expected to have the greatest impact on research, early detection of disease, prevention of unnecessary doctor's visits, discovery of new drugs and more accurate calculation of health insurance rates.

Healthcare Data Analytics Technologies
- Artificial intelligence tools
- Cloud computing platforms
- Block chain networks
- Health information exchanges
- Machine learning models

Tools used in analytics:
- Software that acquires data from sources such as patient surveys, case files and machine-to-machine data transfer
- Programs that clean, validate and analyze the data in response to a specific research question
- Software that builds on the results of the analysis to suggest various actions to achieve specific healthcare goals.

Data Analytics and Nursing Implications
- The main goal of nursing care management is to co-ordinate the managerial and clinical dimensions of nursing work process.
- The nurse administrators have to co-ordinate the facilities and human resources in order to provide quality patient care and enhance the performance of the nursing team.
- Nurse managers should manage in each unit/ward clinical and administrative activities. This includes management of resources, maintaining healthy environment in the ward, patient classification, improving patient safety and health outcomes, workload planning, staffing, scheduling, recruitment of nurses, evaluation of care, maintaining reports and records.
- To fulfill the above roles, nurse managers should analyze situations and take proper and effective decisions for which they require extensive information. That data should be integrated with other hospital information systems to extract the required data.
- Information systems support decision-making among nurse managers in a variety of ways such as through data access, use of data management tools, and statistical analysis.

In addition to collecting, analyzing and interpreting data, analytics software must secure the data and the analysis results. While doing so it must also be ensured that the healthcare professionals will benefit from the insights, have ready access to information in a form they can easily use in their work.

Unit 8 | Using Information in Healthcare Management

REVIEW QUESTIONS

Long Essays (10 Marks)
1. What is the meaning of nursing information system? Describe benefits of NIS.
2. Define nursing informatics. Explain the need for nursing informatics.
3. Define nursing informatics. Explain standards of nursing informatics.
4. Explain competencies and skills required for a nurse informaticist.
5. Explain importance of nursing informatics.
6. What are the roles and responsibilities of informatics nurse?
7. Describe types of health care analytics.
8. Benefits of data analytics in healthcare.

Short Essays (5 Marks)
1. Purposes of nursing information system.
2. Components of nursing information system.
3. Describe strategies to implement nursing information system.

Short Answers (2 Marks)
1. Nursing information system.
2. What is the meaning of nursing informatics?
3. Health care data analytics.

MULTIPLE CHOICE QUESTIONS

1. **Nursing information includes:**
   a. Data used by medical professionals
   b. Data used by nurses
   c. Data in electronic health records
   d. Data in electronic medical records

2. **Electronic health record includes all of the following, *except*:**
   a. It is a digital record of health information
   b. It contains past medical history
   c. It includes progress notes
   d. It includes healthcare professionals' information

3. **Electronic medication administration record means:**
   a. It automatically tracks medications from order to administration
   b. It generates a list of possible medications available in the hospital
   c. It is a tool to enhance drug decision making
   d. It is a computerized drug storage device

4. **What is automated dispensing cabinets?**
   a. It automatically tracks medications from order to administration
   b. It generates a list of possible medications available in the hospital
   c. It is a tool to enhance drug decision-making
   d. It is a computerized drug storage device

5. **What is clinical decision support system?**
   a. These are range of tools to enhance decision making
   b. It displays recommended interventions for selected diagnosis
   c. These are range of tools to increase patient safety
   d. These are range of tools to improve medication administration

6. **What are electronic sign-out and hand-off tools?**
   a. These are notification alerts and reminders for providing care
   b. These are programs that help in planning patient care
   c. These pass specific information from one nurse official to another
   d. These are clinical guidelines for improving patient safety

7. **Shift modules are:**
   a. Automated nurse scheduling systems
   b. Automated medication tracks
   c. Automated templates and order sets
   d. Automated work lists

8. What is healthcare data analytics?
   a. It is a process of data acquiring
   b. It is a process of data management
   c. It is a process of data interpretation
   d. It is a process of data acquiring, managing and interpreting

9. Descriptive analytics:
   a. It provides simple summaries of observations
   b. It forecast outcomes
   c. It determines potential solutions
   d. It tests a hypothesis

10. Predictive analytics:
    a. It provides simple summaries of observations
    b. It forecast outcomes
    c. It determines potential solutions
    d. It tests a hypothesis

11. Prescriptive analytics:
    a. It provides simple summaries of observations
    b. It forecast outcomes
    c. It determines potential solutions
    d. It tests a hypothesis

12. Discovery analytics:
    a. It provides simple summaries of observations
    b. It forecast outcomes
    c. It determines potential solutions
    d. It tests a hypothesis

ANSWER KEY

| 1. b | 2. d | 3. a | 4. d | 5. a | 6. c | 7. a | 8. d | 9. a | 10. b |
| 11. c | 12. d | | | | | | | | |

Information Law and Governance in Clinical Practice

UNIT 9

INTRODUCTION

Healthcare informatics is a rapidly developing field of science which underlies the fusion of health care, information technology, and administration. It guides all aspects of patient health experience including clinical care, nursing, pharmacy, and public health. It deals with the storage, retrieval and use of biomedical data, information and knowledge for problem-solving and decision-making in health care.

Key ethical issues in medicine, nursing, psychology, and social work though are well noted, those related to health informatics are little known. Health informatics now constitutes a source for some of the most important ethical debates in health care profession. There is a growing interest in bioethics and computer-related ethics to orient decision-making in health care informatics.

Information Laws in India (Laws and Acts Related to Health Informatics in India)

In India no specific legislation exists regarding disclosure of medical records. According to the Indian Medical Council Regulations, every medical professional is obligated to maintain physician-patient confidentiality. Any physician disclosing personal information about his or her patients could be held guilty of professional misconduct. Physicians are however allowed to disclose patient information to public health authorities in limited circumstances such as in case of a serious and identified risk to a specific person or community.

Right to Privacy in India

The Supreme Court has on several occasions emphasized that the right to privacy is not an absolute right. The court has chosen a case-by-case approach in the interpretation of the right to privacy. In some instances, the court has allowed a hospital to inform the HIV-positive status of the patient to his/her spouse. The rationale behind disclosure in such cases is to prevent spreading of infectious diseases. In India, the judiciary has leaned towards favoring public interest over individual privacy.

In 2007, the Bombay High Court allowed disclosure of a prisoner's medical condition in response to an RTI application. It was further stated that determination of justifiable disclosure would be made on a case-to-case basis.

The judicial trend observed in these cases has led to a gradual erosion of the principles of personal liberty, autonomy and privacy. Supreme Court's case-by-case approach to defining privacy does not provide safeguards required for a strong data protection regime that respects individual autonomy.

The court has ruled that information contained in a public record cannot be protected under the right to privacy. Since public records could include hospital records, prison records and any other information collected by a state body, this ruling may have the effect of bypassing any authorization requirement for collecting patient data already contained in public records.

Though India does not have dedicated data protection laws, certain provisions of the Information Technology Act 2000 and Information Technology (Reasonable Security Practices and Procedures and Sensitive Personal Data or Information) Rules 2011 deal with the protection of personal information and sensitive personal data that includes health data as well. Currently, a patient's personal information which includes health information is treated as sensitive personal data or information (SPDI) under the Information Technology (Reasonable Security Practices and Procedures and Sensitive Personal Data or Information) Rules 2011. Some of the protection Acts related to information technology are depicted in **Figure 9.1**.

Information Technology Act

- Information Technology Act, 2000 has had several amendments in the last couple of years that have expanded and changed the law in accordance with the latest technological innovations.
- IT rules introduced in 2011 defined sensitive personal data for the first time in India. The rules stipulated that a body corporate/organization collecting such sensitive personal data shall obtain written consent from the provider of said data.
- The data can only be collected for a lawful purpose, which is connected to the working of the body corporate. The body should also make sure that the data provider is made aware of the fact that such information is being collected.
- The provider should be made aware of the reasons for which such information is being collected and of the identity of persons who intend to receive such information.
- There are very few instances in which sensitive personal data can be disclosed to a third party.
- Government agencies can collect such information without prior consent subject to the condition that information is collected for certain specified purposes alone and that those purposes are made known to the individual.
- Information Technology Amendment Act, 2008 describes that 'body corporate' is liable for any negligence in the implementation or maintenance of reasonable security practices and procedures.
- In case any person wrongly suffers a loss, the body corporate would legally be responsible to compensate the person by way of damages.
- Rule 8 of the IT Rules also imposes a duty on the body corporate to ensure compliance with practices and procedures in securing personal information.

Personal Data Protection Bill 2019 (PDP)

Government of India introduced the PDP bill in Lok Sabha in 2019. This bill regulates the protection and privacy of data in both digital and non-digital forms. This legal framework is applicable to processing, storage and transfer of personal data across sectors of the

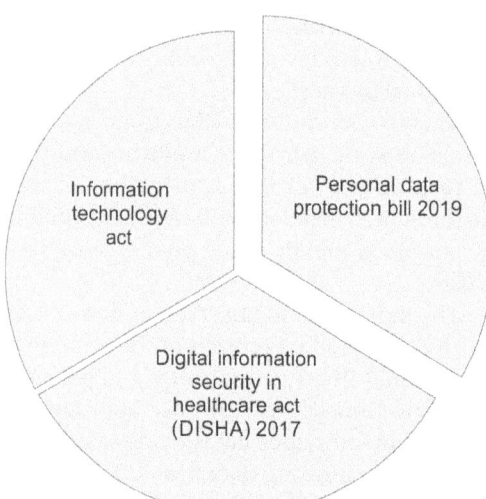

Fig. 9.1: Protection acts related to information technology

economy, academia, industry, and society. The framework classifies data into 3 broad categories: personal data, sensitive personal data (SPD), and critical sensitive personal data.

Personal data: It includes characteristics, traits or attributes of identity that can be used to identify an individual.

Sensitive personal data: It includes financial data, biometric data, caste, religion or any other data specified by the government.

Critical sensitive personal data: It includes such personal data as may be notified by the central government. For example, military or national security data.

- This Bill is applicable to processing of personal data by the government, companies in India, foreign companies dealing with personal data of individuals in India.
- This Bill sets out certain rights of the individual which include right to seek correction of inaccurate, incomplete or out-of-date personal data, restrict disclosure of their personal data by a fiduciary if it is no longer necessary or consent is withdrawn.
- This Bill empowers the Data Protection Authority to take action against anyone who does not comply with the bill of the regulations made by either the authority or the government.
- Processing or transferring personal data in contravention of the Bill is punishable by a fine of Rs. 150 million, or 4 percent of the annual turnover of the data fiduciary, whichever is higher.
- Failure to conduct a data audit is also punishable.
- Furthermore, re-identification and processing of de-identified personal data without proper consent are punishable by up to three years in prison, a fine or both.
- It is very important that citizens' privacy is prioritized as the ultimate goal of data protection system.

Digital Information Security in Healthcare Act (DISHA): This act enables digital sharing of personal health records with hospitals and clinics and between hospitals and clinics. It is the basis for creation of digital health records in India. This act standardizes and controls the processes of collecting, storing, sharing, and using the digital health data. This standardization will help in ensuring that digital health data remains private, confidential and secure.

HIPAA stands for Health Insurance Portability and Accountability Act 1996

HIPAA is a United States of America (USA) legislation that provides data privacy and security provisions for safeguarding medical information. It sets a standard for patient data protection.

Objectives

- To create confidentiality systems within and beyond healthcare facility
- Keeping protected health information private

Goals

- To limit the use of protected health information to those with a "need to know".
- To penalize those who do not comply with confidentiality regulations.

Five main rules of HIPPA:
1. Privacy rule
2. Security rule
3. Transaction and code set rule
4. Unique Identifiers rule
5. Enforcement rule

HIPAA contains five sections or titles:
1. **Title I—HIPAA Health Insurance Reform:** It protects health insurance coverage for workers and their families who change or lose jobs. It prohibits group health plans from denying coverage to individuals with specific diseases and pre-existing conditions and from setting lifetime coverage limits.
2. **Title II—HIPAA Administrative Simplification:** It prevents health care fraud and abuse; medical liability reform;

administrative simplification that requires the establishment of national standards for electronic health care transactions.
3. **Title III—HIPAA Tax-Related Health Provisions:** It includes tax-related provisions and guidelines for medical care.
4. **Title IV—Application and Enforcement of Group Health Plan Requirements:** It defines guidelines for group health plans, health insurance reform, including provisions for individuals with pre-existing conditions and those seeking continued coverage.
5. **Title V—Revenue Offsets:** It governs company owned life insurance policies and the treatment of those who lose their U.S. citizenship for income tax purposes.

Legal exceptions when health care professionals can breach confidentiality without permission:
- Gunshot wounds
- Stab wounds
- Injuries sustained in a crime
- Child/elderly abuse
- Infectious, communicable or reportable diseases

HIPPA protects the following data:
- Written, spoken or electronic data
- Transmission of data within and outside a health care facility
- Applies to anyone or any institution involved with the use of healthcare related data

Governance Structure in India
- Ministry of Health and Family Welfare (MoHFW) conceived the idea of National Digital Health Mission (NDHM).
- This visionary project of the Government of India stemming from the National Health Policy, 2017 is intended to digitalize the entire healthcare ecosystem of India.
- The National Digital Health Blueprint, 2019 recommends that a federated architecture be adopted instead of a centralized architecture for the management of health data to ensure interoperability, technological flexibility and independence across the National Digital Health Ecosystem (NDHE). The main aim is to ensure that the personal and health data of all individuals in India are adequately protected.
- The governance structure for the NDHE shall be as specified by the NHA, which shall lead the implementation of the NDHM.
- In addition, the governance structure shall consist of such committees, authorities and officers at the national, state and health facility levels to implement the NDHM.
- It shall also consist of a data protection officer who shall be a government officer and in addition to the functions identified under this policy communicate with regulators and external stakeholders on matters concerning data privacy and serve as an escalation point for decision-making on data governance and other matters concerning data.
- It is envisaged that the MoHFW and the Ministry of Electronics and Information Technology shall also provide overall guidance to the National Health Authority (NHA) on relevant aspects of NDHM.

Fundamental Ethical Principles Related to Health Informatics

In the present scenario, healthcare informatics plays an important role in the maintenance and delivery of care. As technology becomes more entangled with medicine, there will be more ethical concerns with its use in health care.

Ethics deals with decisions about right versus wrong, good versus bad. An ethical conflict is opposition between moral ideas or interests. For example, the HIV treatment data project aims to create a website that contains patient testimonials on antiretroviral drugs. On one hand the privacy of patients' needs to be preserved, but doing so would make the testimonials ineffective in reaching out to help other HIV patients. More importantly, the necessity to do good to others can be seen in conflict with the patients' need for privacy.

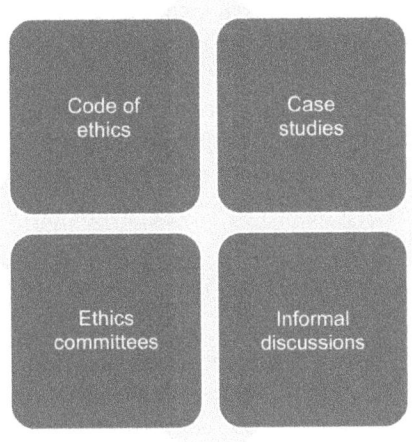

Fig. 9.2: Ethical resources

To help resolve such issues and answer the hard questions various ethical resources such as code of ethics, case studies, ethical committees, etc., are available **(Fig. 9.2)**. These help in determining the course of action to be taken.

1. **Code of ethics:** Ethical codes are formal documents that list ethical principles and duties. Members of the profession or organization are required to adhere to the principles of these codes to guide their ethical conduct. In addition these codes serve to correct any wrong notions about ethical principles.
2. **Case studies:** These are often available references similar to ethical conflicts and situations in the past that may have been resolved in a certain manner. These cases can be applied as jurisprudence.
3. **Ethics committees:** Organizations can have committees and trained staff to discuss and resolve ethical issues. These may include ethics boards or ethics professionals that are contacted for consultation when ethical conflicts occur.
4. **Informal discussions:** Discussions with colleagues or peers can lead to informal advice about how an ethical conflict can be resolved.

Code of Ethics in Health Informatics

Various national and international codes of ethics are as follows:
- **World Health Organization:** WHO eHealth code of ethics specifies guidelines for health-related websites.
- **International Medical Informatics Association (IMIA):** This association provides a Code of ethics for health informatics professionals. It describes duties of health informatics professionals from three perspectives: fundamental ethics principles, informatics ethics principles, and rules of ethical conduct in health informatics.
- **British Computer Society (BCS):** BCS code contains the same material as the IMIA code.
- **Canada's Health Informatics Association (COACH):** Known as Digital Health Canada, the association connects, inspires and educates digital health professionals who are creating the future of health in Canada.
- **American Health Information Management Association (AHIMA) and American Medical Informatics Association (AMIA):** These codes focus more on duties of health informatics professionals expected towards key stakeholders in health care.

International Medical Informatics Association

International Medical Informatics Association (IMIA) revised the code of ethics for health informatics professionals in 2016.

Health Information Professionals (HIP) are individuals who in their professional capacity provide health informatics services and therefore occupy a special position in modern health care. Given the ethically sensitive nature of health data and of health information, it is appropriate that the conduct of HIPs be guided by a Code of Ethics that identifies major lines of responsibility. The rules of ethical conduct fall into six general rubrics each with several subsections.

Subject-centered Duties
- HIPs have a duty to ensure that the potential subjects of electronic health records are aware of the existence of systems, programs, protocols or devices whose purpose is to collect and/or communicate data about them.
- HIPs have a duty to ensure that appropriate procedures are in place so that electronic health records are established, maintained, stored, used, linked, manipulated or communicated only with the voluntary, competent and informed consent of the subjects of such records.
- HIPs have a duty to make subjects of electronic health records aware of who has established them and who maintains them, what is contained in them, the purpose for which they are established, the individuals, institutions or agencies who have access to them or to whom they (or an identifiable part of them) may be communicated, where the records are maintained, the length of time they will be maintained, and the ultimate nature of their disposition.
- Health Information Professionals have a duty to ensure that the subjects of electronic health records are aware of any rights they may have with respect to access, use and storage, communication, linkage and manipulation, quality and correction, and disposition of their electronic health records and of the data contained in them.
- HIPs have a duty to ensure that all reasonable and appropriate measures are in place to safeguard the security, integrity, material quality, usability, and accessibility of electronic health records.

Duties Towards Health Care Professionals (HCPs)
- HIPs have a duty to assist duly empowered HCPs who are engaged in patient care or planning in having appropriate, timely and secure access to relevant electronic health records (or parts of thereof), and to ensure the usability, integrity, and highest possible technical quality of these records; and to provide those informatic services on which the HCPs rely to carry out their mandate.
- HIPs should keep HCPs informed of the status of the informatic services on which the HCPs rely and immediately advise them of any problems or difficulties that might be associated with or that could reasonably be expected to arise in connection with these informatic services.

Duties Towards Institutions, Employers and Agencies
- HIPs owe the institutions, employers or agencies with whom they are professionally associated a duty of competence, diligence, integrity, and loyalty.
- HIPs have a duty to take all reasonable steps to ensure that the informatic products, services, tools or devices they recommend to the institutions, employers or agencies with whom they are associated in a professional capacity are suitable, reliable, effective, and qualitatively appropriate so as to allow the latter to meet their respective obligations.
- HIPs have a duty to take all reasonable steps to ensure that the informatic protocols or procedures they recommend to the institutions, employers or agencies with whom they are associated in a professional capacity are suitable, reliable, effective, and qualitatively appropriate so as to allow the latter to meet their respective obligations.

Duties Towards Society
- HIPs have a duty to facilitate the collection, storage, communication, use, linkage, and manipulation of health care data that are legitimately used in research or that are necessary for the planning and providing of health care services on a social scale.
- HIPs have a duty to educate the public about the various issues associated with the nature, collection, storage, use, linkage, and manipulation of health-related data and also make the society aware of the associated problems, dangers, implications or limitations.

- HIPs will refuse to participate in or support practices that violate human rights.
- HIPs will be responsible in setting the fee for their services and in their demands for working conditions, benefits, etc.

Self-regarding Duties of HIPs

- HIPs have a duty to recognize the limits of their competence
- HIPs have a duty to consult when necessary or appropriate
- HIPs have a duty to maintain competence
- HIPs have a duty to take responsibility for all actions performed by them or under their control or authority
- HIPs have a duty to avoid conflict of interest
- HIPs have a duty to give appropriate credit for work done
- HIPs have a duty to act with honesty, integrity, and diligence

Duties Towards the Profession

- HIPs have a duty to always act in such a fashion as not to bring the profession into disrepute.
- HIPs have a duty to assist in the development of the highest possible standards of professional competence, to ensure that these standards are publicly known, and to see that they are applied in an impartial and transparent manner.
- HIPs will refrain from impugning the reputation of colleagues, but will report to the appropriate authority any unprofessional conduct by a colleague.
- HIPs have a duty to assist their colleagues in living up to the highest technical and ethical standards of the profession.
- HIPs have a duty to promote the understanding, appropriate utilization, and ethical use of health information protocols and technologies, and to advance and further the discipline of Health Informatics.

Functions of Ethical Principles and Ethical Codes

- Similar to other codes of ethics, informatics offers recommended ethical guidelines to clinicians and other health care professionals.
- All these ethical principles provide insight into the duties and responsibilities of clinicians, administrators and other healthcare personnel when dealing with patient-related content.
- These principles provide guidance depending on the nature, context, and specific details of each individual situation.
- Informatics code of ethics functions as a gold standard against which actions of professionals can be compared.
- The code of informatics ethics offers patients and the general population an established statement of standards which may mold professionals' actions and behaviors.
- Ethical codes provide a simplified framework that allows ethical conflicts in health informatics to be resolved.

Health Informatics Ethics

Health informatics refers to the use of computers to enhance the way health information is processed. The three aspects of health informatics are: health care, information, software.

- **Healthcare:** Health informatics is referred to in the context of healthcare. Information systems are developed in health care to facilitate easy delivery of care.
- **Information:** Health informatics deals with processing information efficiently. A large amount of patient information requires to be stored for future reference and retrieved as and when required. This can be achieved through electronic medical records. The transfer of information between healthcare organizations needs to be handled with utmost care and safety.
- **Software:** Information can be processed, stored and retrieved effectively using appropriate software. Organization wise software systems are needed to manage information in clinics and hospitals.

With the above components serving as a base for health informatics, ethical dimensions in each of the components can be explained.

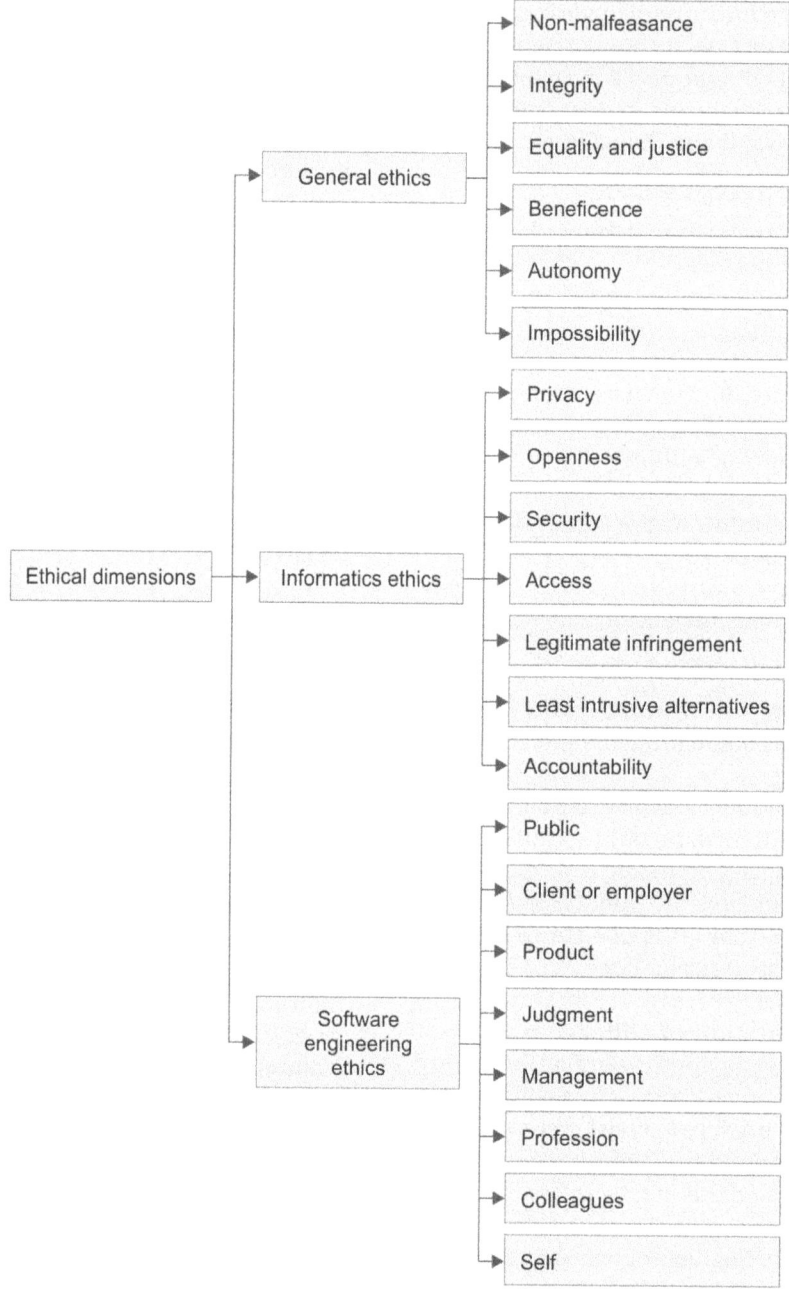

Fig. 9.3: Ethical dimensions of health informatics

Health informatics professionals need to adhere to these three ethical dimensions of their profession: general ethics, informatics ethics, software engineering ethics (**Fig. 9.3**).

1. **General ethics:** Our social interactions are usually guided by general ethics. It is also the first dimension to health informatics. General ethics have six major principles

which need to be adhered to by every member of the society.

a. *Principle of Non-Malfeasance*: All persons have a duty to prevent harm to others without undue harm to themselves. All members of the society are expected to value life and protect it by not engaging in activities that cause harm.
b. *Principle of Integrity*: We have a duty to fulfill our obligations to the best of our abilities. Every member of the society is expected to be honest.
c. *Principle of Equality and Justice*: All persons have a right to be treated equally. Members of the society ought to treat their fellow members equally and without any discrimination. It implies equitable resource allocation and fairness in decision-making.
d. *Principle of Beneficence*: All persons have a duty to advance the good of others. A member of the society does not seek just his or her own good but the general good and advancement of the society as a whole. Beneficence provides care that benefits the patient and prevents harm.
e. *Principle of Autonomy*: All persons have a fundamental right to self-determination. Members of society ought to be given independence in making decisions and judgments. Respect for autonomy allows individuals the capacity to choose on their own.
f. *Principle of Impossibility*: All rights and duties hold subject to the condition that it is possible to meet them. In-line with the principle of impossibility, a surgeon performs the operation to the best of his or her agreement.

2. **Informatics ethics:** It is the second dimension to health informatics ethics. It deals with ethical behavior required of anyone handling data and information. The seven principles stated in the BCS/IMIA code to define informatics ethics are:

a. *Principle of Privacy*: Everyone has a right to privacy of their own information. Every person has the right to decide how much information they wish to disclose about themselves and what information they wish to withhold. Furthermore, individuals have a right to control what information is being collected and how it is stored, accessed, used, communicated, manipulated, and linked.
b. *Principle of Openness*: Data collection about any person must be done transparently. This implies that the person about whom the data is being collected needs to be informed of the intent for collecting data and what the data will be used for.
c. *Principle of Security*: Data collected must be protected by all reasonable and appropriate measures against loss, degradation, unauthorized destruction, access, use, manipulation, linkage, modification, and communication. Once the data is collected it must be safeguarded against unauthorized access by other parties. In addition, the data needs to be protected against manipulation, both malicious and unintentional.
d. *Principle of Access*: Everyone has a right to access and correct their own data. The subjects of electronic health records have a right of access to those records and the right to correct, use, manipulate, link, modify, and communicate.
e. *Principle of Legitimate infringement*: The individuals' right to privacy and access may be infringed upon if doing so would be for the larger good of society.
f. *Principle of Least intrusive alternatives*: Any legitimate infringement must be done with minimum interference to the rights of the people affected. Legitimate infringement of an individuals' data does not give free reign.

g. *Principle of Accountability*: Legitimate infringement must be reported to the person affected in due time.
3. **Software engineering ethics:** The third dimension to health informatics ethics is software engineering ethics. These are related to activities carried out by software developers that have the potential of affecting end users. Software engineers need to be ethically responsible, especially when the sensitive data involves health-related information. The code of ethics for software engineers contains the following eight ethical principles:
   a. *Public*: Developers while carrying out activities with best interest of the society in mind, should also be aware of the social impact of software systems in the process of developing them as well as their eventual usage.
   b. *Client or employer*: Developers though are obliged to carry out activities in the best interest of their employers and clients, they should balance it with their duties towards the public. They should maintain client information private and confidential.
   c. *Product*: Developers while striving to build products that are not sub-standard should ensure that the expected professional standards are met. They should make certain that the product is thoroughly tested and debugged and unsolved problems well documented.
   d. *Judgment*: Integrity and independence should be adhered to while making decisions related to software development. Developers should avoid situations in which their clients have conflict of interest either internally or with other parties.
   e. *Management*: Managers and leaders should subscribe to ethical approaches in software development. Realistic and effective costs, schedules and procedures should be promoted.
   f. *Profession:* Reputation of the software engineering profession should be advanced. Developers should promote and facilitate education of software engineering and point out anyone who violates profession's standards and codes.
   g. *Colleagues*: Colleagues are to be supported and treated fairly. This includes support in development as well as in understanding of the profession's codes.
   h. *Self:* Re-training and improvement is to be pursued by the software developer. Developers should not encourage others directly or indirectly to perform actions that violate the profession's code.

PRIVACY AND CONFIDENTIALITY IN ELECTRONIC HEALTH-RELATED DATA

Before the introduction of electronic health records there existed a confidentiality guarantee for the privacy of patient-physician relationship. Safeguarding of confidentiality did not seem to be problematic as conventional means of communication such as paper, pencil, typewriter, telephone, etc., were being used. This scene has now changed with the introduction of electronic data processing in hospitals through health information system.

Health Big Data

Emerging technologies such as electronic health records, smartphones and wearable devices collect huge amounts of health data from the consumers. Big data in healthcare is a term used to describe massive volumes of information created by the adoption of digital technologies that not only collect patient's records, but also help in managing hospital performance. This big health data is too large and complex for traditional technologies to process and as such mostly processed by machine learning algorithms and data scientists.

Health big data helps in personalized medicine. Secondary use of health data can support clinical decision-making, extract knowledge about diseases, genetics and medicine. It also improves patient's health care experience, reduces health care costs and supports public health policies.

As health big data contains a great deal of personal and confidential information, it not only has a huge potential value of secondary use but also a serious privacy disclosure concern. Hence, there is an urgent need to protect consumer privacy, security, and confidentiality. The need for promoting data protection policies and protecting health-related personal information becomes very crucial.

Digital Health Data

Digital health data is actually the information about an individual in an electronic form. This data may be related to:
- Physical or mental health
- Health service provided to the individual
- About an organ or blood donated by the individual
- A clinical establishment used by the individual

Digital health-related information is highly sensitive. If compromised, lost or exposed it can cause harm, lead to violence, discrimination or even embarrassment to individuals. At times it can be put to illegal use by unauthorized entities to judge and make decisions about the physical and mental conditions, sexual orientation, alcohol consumption, abortion, HIV status, etc. The Indian government thus wants to ensure that all the digital health data of consumers in India remains secure and private.

Sensitive Personal Data

The following personal data is considered sensitive and is subject to specific processing conditions:
- Personal data revealing religion, race, caste or tribe or ethnic origin or philosophical beliefs
- Data pertaining to religious or political belief or affiliation information
- Data containing financial information such as details of bank accounts, credit cards, debit cards or any other payments
- Genetic, physical, psychological and physiological data, sexual data and sex life information
- Data pertaining to transgender status, intersex status
- Biometric data

Health Data Management Policy in India

Health data management policy was approved by the Government of India on 14th December, 2020 as a part of the National Digital Health Mission. The main focus of this policy was to incorporate security and privacy by designing principles into the proposed digital health framework and defining minimum standards for data protection.

Key Points of the Policy

- The policy acts as a guidance document across the National Digital Health Ecosystem (NDHE).
- The data collected across NDHE will be stored at the central level, the state or Union territory level and at the health facility level.
- The policy sets out minimum standards for data privacy protection.
- Authenticity of doctors under this policy will be taken care of by the digidoctor platform under which each and every doctor will be approved by the legitimate council.
- Health care providers under this policy will be connected by a single platform.
- The policy is an initiative to connect all the individual digital health systems with each other, create an ecosystem to facilitate the access of data from one system to another.
- Access to data is provided to ensure quality healthcare.
- Doctor from any hospital can access patient's data but only if he/she gives the consent for accessing explicit information.

- Health care providers shall be in a position to see patient's health status from any part of the country but only with patient's due consent. It is also possible to give partial consent. The patient may provide the doctor consent to view a certain health record and may restrict the doctor from viewing other records.
- **Consent manager:** For consent, an electronic system called the consent manager will be introduced wherein every request for the data will be followed up by the consent manager that will verify the identity of the person seeking data and providing the data. It will also ensure that access to data is provided only after receiving appropriate consent.
- Partial consent will be required if a person has to provide data only for a particular medical condition. The person will be able to withdraw the consent from the record he does not want to show. Also the consent will be provided for a particular period of time only.

The effort of the Indian Government in trying to digitize the medical sector by bringing in the digital health management policy is a milestone in the field of medicine. This can revolutionize the management of individual data towards providing improved medical facilities.

Telemedicine is a pioneer in digital treatment of patients. Though a cost-effective tool, concerns related to patient data security and lack of any solid data protection act stand as a big challenge which should be the key area of focus.

Ethical Priorities of Electronic Health Records

The rapid development and application of health information technologies enable medical organizations to store, share and analyze large amount of personal health and biomedical data. The internet and electronic data collection provides easier access to and dissemination of health information as more and more health information becomes available in electronic form.

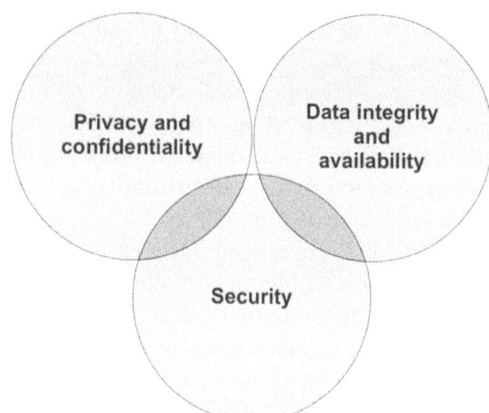

Fig. 9.4: Ethical priorities for electronic health records

There are three major ethical priorities for electronic health records (**Fig. 9.4**):

Privacy and confidentiality: Privacy is the right of the individuals to keep information about themselves from being disclosed to others. Confidentiality relates to non-disclosure of information. The following standards need to be adhered to for maintaining privacy and confidentiality:
- Patient information should be released to others only with patient's due permission or be allowed by law.
- Information can be released for treatment, payment or administrative purposes without patient's due authorization.
- The patient too has a legal right to view, obtain a copy of and amend information in his or her health record.
- The key to preserving confidentiality is making sure that only authorized individuals have access to information.
- The practice administrator identifies the users, determines what level of information is needed and assigns usernames and passwords.
- Basic standards for password maintenance such as the requirement of changing passwords at set intervals, setting a minimum number of characters and prohibiting the reuse of passwords are practiced.

- Two-tier approach to authentication by adding a biometrics identifier scan such as palm, finger, retina or face recognition is followed.
- Extensive training, strong privacy and security policies and procedures are essential to securing patient information.

Security: It encompasses detecting and preventing the use of computers without owner's authorization. Data security exists when data are protected from accidental or intentional disclosure to unauthorized persons or accidental alteration. Computer-based protective safeguards include:

- Hardware (e.g., memory protection)
- Software (e.g., audit trails, log-on procedures)
- Personnel control (e.g., badges or other mechanisms to control entry or limit movement)
- Disaster preparedness (e.g., sprinklers, tape vaults in case of fire, flood, etc.)
- Procedures (e.g., assigning passwords)
- Administration (e.g., auditing events, disaster preparedness, security officer)

The intent of these safeguards is to provide high assurance that the system, its resources and information are protected against harm.

Data integrity and availability: Integrity assures that the data is accurate and has not been tampered with. Poor data integrity results from documentation errors. Making user-friendly software improves data integrity. If the system is hacked or becomes overloaded with requests, information therein may become unusable. To ensure availability, electronic health record systems often have redundant components. The system switches to a backup component in the event a problem is experienced.

NURSES' RESPONSIBILITIES IN LEGAL AND ETHICAL ASPECTS OF DIGITAL HEALTH

Nancy J. Brent has listed the following legal aspects for nurses to bear in mind:

- The highest priority of health informatics management team must be patient safety.
- Health information management procedures must be established and team members trained.
- Information must be held as securely as possible.
- Password and other login credentials must be not shared among other team members.
- Protection of patient's rights and progress towards better health outcomes depend upon the health professional's depth of knowledge regarding health informatics.
- In health care setting sensitive personal data of patients must be well protected in terms of confidentiality and privacy.
- A nurse should keep the following in mind while documenting patient digital data:
  - Data should be processed fairly, and lawfully
  - It should be adequate, relevant and necessary
  - It should be processed for lawful purposes only
  - It should be accurate and up-to-date
  - It should be in accordance with the rights of the individual as per the existing laws
  - Appropriate security measures must be adhered to
- A nurse must be aware of information security safeguards, protection of personal health information against loss and theft, unauthorized access, disclosure, copying, use, and modification. The need for accuracy in digital documentation is relevant particularly in the delivery of healthcare.
- A nurse protects the right to information of patients, enquires the purpose for which patient information is being collected, used and disclosed. The patient should be assured about its accuracy, and amend inaccurate or incomplete information.
- A nurse understands the importance of consent because an organization should be able to demonstrate that it is in compliance with existing laws and that the patient can reasonably be expected to know that information about him was going to be collected and used for defined purposes.

- The nurse is accountable for information being collected, recorded, storing, and disclosure.
- Personal health information should not be collected indiscriminately. There have been instances where data fields such as religion and race were collected in patient records even though they had little or no bearing on treatment and care.
- Points to be kept in mind while processing digital data:
  - Beware of threats related to hackers and crackers, terrorists, viruses, flooding sites, power fluctuations, and revenge attacks.
  - Troubles can arise by visiting pirated websites, poor password management, compromised devices, fires and natural disasters, human error, and unauthorized insider access.
  - Choose passwords that are 8–12 characters long, avoid obvious passwords, keep the password private and do not change or share it frequently.
  - Do not post or write down passwords, leave computers or applications running when not in use, re-use the same password for different systems, and use the "browser save" feature.

TELENURSING PRACTICE GUIDELINES IN INDIA

Telemedicine is a boon for health care providers in bridging the treatment gap between rural and urban India. The Indian government through its flagship scheme, the Pradhan Mantri Jan Arogya Yojana (PMJAY) popularly known as Ayushman Bharat Yojana Scheme took the initiative to connect health and wellness centers with district hospitals and medical colleges digitally so as to enable access to specialist services. E-Sanjeevani is a telemedicine service that is implemented under Ayushman Bharat health initiative at Health and Wellness Centers.

Telenursing Initiatives in India

According to International Council of Nurses (ICN, 2009) telenursing is 'the use of telecommunications technology in nursing to enhance patient care'. It involves the use of electronic channels such as wire, radio and optical to transmit voice, data and video communication signals. Telenursing though in its nascent stage continues to grow as a valuable method for providing nursing, especially in India. Following are the few initiatives of telenursing in India:

- Indian Nursing council has been using telenursing for running its PhD program since 2006.
- Department of Nursing at NIMHANS has been training and conducting patient case discussions with District Mental Health Program (DMHP) nurses in Karnataka and Bihar through telenursing since 2017.
- PGIMER Chandigarh is educating nurses from Nepal and Afghanistan through telenursing.
- During COVID-19 pandemic, nurses conducted webinars all over India to create awareness among nursing professionals.

Telenursing can have a significant impact on overcoming some of the health care challenges such as access to care, cost-effective care delivery and unequal distribution of health care providers.

NIMHANS Telenursing Practice Guidelines in India

The present telenursing guidelines were developed by faculty at NIMHANS in association with telemedicine society of India and the Trained Nurses Association of India. These guidelines are based on Code of Ethics and Professional Conduct for nurses in India.

Purposes

- To provide a clear direction for registered nurses to practice telenursing within their professional boundaries.
- To help nurses collaborate with specialist doctors, professional colleagues, and other health care team members in offering the best possible care on time.
- To act as a framework for enabling nurses adhere to ethical and professional norms

and direct them to be accountable for the care offered by them.
- To enable the nurses sustain professional, legal and ethical integrity in offering telenursing care.

Scope

- These guidelines are intended for registered nurses and registered auxiliary nurse midwives (RN & R. ANMs) under the INC Act 1947.
- Telenursing and telemedicine include all channels of communication with the patient that leverage information technology platform including voice, audio, text, and digital data exchange.
- These guidelines can also be utilized to educate health care workers in various aspects to update their knowledge.

Qualifications Required to Practice Telenursing in India

- At the National Institute of Mental Health and Neurosciences, Bengaluru registered nurses must undergo an online course/training on the practice of telenursing.
- Registered nurses are entitled to provide telenursing consultation to patients from across India both in private and public health establishments.
- Registered nurses who practice telenursing shall uphold the same professional and ethical norms, laws and clinical standards consistent within the scope of professional organizations [Indian Nursing Council Act, Code of ethics and professional standards for nurses in India and position statements by Trained Nurses Association of India (TNAI)].

Professional Responsibility and Accountability

- Seek help and share knowledge
- Identify learning needs as technology is ever-changing in the field of health care
- Be clear about professional roles and responsibilities and be consistent with standards and guidelines
- Report unprofessional or unsafe behavior of their professional colleagues to the authority
- Be aware of professional responsibility when using social media such as Facebook, WhatsApp, Videoconferencing, etc.
- Act as an advocate on behalf of their patients and ensure that their rights and interests are protected
- Maintain professional boundaries with their patients
- Respect other health team members

Legal and Ethical Considerations

- Ask the patients how they would like to be addressed
- Ensure the presence of family members while carrying out visual physical examination by the registered medical practitioner
- Maintain confidentiality of patient related information. Inform the patient that other health care team members who are directly involved in their care will have access to their personal health information
- Listen to patients' concerns and involve them in treatment decisions
- Empower the patients by providing appropriate information on their health condition
- Ensure that the patient understands what they are consenting to undergo
- Safeguard the area where audio or visual images are received from passers-by, casual intruders and unauthorized personnel

Documentation

- Ensure that documentation is done at the end of each telenursing consultation
- Confirm that documentation reflects the nursing process
- Follow the principles of documentation (accurate and relevant, complete, up to date, organized logically and sequentially)
- Ensure that the documentation of patient care begins with date and time and ends with nurses signature, RN/RM registration number and designation

Guidelines for Telenursing Practice

The following elements need to be considered before commencing the telenursing consultation:
- Context
- Identification of RN and patient
- Mode of communication
- Consent
- Assessment and communication of patient, related information with RMP
- Patient management
- Professional accountability and responsibilities of the registered nurse

Context

Registered nurses should exercise their clinical skills and professional judgment to decide whether a telenursing consultation is appropriate in a given situation or in-person consultation is needed in the interest of the patient. In this phase, the RN should make initial assessment of the patient and communicate with the registered medical practitioner. After discussing with RMP, the RN helps patients in deciding the type of care suitable for them. Whatever the context or situation, the registered nurse should uphold the same standard of care as in-person consultation.

Identification of the registered nurse and the patient

- In telenursing consultation, both patients and nurses need to know each other's identity. Nurses should verify and confirm patient's identity before using a checklist or a form to acquire patient details.
- The RN should ask for valid documents to confirm their age, height, weight, etc. She should confirm the presence of adults when children below the age of 18 years are being teleconsulted.
- The RN should obtain consent from patient/family members to transmit patient related data to RMPs and other health team members.
- The RN should display her identity information in all electronic communications.

Mode of Telenursing

- The most commonly used modes of communication are video, audio or text.
- Mode of communication should be based on patient's symptoms and preferences of health care providers.

Patient Consent

Patient consent is necessary for teleconsultation. Consent can either be implied or explicit. If the patient himself initiates telemedicine consultation, consent is implied. Explicit patient consent is required if a registered nurse or RMP or family member initiates the telemedicine consultation. Explicit consent can be in the form of an email, text, audio or video message.

Assessment and communication of patient related information with RMP:
- RN should collect patient history based on protocols and guidelines.
- RN should make a detailed assessment of patients based on written protocols. This information can help the RMPs to rule out emergencies and ensure positive patient outcomes.
- In case physical examination or in-person consultation is critical for the patient, RN should facilitate the same with the RMP.
- RN should maintain all patient records including case history, investigation reports, images, treatment prescriptions, and care details.

Patient management: Clinical care, health education and counseling, medication.
- Nursing management of patient includes- clinical care, providing information and health education related to the disease condition, counseling, reinforcing treatment regimen as prescribed by the doctor.
- The RN often initiates teleconsultation with the RMP to provide best possible care to the patient.
- The RN should offer nursing care to patients as per suggestions given by the RMP.
- Few of the nursing care activities include monitoring vital signs, distribution of

medications as prescribed by the RMP, wound dressing, suture removal, administration of IV fluids and medicines, and facilitating referrals to other health team members.
- The RN should educate patients on lifestyle changes, diet, stress management techniques, etc., and empower patients by providing necessary information about the disease condition. They should use educational videos to educate patients.
- The RN should provide information about disease condition, importance of medication adherence, follow-up visits, investigations that need to be done before the next visit with RMP and emotional support to patients and family members, etc.
- The RN should provide information about diet, dose and route, time frequency of the medications as prescribed by the RMP.
- The RN should receive a signed prescription or e-prescription issued by the registered medical practitioner and be able to transmit it in various digital formats to the patient via email or any other messaging platform.
- In case the RN is transmitting e-prescription directly to a pharmacy, explicit consent of the patient must be ensured which will entitle him to get the medicine dispensed from pharmacy of his choice.
- RN should document the care provided to the patients in their health records.

Professional Accountability and Responsibility of the Registered Nurse

- **Nursing ethics, data privacy and confidentiality:**
  - Principles of nursing ethics including professional norms for protecting patient privacy and confidentiality as per the INC act shall be binding and be upheld and practiced.
  - Registered nurses would be required to fully abide by the Indian Nursing Act 1947 and with the relevant provisions of the IT act, data protection and privacy laws or any applicable rules notified from time to time for protecting patient's privacy and confidentiality and regarding the handling and transfer of such personal information regarding the patient. This shall be binding and be upheld and practiced.
  - RN will not be held responsible for breach of confidentiality if there is reasonable evidence to believe that the patient's privacy and confidentiality have been compromised by a technology breach or a person other than the RN. The RN should ensure that a reasonable degree of care is undertaken while hiring such services.
- **Misconduct:** The RN is legally liable if their actions willfully compromise patient's care or privacy and confidentiality or violation of prevailing laws. Some examples of misconduct in telenursing practice are as follows:
  - RNs insisting on telemedicine while the patient is willing to travel to a facility or requests an in-person consultation
  - RNs misusing patient images and data that are especially private and sensitive (e.g., RN uploads explicit pictures of the patient on social media, etc.)
  - RNs issuing prescription, giving inappropriate advice out of their professional boundaries
  - RNs are not permitted to solicit patients for telenursing through advertisements or inducement.

REVIEW QUESTIONS

Long Essays (10 Marks)
1. Write detailed notes on information laws in India.
2. Narrate fundamental ethical principles related to health informatics.
3. Write a detailed note on ethical dimensions of health informatics.
4. What are the nurse's responsibilities in legal and ethical aspects of digital health?
5. Describe telenursing practice guidelines in India.
6. Describe privacy and confidentiality in electronic health-related data.
7. Explain health data management policy in India.
8. What are the ethical priorities of electronic health records?

Short Essays (5 Marks)
1. Right to privacy in India.
2. Explain protection act related to information technology.
3. Describe information technology act.
4. Describe personal data protection bill 2019.
5. Explain digital information security in healthcare act (DISHA-2017).
6. Explain governance structure in India related to information law.
7. Write a brief note on international medical informatics association.
8. Explain principles of general ethics.
9. Describe informatics ethics.
10. Explain code of ethics for software engineers.
11. Explain telenursing initiatives in India.

Short Answers (2 Marks)
1. Health big data
2. Digital health data
3. Sensitive personal data
4. Privacy and confidentiality
5. Security
6. Data integrity
7. Data availability
8. E-Sanjeevani
9. HIPAA
10. DISHA-2017

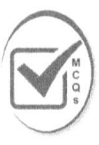

MULTIPLE CHOICE QUESTIONS

1. Which of the following bills in India regulates the protection and privacy of data in both digital and non-digital forms?
   a. Personal data protection bill
   b. DISHA act
   c. HIPAA act
   d. Information technology act
2. Which of the following includes personal data?
   a. Height of the person
   b. Religion of the person
   c. National security data
   d. Caste of the person
3. Which of the following includes personal sensitive data?
   a. Height of the person
   b. Religion of the person
   c. National security data
   d. Skin color of the person
4. Which of the following includes critical sensitive personal data?
   a. Height of the person
   b. Religion of the person
   c. National security data
   d. Caste of the person
5. Which of the following acts standardizes and controls the process of collecting, storing, sharing and using digital health data?
   a. Personal data protection bill
   b. DISHA act
   c. HIPAA act
   d. Information technology act

Unit 9 | Information Law and Governance in Clinical Practice

6. Which of the following acts is a legislation of the United States of America?
   a. Personal data protection bill
   b. DISHA act
   c. HIPAA act
   d. Information technology act

7. What is code of ethics?
   a. It includes ethical principles and duties
   b. It includes ethical conflicts and situations
   c. It includes ethics committee responsibilities
   d. It includes general guidelines of organization

8. All the following are general ethics, except
   a. Non-malfeasance
   b. Security
   c. Beneficence
   d. Autonomy

9. All of the following are informatics ethics, except
   a. Equality and justice
   b. Privacy
   c. Openness
   d. Access

10. All of the following are software engineering ethics, except
    a. Judgment
    b. Management
    c. Profession
    d. Accountability

11. What is health big data?
    a. Data related to physical and mental health
    b. Huge health data from the consumers
    c. Personal data revealing religion, race or ethnic origin
    d. Biometric data

12. Which of the following denotes right of the individuals to keep information about themselves from being disclosed to others?
    a. Security
    b. Privacy
    c. Integrity
    d. Availability

13. Which of the following denotes protection from accidental and intentional disclosure to unauthorized persons?
    a. Security
    b. Privacy
    c. Integrity
    d. Availability

14. Which of the following denotes data is accurate and has not been changed?
    a. Security
    b. Privacy
    c. Integrity
    d. Availability

15. Which of the following is related to e-Sanjeevani?
    a. Telemedicine services under Ayushman Bharat initiative
    b. Telenursing services to rural people
    c. Telenursing practice guidelines
    d. Telemedicine practice guidelines

ANSWER KEY

1. a	2. a	3. b	4. c	5. b	6. c	7. a	8. b	9. a	10. d
11. b	12. b	13. a	14. c	15. a					

Health Care Quality and Evidence Based Practice

UNIT 10

INTRODUCTION

Quality is the degree to which health services for individuals and population increase the likelihood of desired health outcomes and that which are consistent with current professional knowledge.

Quality improvement is a framework used to improve care in a systematic manner. It seeks to standardize processes and structure to improve outcomes for patients, health care systems and organizations.

Quality Improvement

Quality improvement is defined as the combined and unceasing effort of health care professionals, patients and their families, researchers, planners and educators to make changes that will lead to better patient health outcomes, system performance (care) and professional development.

Advantages of Quality Improvement for Health

- Ensures proper usage of resources
- Confirms use of latest scientific knowledge and new technologies in treatment
- Ensures that people with disorders receive the care they need
- Helps to build trust in the effectiveness of the system
- Assists in overcoming barriers to appropriate care at different levels
- Provides an opportunity to improve health care in a systematic way

As significant focus has been placed on enhancing the quality of health care services, patient safety outcomes and cost control in the health care system framework a more prominent emphasis was placed on evidence-based practice (EBP) which was recognized as crucial for promoting quality care and health care excellence.

Role of Nurse to Ensure Quality Health Care

Nurses actively participate in the formal organizational evaluation of overall patterns of care through a variety of quality improvement activities (Baker et al., 2000; Williams, 1998).

- Interprets own professional strengths, role and scope of ability to peers, patients and colleagues.
- Incorporates professional/legal standards into practice.
- Acts ethically to meet the needs of patients.
- Assumes accountability for practice and strives to attain the highest standards of practice.
- Engages in self-evaluation concerning practice and uses evaluative information including peer review to improve care and practice.
- Collaborates and/or consults with members of the health care team about variations in health outcomes.

- Uses an evidence-based approach to patient management that critically evaluates and applies research findings pertinent to patient care management and outcomes.
- Evaluates patient's response to the health care provided and effectiveness of care.
- Uses the outcomes of care to revise care delivery strategies and improve quality of care.
- Accepts personal responsibility for professional development and maintenance of professional competence and credentials.
- Considers ethical implications of scientific advances and practices accordingly.

Nurses play an essential role in identifying opportunities for improvement, collecting data for analysis of the current process, evaluating the effectiveness of new processes, and representing nursing perspective in the improvement of team's deliberations.

Evidence-Based Practice (EBP)

Evidence-based practice is the meticulous and thoughtful use of current best evidence to guide health care decisions. Evidence-based nursing (EBN) is the process of integrating clinical knowledge, judgment, expertise skills and individual preferences with the best available clinical evidence (Box 10.1).

Evidence-Based Nursing involves identifying sound research findings and implementing them in nursing practices so as to improve quality of patient care. The main goal of EBN is to provide high quality and cost-efficient nursing care.

Definitions

Evidence-based practice is the conscious, explicit and judicious use of current best evidence in making decisions about the care of individual patients. —(Sackett 1996)

Evidence-based practice (EBP) is a problem-solving approach to the delivery of health care that integrates the best evidence from studies and patient care data with clinician expertise and patient preferences and values. —(Fineout-Overholt E, 2010)

Scope of EBP

EBP in nursing not only helps in taking decisions about patient care but also extends to

- Identifying knowledge gaps
- Finding scientifically evaluated knowledge
- Condensing the evidence to assist clinical expertise

EBP has become a suitable framework and a prominent care model that has been recognized for facilitating the transfer of research evidence to clinical practice. EBP improves patient outcomes, nurses' efficiency and cost-effective care delivery for organizations.

Relevance of Evidence-based Practice in Providing Quality Health Care (EBP and Quality Improvement)

- Components of evidence-based medicine and quality improvement are complementary. While evidence-based medicine justifies clinical decisions with evidence, quality improvement is translational; putting evidence-based medicine into practice in health care systems.
- Quality improvement becomes difficult to justify or measure and arguably does not work without evidence.
- Implementing EBP and Quality improvement are recognized as crucial competencies for which each health care professional should contribute.
- Clinical research, EBP and quality improvement are separate but interrelated areas of investigation.

Box 10.1: Evidence-based nursing practice integrates

- Best evidence available
- Nursing expertise
- Values and preferences of the individuals, families and communities

- EBP was considered the gold standard and a problem-solving approach to deliver safe and high-quality patient care.
- Quality improvement was found to be a vital contextual organizational factor for the adoption of EBP as it could be used to validate the introduction of EBPs, while clinical research offered empirical evidence for EBP.
- To significantly influence the improvement of quality in health care there is a need to apply evidence-based practice.
- Without EBP, health care providers are at a risk for variances in care that could seriously affect patient outcomes.

Benefits of EBP

- **For patients**
  - Provides high-quality cost-effective nursing care
  - Results in better patient outcomes leading to greater patient satisfaction
- **For nurses**
  - By reading all published literature in the specialized area the nurse can keep herself abreast with the latest information
  - Increases efficiency in providing care to the patients
  - Provides rationale to all nursing interventions thereby helping in the development of the profession
  - Nurses can communicate effectively with patients and other health care team members about the rationales for decision-making and care plan
  - Provides legal accountability for practice
  - Resolves problems in the clinical setting
  - Achieves excellence in care delivery, at times even exceeding quality assurance standards
  - Introduces innovation
  - Reduces the variations in nursing care
  - Unnecessary practices are eliminated and ineffective practices replaced with effective ones
  - Assists with efficient and effective decision-making thereby building confidence
- **For health care organization**
  - Helps the hospital in achieving Magnet status. The Magnet Recognition Program acknowledges quality patient care, nursing excellence and innovations in nursing practice. Being a magnet facility patients are assured of excellent nursing service.
  - Since care is delivered based on best evidence, it is less likely to attract litigation and able to defend the care provided.
  - Allows scrutinizing of practice for effectiveness. This process results in significant cost savings.
- **For community**
  - Resources are preserved by not wasting them on implementation of ineffective interventions.
  - Ensures most effective care and limits the amount of disability and suffering from people.

Role of Informatics in Evidence-based Practice

The majority of clinical practice is based on a small amount of data, primarily textbooks, outdated research or case studies, fragmentary reviews. Because of lack of awareness or understanding of the available data, proven therapies with substantial evidence are not used. Also clinicians frequently do not believe that outcomes reported in clinical trials can be easily translated into clinical practice.

Development of outcome research studies as well as the growing interest in health care costs contributed to the push for a more logical approach to clinical decision-making. Technology advances helped health care professionals to critically appraise and utilize peer-reviewed published data in a systematic manner. An increase in patient requests for information and a loss of trust in health care practitioners all contributed to the growing relevance of evidence-based procedures.

Current trends in health care are the application of evidence-based practice through the development of research and information technology/informatics. The main advantage of EBP is to improve patient care by choosing best clinical practices. The ultimate goal is to shift health care decisions and actions to a more scientific based level. Informatics is a key factor in the development of evidence-based practice in nursing and other health care disciplines.

Finding Evidence Using Technology Support

- Evidence-based medicine (EBM) is a more scientific approach that avoids the use of unapproved and unsystematic data. Evidence-based practice ensures the connectivity between clinical expertise and research evidence. Evidence-based practices strengthen the link between knowledge and decision-making while also adding science and professionalism to the diagnosis, treatment and patient care processes.
- More software, toolkits, journals, digitalized research chapters are the simplest forms of technology development in health care sector. This frequently necessitates the examination of a huge amount of complex data. As a result, health care managers in charge of implementing information systems and EBM policies and guidelines need to understand EBM ideas as well as the capabilities and limitations of various IT solutions for EBM.
- In the practice of evidence-based medicine, information technology is critical because it allows health care practitioners to access and analyze clinical evidence as they develop patient care plans.
- Digital health technology offers important opportunities to optimize both evidence-based delivery and clinical literature review.
- Health information technology increases patient-centered decision-making, quality of patient care and safety.
- Technology by connecting patients to community and educational programs improves health literacy.
- Despite their potential the use of such digital technologies in evidence-based practice and research faces major data quality, privacy and regulatory concerns.
- Health informatics paves way for managing and accessing clinical data. It helps health care professionals to seek related information at essential times.
- Internet of Things, Machine Learning, Deep Learning, etc., are now the current trend for data management. They provide daily updates on the evidence that are made out of particular case subjects.
- An increasing amount of clinical data and database creates more obstacles for health professionals in realizing appropriate information. Therefore, a need for efficient management of the information is important. Updating to the current technology becomes an essential need.
- EBP and Information and communication technology is crucial to ensure that doctors and nurses provide care based on current and appropriate evidence.

Steps in Evidence Based Nursing and Role of Informatics

To practice evidence-based nursing, nurses must not only recognize and appreciate the concept of research but also know how to evaluate the research findings accurately. These skills should be integrated into the nursing curriculum and made a part of their professional training. There are six steps in EBP in nursing (**Box 10.2**).

Box 10.2: Steps in EBN process

- Select a research problem
- Form a team
- Retrieve evidence
- Evaluate the evidence
- Apply the evidence
- Evaluate the efficacy

1. The EBP process begins with selecting a clinical problem. The nurse can select a clinical problem by reviewing the evidence found in research articles and sources. Technology can be very helpful at this stage to review information.
2. Forming a team is paramount in successful implementation and evaluation of EBP. Through informatics the team members can communicate effectively and educate the co-workers, clarify doubts and clear any misconceptions to improve the outcomes.
3. Once the clinical problem is finalized, relevant literature must be extensively reviewed. This process begins by using appropriate electronic databases and performing effective online searches using computers. Computer networks allow knowledge to be shared in multiple ways. The World Wide Web (WWW) is a network program which makes it possible to gather information from many sources and also share information around the globe. Smart phones add another layer of information gathering and storage via telephone and global positioning system (GPS) technology thus preserving the ability to access and disseminate information.
4. Once the literature is located, the article needs to be evaluated. Not all evidence is equal nor will all evidence be applicable to a particular clinical setting. Technological advances and tools address the validity of the study, reliability of the results and applicability to the particular patient care setting.
5. Once the literature is analyzed using a systematic approach, the next step is putting the EBP process into practice. A timeline for the project is essential to keep it on track. The timeline plan can be made using an Excel spreadsheet or a software specific for project planning. Following the timeline and sharing the project results during implementation help other nurses to remain engaged in practice change.
6. Next step involves evaluating the evidence. Standardized computer terminology and databases provide an opportunity to evaluate evidence-based practice. Outcome data is available from electronic hospital records, disease-specific registers and other quality care databases.

Nursing Informatics and EBP

Nursing informatics is a specialty that integrates nursing science, computer science and information science to manage and communicate date, information, knowledge and wisdom in nursing practice. Nursing informatics continues to be a growing field as nurses' face ever changing and challenging practice situations. Competency in nursing informatics not only strengthens nurse's clinical decision-making skills but also enhances their practice skills. The advantages of use of informatics for nurses are as follows:

- Informatics helps nurses to get quicker access to patient information, improve overall efficiency and reduce potential errors.
- Nursing informatics has the potential to improve nursing practice and better patient outcomes.
- Information processing has been a vital part of nursing. Information processing and communication are involved in all nursing activities such as obtaining and recording information about patients, communicating among health care professionals, accessing medical literature, selecting diagnostic procedures, interpreting laboratory results, collecting clinical research data.
- Information and communication technology advancement has made it possible to harness technology for quickening all these activities and accessing a digitally stored pool of literature and statistics. It not only assists in decision making but also provides a platform for nurses to record and plan individual patient care.
- This advancement in access to quality data, information and knowledge can be a very valuable resource for practicing evidence-based nursing.

Unit 10 | Health Care Quality and Evidence Based Practice

REVIEW QUESTIONS

Long Essays (10 Marks)
1. What is quality improvement? List advantages of quality improvement for health. Describe role of a nurse in ensuring quality health care.
2. Define evidence-based nursing practice. Detail on scope and its relevance in providing quality health care.

Short Essays (5 Marks)
1. Describe benefits of EBP.
2. Explain role of informatics in evidence-based practice.
3. Nursing informatics and EBP.

MULTIPLE CHOICE QUESTIONS

1. Which of the following meanings is related to evidence based nursing?
   a. It is the process of integrating clinical knowledge, judgment expertise skills and best available clinical evidence to provide quality care
   b. It is the process of integrating clinical knowledge, judgment expertise skills and individual preferences with the best available clinical evidence to provide quality care
   c. It is the conscious, explicit and judicious use of research resources to provide patient care
   d. It is an approach to delivery of health care that integrates current research resources and personal judgement of health care professionals to provide best patient care services

2. Which of the following is the first step in EBN?
   a. Form a team
   b. Evidence retrieval
   c. Select a research problem
   d. Evaluate the efficacy

3. In which of the following steps of EBN are the research articles evaluated?
   a. Evidence retrieval
   b. Apply evidence
   c. Evaluate the evidence
   d. Evaluate the efficacy

ANSWER KEY

1. b   2. c   3. c

Index

Page numbers followed by *b* refer to box, *f* refer to figure and *t* refer to table.

A

Academic record keeping 8
Accelerates research 67
Accomplishes health priorities 162
Accountability 83
Accreditation standards 67
Accuracy 12
Acquisition 60
Activities covered under e-health 164
Administrative control 22
Administrative data 70
Administrative documentation 55
Administrative functions 66
Administrators, role of 128
Advanced telehealth 193
Allocates appropriate resources 72
Alternative billing concepts codes 151
American Health Information Management Association 205
American Medical Association 150
American Medical Informatics Association 64, 194, 205
American Nurses Association 153, 179
American Nurses Credentialing Center 191
American Nursing Informatics Association 194
American Society of Healthcare Risk Management 129
Analyzing clinical data 197
Ancillary information system 86
Angiography 86
Apps, types of 171
Architectural building blocks, five-layered system of 107
Architectural principles, set of 107
Arithmetic and logic unit 2
Arogyasree 169
Artificial intelligence tools 198
Asynchronous telemedicine 169
Automated calling systems 173
Automated medication dispensing cabinets 119, 185
Automated processes 83, 136
Automatic staff scheduling 186

Autonomy, principle of 209
Ayushman Bharat Digital Mission 175
    components of 176, 176f
Ayushman Bharat Scheme 167
Ayushman Bharat Yojana Scheme 214

B

Bar code technology 120
Beneficence, principle of 209
Better staff management 187
Bibliographic database 40, 41
    strategies for 41f
Biometric data 70
Block chain networks 198
Blood
    clots 116
    glucose monitors 175
    pressure monitors 175
    vessels 174
Blueprint include 107
Body temperature monitors 175
Boolean operators 42
    concepts of 42f
British Computer Society 205
Broadband 33
Browser 33, 33t

C

Cable 34
Canada's Health Informatics Association 205
Capturing rich patient data 101f
Cardiac arrhythmia devices 175
Cardiovascular information system 85
Cardiovascular picture archiving and communication systems 86
Care
    current standards of 180
    delivery of 66
    impersonalization of 67
    outcomes of 122
    plan 15, 85
    quality of 51, 87, 192

Catastrophes, plans for 130
Centers for Disease Control and Prevention 49, 150
Centers for Health Informatics 167
Central processing unit 2, 3
Child abuse 204
Client server architecture 80, 81f
Clinical care classification system 151, 152
Clinical data 69
Clinical decision support 62, 76, 85
    systems 120, 186
Clinical documentation 55, 84
Clinical information system 63, 83, 84
    areas of 84f
    barriers of 88, 88f
    benefits of 86, 86f
    information flows of 84
    infrastructure of 84
    major areas of 84
Clinical knowledge and decision-making 140
Clinical research 87, 163
    informatics 63
Closed sources software 45
Cloud architecture 81
Cloud based health information systems 62
Cloud computing platforms 198
Cognitive psychology 115
Commercial websites 35
Common desktop applications 118
Common surgical procedures 174
Communicable diseases 204
Communicate plan 133
Communication 17, 61, 66, 95
    lack of 97
    systems 82
    technology 162
    tool 28
Compatible learning style 7
Comprehensive primary health care 167
Computed tomography 60, 86
Computer 1
    application, forms of 8
    assisted learning 8
        advantages of 10f
        limitations of 10f
        modes of 9f
    based system 92
    breakdown 96
    classification of 4
    components of 1, 2f
    features of 5
    generated nursing care plans and critical pathways 185
    historical perspectives of 5
    importance of 12
    influence of 1
    parts of 2, 3f
    peripherals 80
    role of 12, 13, 14f, 18
    skills 179
    systems 80
    use of 6, 12, 12t
Computerized care documentation 121, 184
Computerized physician order entry 120
Confidentiality 97, 210, 212
Consent management 107
Consumer health informatics 63
Control unit 2
Co-ordinates patient care 193
Core systems 82
Coronary artery bypass 174
Cost constraints 96
Cost effective 83
    care 162
Cost reduction 71, 95
Course record management 8
COVID-19 pandemic 214
Critical sensitive personal data 203
Current procedural terminology 150
Cyber security
    issues 96
    risks 67

D

Data 69, 142
    aggregation 136
    analytics 198
        benefits of 196, 196f
    change, principle of 105
    complex forms of 92
    encryption 105
    exchange 104
    induced observations 145
    integrity 105, 213
    management 77
    matrix code 121
    privacy 105, 217
    resources 80
    security 105
    sources 77
    types of 69
    use of 68, 69
Decision making 15, 143, 147
Decision support systems 61
Delivering health care services 163

Desktop 22
　computers 5
　information systems 180
Diagnostic procedures 55
Digital certificate 105
Digital health 107
　data 211
　ethical aspects of 213
　National Digital Health Blueprint outlines
　　　six pillars of 107
　services 168, 168f
Digital information security in
　　　healthcare act 109, 203
Digital infrastructure 168
Digital slate 11
Digitalize healthcare documents 146
DirectX, addition of 22
Disaster management 170
Discovery analytics 196
Display 20, 61
Distance learning 7
Distributed system 81
District mental health program 214
Doc-to-print 24
Document camera 11
Documentation 16, 215
Drug administration 188
Duties towards
　health care professionals 206
　institutions, employers and agencies 206
　profession 207
　society 206

■ E

Education 67, 161, 163, 170
Educational resources 145
Educational websites 35
Effective health care 69
Effective record-keeping system 95
Effective teaching experience 7
Efficient decision-making 187
e-health 158, 164f
　benefits of 161, 161b
　characteristics of 160, 160b
　core areas of 159
　goals of 160
　government-led initiatives 164
　infrastructure 167
　purposes of 160
　services 162
e-hospital 165
e-learning modules 10

Electrocardiograph 60
Electronic
　databases 38, 39t
　health record 17, 63, 65, 68, 75, 90, 91, 91t, 97,
　　　107, 122, 165, 175, 177, 179, 180, 184, 190
　　adoption 107, 108
　　ethical priorities of 212
　　model 110, 111f
　　standards 103
　　system, components of 111
　　trends in 91
　learning 10, 175
　medical record 18, 76, 90, 91, 91t, 106, 179, 180
　　need for safety of 98
　medication administration record 85, 184
　patient record 75
　personal record 75
　physician orders 120
　records
　　benefits of 94f
　　implementation of 96
　sign-out and hand-off tools 120, 186
E-mail 35
　management 173
Emergency department information systems 85
Enhanced academic performance 6f, 7
Entertainment websites 35
e-office 166
e-pharmacies 175
Epidemiological surveillance 170
e-prescription 105, 120
Ethical codes, functions of 207
Ethical issues 97
Ethics 161
　code of 205
　committees 205
Evidence-based medicine 223
Evidence-based nursing 221
　practice integrates 221b
　steps in 223, 223f
Evidence-based practice 220-222
　benefits of 222
　relevance of 221
　scope of 221
Excellent virus protection 21
External legislations 132

■ F

Facilitates
　compliance 137
　organizational change management 192
　strategic planning 79

Fairness 8
Fan 4
Financial systems 82
Flexible design 136
Font styles and formatting 25
Food and Drug Administration 151
Formal decision support 145
Functioning, mode of 81
Fundamental ethical principles 204

G

Gallbladder removal 174
Games 9
Geographical information system 170, 177, 178
Global information systems 92
Global positioning system 224
G-mail 35
   screenshot of 36f
Google
   chrome 31
   drive 35
   forms, outlook of 37f
Gradual implementation 127
Graphical user interface 20
Graphics
   card 20
   processing unit 4
Graphs 27
Grid architecture 81
Gross domestic product 107
Group health plan requirements,
   enforcement of 204
Gunshot wounds 204

H

Hard disk
   drive 4
   space 20
Hardware
   equipment 11
   problems 101
   resources 80
Health 163
   administration 134
   analytics 107
   and wellness centers 167
   big data 210
   facility registry 176
   insurance 203
   kiosks 173
   literacy program 165
   population support 71
   portals 173
   promotion of 177
   record 103, 176
   research 163
Health care 74, 94f, 123, 129f, 145, 146f, 162, 196, 196f, 207
   adverse events in 116
   analytics 136
      types of 195
   associated infections 116
   common procedure coding system 150
   costs, reduction in 196
   data
      analytics 70, 194, 195f, 198
      evaluation of 194
      management, benefits of 71, 71f
      presentation of 194
      types of 69f
   delivery 170
      minimum level of 109
   informatics 201
   knowledge management 143
      activities of 144, 144f
      goals of 144
      modalities of 145
      types of 144, 144f
   management 170
      using information in 183
   organization 222
      management of 194
   professional 52, 60, 162
      registry 176
      role of 127
   providers 123
   quality 65, 220
   risk management 129, 136
      and technology 135
      plan 132, 133f
   sector 69
   terminology standards, classification of 149
Health data management 163
   policy 211
Health informatics 59, 149, 204, 205
   applications of 63, 63f
   benefits of 64, 65b
   central concepts in 69f
   elements in 60, 60f
   ethical dimensions of 208f
   ethics 207
   limitations of 67f
   need for 64
   objectives of 64
   principle of 59, 64

Health information
  and technology 149
  exchanges 198
  governance 126
  professionals 205
    self-regarding duties of 207
  system 61, 62, 75, 76
    benefits of 77, 78f
    components of 76, 76f
    essentials of 63, 79
    historical development of 74
    types of 61, 62f
  technology 68, 115, 118
    advantages of 122, 122f
    importance of 122
Health Insurance Portability and Accountability Act
  administrative simplification 203
  five main rules of 203
  health insurance reform 203
  tax-related health provisions 204
High turnover rate 125
High-level privacy 94
High-quality patient care, delivery of 124
Hip replacement 174
Home health care classification 152
Hospital administration 55
Hospital electronic medical records 91
Hospital information system 17, 81, 82f, 165, 183
  elements of 82, 83f
  features of 83f
  need for 77
  parts of 82f
Hospital management information system 50, 163
  goals of 51
  importance of 51, 52f
  softwares 56, 56f
  tasks of 51, 52f
Hospital risk management process 135, 135f
Hospital stays, reduces length of 66
Human factors engineering 115
Human infrastructure 168
Hyper text
  markup language 31
  transfer protocol 32
Hysterectomy 174

I

India Health Information Network
  Development 164
Indian Nursing Council 10
Infectious diseases 204
Informal discussions 205

Informatics
  ethics 209
  knowledge 180
  limitations of 123, 123f
  nurse 189
    competencies required for 179
    responsibilities of 194
    role of 194
    specialist 189
  role of 222
  skills 180
Information 10, 52, 69, 70, 74, 142, 207
  and communication technology 10, 59, 158
  collection 70
  easy access to 93
  e-mail exchange of 172
  laws 201
  model 104
  processing 59
  products 77
  science of 59
  security management 105
  system 74
    architecture 79, 80
    basic types of 61f
    components of 80, 80f
    engineering of 59
  technology 180, 202, 202f
    act 202
    use of 118
  transfer 70
  use of 162
Infrastructure issues 107
Inpatient clinical information system 84
Input unit 1
Insta 56
Insurance processing 173
Integrated disease surveillance program 165
Integrity, principle of 209
Intensive care unit information system 85
Interactive health communication and
    disease prevention 170
Interactive voice response systems 173
Interface terminologies 151
International Classification for Nursing
    Practice 151, 152
  elements of 152
International Council of Nurses 153, 214
International Medical Informatics
    Association 68, 205
International Standards for Electronic
    Health Record 106
Internet 30, 32, 32t

connection 32
   modes of 33f
  sites 34
   types of 34f

K

Keyboard 2
Kidney transplant 174
Knowledge 51, 69, 142
  acquisition 143
  creation 70, 143
  management 140, 148
   benefits of 145, 146f
   components of 141, 141f
   concepts of 141f
   dimensions of 143
   process of 142f, 143, 143f, 145
   role of 147
   stages of 142, 142f
   tools 143

L

Laboratory information system 86
Laptops 5
LaQshya 167
Learning 6
  management system 11
  time, optimal use of 7
Least intrusive alternatives, principle of 209
Legacy system, integration of 88
Legitimate infringement, principle of 209
Libreoffice 48
Literature search 36
  evidence-based databases of 39t
  methods of 38, 38f
  process of 43
  purposes of 37
  strategies 40f
  web-based methods of 39t
Local area network 5, 80
Low public health expenditure 107
Lowers administrative burden 162

M

Machine learning models 198
Magnetic resonance imaging 60
Mainframe 5
  architecture 81
Malpractice liability concerns 96
Management information system 61, 132
Manpower challenges 102
Master patient index 62

Medcin 150
Medical devices 118
  interfacing 105
Medical documentation systems 83
Medical errors
  circumvention of 79
  lowers risk of 122
  reduction in 93, 146
Medical knowledge 144
  advancement of 72
Medical professionals 146
Medical research 71, 197
Medical support systems 83
Medical system software applications 118
Medical virtual assistants 172
Medication errors 19, 116
Medicine
  improves practice of 122
  systematized nomenclature of 150
Memory 4
  unit 2
Mesh page, outlook of 41f
Mhealth 171
  application of 172, 172f, 173
Mic 4
Microsoft internet explorer 31
Microsoft office 20, 24
  excel 20, 26, 27, 45
   features of 27
   interface of 28f
  overview of 24f
  PowerPoint 20, 28, 29
   basics of 30f
   features of 28, 29f
  word 20, 24, 25
   computer shortcut keys for 27t
   features of 24, 24f, 25f
   interface of 26f
Minicomputer 4
Minimized operational expense 79
Minimum data sets 151
Minimum viable standards, lack of 108
Ministry of Health and Family Welfare 160, 169, 204
  telemedicine division of 169
Minitab 46
Misconduct 217
Mobile 33
Mobilize data 101
Modern healthcare environment 79
Monitor 2
  care 130
  regional outbreaks 72
  trends over time 71

Monitoring student progress 6f
Motherboard 3
Mouse 3
Multiple access channels 107
MyHealth app 107

N

National Cancer Network 165
National Council Licensure Examination 8
National Digital Health Authority 109
National Digital Health Blueprint 106, 204, 211
National Digital Health Mission 107, 112, 175, 204
National Drug Code 151
National Drug File-Reference Terminology 150
National Electronic Health Authority 109
National Health Authority 204
National Health Exchange 107
National Health Policy 175, 204
National Health Portal 164, 167
National Informatics Center 164
National Library of Medicine 41, 153
National Medical College Network 166
National Program for Health Care for Elderly 167
National Telemedicine Network 166
National Telemedicine Portal 169
Natural Language Processing 148
Nerves 174
Net books 5
Netscape navigator 31
Network
    connection, flow of 33f
    resources 80
    support 21
Networking systems 82
New medical therapies, development of 123
NITI Aayog 106
Non-clinical data 70
Non-communicable disease program 167
North American Nursing Diagnosis Association
    International 151
    terminology 153
Nurse
    administrator, role of 134
    documentation 187
    informaticist, responsibilities of 180
    responsibilities 213
    role of 134, 179, 220
Nursing
    administration 18, 19, 186
    care performance 148
    education 8, 16, 155
    ethics 217
    implications 198

management minimum data set 151, 154
minimum data set 151, 154
outcome classification 151, 153
practice 1, 13, 14f
Nursing informatics 180, 183, 188, 224
    goal of 189
    history of 191
    importance of 192, 193f
    need for 189
    practice, standards of 191
Nursing information system 183, 184, 188
    benefits of 187, 187f
    components of 184, 185f
    purposes of 183
Nursing interventions classification system 151, 153

O

Occupational safety 134
Omaha system 151, 153
Oncology information system 86
Online
    consultation-telemedicine 166
    registration system 166
    services 166
    software 50
Open document format 48
Open source software 48
    advantages of 48
    disadvantages of 48
Openness, principle of 209
Operational knowledge 145
Optical character recognition 61
Optimal care delivery 181
Organizational leadership 125
Organized and coordinated treatment process 78
Outpatient clinical information system 84

P

Page and margins 24
Partial kidney removal 174
Patient care 122
    delivery system, computer applications for 1
    services, improves quality of 71
Patient classification systems 186
Patient consent 216
Patient data, easy access to 86
Patient education 16
Patient electronic portals 121
Patient empowerment 93
Patient feedback
    data 70
    system 166

Patient health information system 62
Patient identification confidentiality 146
Patient knowledge 144
Patient management 216
Patient records, handling of 55
Patient safety 78, 87, 115, 118, 122, 123
    Initiative
        benefits of 117f
        importance of 117
        issues 116f, 117
        nature of 115
        outcomes, monitoring of 127
Pediatric echocardiography reports 86
Pedometers 175
Performance analysis, hassle-free process of 78
Perioperative nursing data set 151, 154
Personal computer 4, 20
Personal data 203
    protection bill 202
Personal healthcare 105
Personal websites 35
Personalized digital assistant 75
Pharmacy information system 86
Phrase search 42
Physical infrastructure 167
Picture archiving communication system 111
Point-of-care diagnostics 171
Policy 211
    infrastructure 168
Population health management 197
Positron emission tomography 60
Potential privacy 96
Power outages 96
Practice management software 62
Practitioner's clinical experiences 145
Pradhan Mantri Jan Arogya Yojana 106, 214
Pradhan Mantri Surakshit Matritva Abhiyan 167
Precision medicine 71
Predictive analytics 196
Prescriptive analytics 196
Preventive medicine 71
Primary health center 110
Privacy 88, 97, 107, 210, 212
    causes invasion of 124
    principle of 209
    problems 22
Privilege management and access control 105
Processor 20
Promotes precise medicine 123
Public health 162, 169, 170f, 172, 172f
    informatics 64, 176
        concepts of 176
        principle of 177, 177f
        process of 179
        scope of 178
Public private partnership 109
PubMed search 44f

Q

Quality assurance 187
Quality health care 140
Quality improvement 220
    advantages of 220
Quicker access 94

R

Radiation errors 116
Radiology exams 60
Radlex 150
Random-access memory 4, 20
Rashtriya Bal Swasthya Karyakram 167
Reduces medical errors 129, 162
Reduces practice variation 123
Registered nurse
    professional accountability of 217
    responsibilities of 217
Remote monitoring 172
    telemedicine 169
Remote patient monitoring 62
Repetitive manual tasks, automation of 87
Retained surgical items prevention
    technology 120
Revenue offsets 204
Risk management cycle, stages of 130, 130f
Risk management
    advantages of 129
    process
        applications of 128
        functions of 128
Robot assisted surgery 173
Robotic assistance 174
Robotic surgery procedure 174
Rxnorm 150

S

Safety evidence, lack of 125
Safety practices 129
Safety risk identification 127
Satcom based telemedicine nodes 166
Satellite 34
Sciences underpinning nursing informatics 189
Scientific research data 70
Search
    box 23
    engine 32, 33, 33t, 35

Security 88, 97, 213
    challenges 102
    components 99
    patient information 136
    principle of 209
    strategies 99
Self-monitoring health care devices 174, 175
Sensitive personal data 202, 203, 211
Sepsis 116
Share data 101
Shortcuts 21
Sleep apnea monitors 175
Smart audio 11
Smart classroom 10
    components of 11, 11f
Smart pumps 119
SNOMED clinical terms 151
Social knowledge 145
Software 207
    engineering ethics 210
    problems 101
    resources 80
Speakers 4
Specialty information systems 85
Speed 12, 83
Stake-holder involvement 127
Standard nursing terminologies 151
Standardized electronic health record,
    development of 110
Standardized languages, benefits of 155
Standardized software languages 149
Start button 20
Start menu 22
Stata windows view 48f
Statistical packages
    types of 45f
    uses of 44
Statistical software, types of 44
Strategic information management orientation 92
Streamline data collection 109
Strengthens clinical decision-making 193
Sub-health center 110
Super computer 5
Supply management 173
Support clinical research 95
Support clinical treatment decisions 196
Support electronic medical records 93
Supports patient-centered care 188
Surgical console 173
Sustainable development goal 118
Suvarna Health Information Systems 56
Synchronous telemedicine 169

System icons 23
Systematic process 140

T

Tablet and pen 11
Tablet computers 5
Tacit knowledge 145
Taluk Health Center 110
Taskbar 20, 23
Teaching 6
Technological factors 148
Technological flaws compromise patient
    safety 125, 126f
Technology 141
    flaws 126
    optimization 127
    types of 118, 119, 119f
Tedious manual activities, automates of 87
Teleconferencing 172
Telehealth 62, 168
Telemedicine 17, 71, 168, 178
    application 169, 170f
        types of 169, 169f
    consultation center 168
    current scenario of 169
    specialty center 168
    system 168
Telenursing 186
    initiatives 214
    mode of 216
    practice guidelines 214, 216
Teleradiology 166
Terminology standards, benefits of 149
Therapeutic procedures 55
Total kidney removal 174
Touch screen 22
Trained Nurses Association India 215
Transaction processing systems 61
Translational bioinformatics 63
Transport infrastructure 167
Truncation 42
T-test 46

U

Unified medical language system 153
Uniform minimum health data set 154
Uniform resource locator 31
Unique health ID 107
Universal health coverage 106, 118
Unsafe injections practices 116
Unsafe surgical care procedures 116
Unsafe transfusion practices 116
User experience issues 125

V

Venous thromboembolism 116
Video conferencing facility 167
Village resource center 169
Virtual medical assistant 172
    activities of 172, 173f
Vision cart 173
Visual supplement 28

W

Web 32, 32t
    browser 32
    pages 35
Web-based architecture 81
Webcam 4
Websites 34
Wellness management apps 171
Wide area network 5, 80
Wi-fi hotspots 33
Wildcard symbol 42
Windows 20
    basic tools of 22
    features of 20, 20f
Windows 10
    advantages of 21t
    disadvantages of 21t
    hardware requirements for 20
    interface of 23f
    pros and cons of 21
    start-up screen of 22f
Wireless local area network 33
Word processing 25
Work organization 55
World Health Assembly 117
World Health Organization 116, 205
World patient safety day 117
World wide web 31

EU GSPR Authorised Reprsentative
Logos Europe, 9 rue Nicolas Poussin
1700, La Rochelle, France
Phone: +33 (0) 6 67 93 73 78
E-mail: contact@logoseurope.eu

www.ingramcontent.com/pod-product-compliance
Ingram Content Group UK Ltd.
Pitfield, Milton Keynes, MK11 3LW, UK
UKHW050456150426
5217IPUK00025B/1716